Botulinum Toxin Treatment in Clinical Medicine

Bahman Jabbari
Editor

Botulinum Toxin Treatment in Clinical Medicine

A Disease-Oriented Approach

Springer

Editor
Bahman Jabbari, MD, FAAN
Emeritus Professor of Neurology
Yale University, New Haven
CT, USA

ISBN 978-3-319-56037-3 ISBN 978-3-319-56038-0 (eBook)
DOI 10.1007/978-3-319-56038-0

Library of Congress Control Number: 2017949684

Printed on acid-free paper

This Springer imprint is published by Springer Nature
The registered company is Springer International Publishing AG
The registered company address is: Gewerbestrasse 11, 6330 Cham, Switzerland

I also like to dedicate this book to my wife Dr. Fattaneh Tavassoli Jabbari who has done a fair amount of editorial work in this book.

Preface

Over the past four decades, botulinum neurotoxins have made a major impact as effective therapeutic agents for treatment of a variety of medical disorders in clinical medicine. Their indications have now expanded from the field of movement disorders to pain medicine and beyond. In the recent years it has become clear that botulinum neurotoxins can effectively alleviate more than one symptom in a variety of medical diseases ranging from spasticity, muscle spasm and sialorrhea in stroke and spasticity, movement disorders and bladder dysfunction in multiple sclerosis. It is, therefore, time to look beyond single symptom relief and explore specifically how these agents can help a patient with various dysfunctions related to a single disease.

This book provides information on the utility and efficacy of botulinum neurotoxins via a "Disease-Oriented Approach." In the first chapter, Dr. Ornella Rossetto, in a clear and concise language, describes the molecular structure and mechanism of action of various available botulinum toxins. In Chaps. 2–14, the authors explain the role of botulinum toxins in alleviating symptoms of different medical diseases using an evidence-based approach. The use of ancillary techniques (Ultrasound and EMG) to locate the muscles contributing to the symptoms (spasticity or involuntary movement) is discussed by Drs. Katharine E. Alter and Barbara I. Karp in Chap. 15. Chapter 16 of the book provides information on potentially upcoming indications and what is on the horizon.

I am grateful to the help of several people who were instrumental in the development and completion of this book, and to the authors of different chapters who took time from their busy schedules and provided their chapters on time for production. Fattaneh Tavassoli, M.D., provided invaluable editorial assistance. Damoun Safarpour, M.D., and Tahereh Mousavi, M.D., have kindly provided the drawings to illustrate the details of injection sites for several chapters. Carolyn Spence and Michelle FengeHe from Springer provided the most useful guidance and advice throughout the entire project. Foremost, I am much indebted to all patients who, during almost four decades of my practice, supported and helped me learn how I can improve and obtain better results with botulinum toxin therapy in clinical practice.

I hope this book will be of help to clinicians, other health providers as well as researchers, ultimately providing better care to our patients.

July 24, 2017 Bahman Jabbari
Newport Coast, CA

Contents

Botulinum Toxins: Molecular Structures and Synaptic Physiology

Ornella Rossetto

Introduction

Botulinum neurotoxin (BoNT) was identified as the sole cause of botulism over a century ago, after the discovery of the anaerobic and spore-forming bacteria of the genus *Clostridium* [1]. Botulinum neurotoxins are produced by different *C. botulinum* strains, which belong to four phylogenetically distinct groups, and by *C. butyricum* and *C. barati* and are historically classified into seven different serotypes (BoNT/A to /G) based on their immunological properties. Among the seven BoNT serotypes, types A, B, E, and F are associated with botulism in both humans and animals, whereas BoNT/C and /D primarily cause disease in domestic animals. BoNT/G-producing organisms have been isolated from soil but never reported as the cause of botulism. Recently, thanks to the development of next-generation sequencing, many toxin variants named subtypes have been identified within each serotype (distinguished using an alpha-numeric code BoNT/A1, /A2, etc.) and much more are expected to be reported soon [2, 3]. BoNTs bind with high affinity to peripheral cholinergic nerve terminals and enter into their cytosol where they cleave SNARE proteins thus blocking the release of neurotransmitters. The high potency and neurospecificity, the very limited diffusion when locally injected, and the reversibility of action have rendered BoNT/A1 the safest and most efficacious therapeutic for the treatment of a variety of human pathological conditions characterized by hyperfunction of selected nerve terminals. Their clinical use has been continuously expanding since its introduction in the 1970s,

O. Rossetto (✉)
Dipartimento di Scienze Biomediche, Università di Padova,
Viale G. Colombo 3, 35121 Padova, Italy
e-mail: ornella.rossetto@gmail.com

B. Jabbari (ed.), *Botulinum Toxin Treatment in Clinical Medicine*,
DOI 10.1007/978-3-319-56038-0_1

including treatment of movement disorders such as focal and segmental dystonias and spasticity and cosmetic treatments based on the blockade of hyperactive cholinergic motor nerve terminals [4–8]. The ability of the BoNTs to block the cholinergic autonomic nerve endings innervating salivary and sweat glands provided an effective therapy for hypersalivation and hyperhidrosis [9]. In addition to the blockade of the acetylcholine secretion, animal experiments indicate BoNTs induce blockade of transmitters involved in pain perception, transmission, and processing, and this is on the basis of the expanding pain indications of BoNTs recently explored in humans [10]. This review aims to describe the recent structural and mechanistic studies that have advanced our understanding of BoNT entry and trafficking in nerve cells. These achievements, together with the identification of several toxin variants, can be exploited both to explore new clinical applications and to design novel toxin inhibitors that block a step of intoxication common to the different toxin variants.

Molecular Architecture

BoNTs are produced by bacteria together with nontoxic accessory proteins (NAPs) to form high molecular weight progenitor complexes of various sizes (up to 900 kDa) named PTCs. NAPs include a non-toxic non-hemagglutinin component (NTNHA), which forms with the neurotoxins a hand-in-hand shaped heterodimer, and several hemagglutinin components (HAs) or OrfX proteins. The crystallographic structures of PTCs of some toxin serotypes have been recently defined ([11], [12, 13]) and suggest for NTNHA a protective role of the neurotoxin from the hostile gastrointestinal tract environment after toxin ingestion and from the many proteases present in decaying biological materials where BoNT is produced (for review see [1]). Conversely, HA proteins of PTCs present multiple carbohydrate-binding sites which are likely to act as adhesins binding the intestinal mucus layer and the polarized intestinal epithelial cells of the intestinal wall through which BoNTs enter into the lymphatic circulation and then in the blood circulation [14, 15].

Despite existence of a high number of isoforms, all BoNTs are structurally similar and consist of two chains linked by a unique disulfide bond: a light chain (L, 50 kDa) and a heavy chain (H, 100 kDa). The complete crystallographic structures of three BoNTs (A1, B1, and E1) [16–18] reveal a modular architecture comprising three domains, which are functionally linked to the multi-steps mechanism of neuron intoxication by BoNTs (Fig. 1). The L chain is a zinc-metalloprotease that specifically cleaves the three SNARE proteins necessary for neurotransmitter exocytosis; the N-terminal HN domain assists the translocation of the L chain across the membrane of intraneuronal acidic vesicles into the cytosol; the C-terminal HC domain is responsible for presynaptic binding and endocytosis and consists of two sub-domains (HC-N and HC-C) with different folding and membrane binding properties.

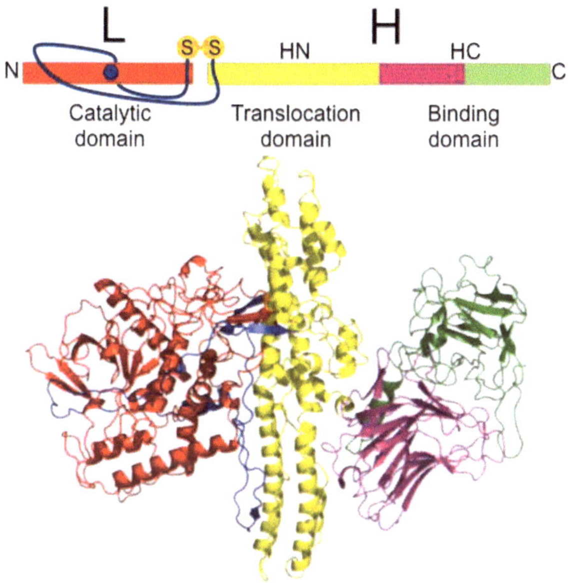

Fig. 1 Molecular structure of BoNT/A1. Schematic drawing and crystal structure of BoNT/A1 (PDB ID: 3BTA) [16] showing the organization of the three toxin domains: the binding domain which consists of the neurospecific binding HC-C sub-domain (*green*) and the lectin-like HC-N sub-domain (*purple*), the translocation HN domain (*yellow*), and the metalloprotease L domain (*red*). A peptide belt (shown in *blue*) surrounding the L domain, the atom of zinc at the center of the catalytic domain (*blue ball*) and the inter-chain disulfide bond (*orange*) linking the L and HN domain are also shown

Mechanism of Action

The structural organization of BoNTs has been designed by the evolution to deliver the catalytic L chain into the host cell cytosol through a mechanism of nerve terminal intoxication which can be conveniently divided into five major steps: (1) binding to nerve terminals, (2) internalization within an endocytic compartment, (3) low pH driven translocation of the L chain across the vesicle membrane, (4) release of the L chain in the cytosol by reduction of the interchain disulfide bond, and (5) proteolytic cleavage of SNARE proteins with ensuing blockade of neurotransmitter release and neuroparalysis (Fig. 2).

Binding to Nerve Terminals

After entering the lymphatic and blood circulations, the C-terminal part of the HC domain (sub-domain HC-C, 25 kDa) mediates the interaction of BoNTs with unmyelinated areas of motor neurons at the neuromuscular junction (NMJ), ensuring a rapid and strong interaction of the toxin with peripheral cholinergic nerve endings

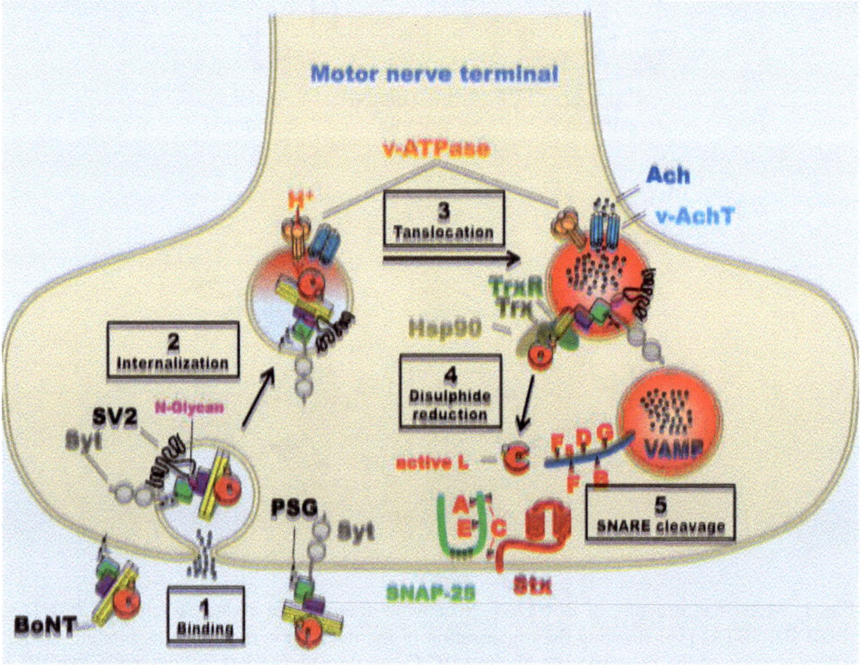

Fig. 2 Multi-steps mechanism of nerve terminal intoxication by botulinum neurotoxins. The first step (1) is the binding of the HC domain (*green*) to a polysialoganglioside (PSG) receptor of the presynaptic membrane (*gray* and *black*), followed by binding to a protein receptor. The currently known protein receptors are: (a) synaptotagmin (Syt, *gray*) for BoNT/B1, /DC, and /G; (b) glycosylated SV2 (*black* with its attached N-glycan in fuchsia) for BoNT/A1 and /E1. Syt may be located either within the exocytosed synaptic vesicle or on the presynaptic membrane. The BoNT is then internalized inside SVs. The acidification of the vesicle, operated by the v-ATPase proton pump (*orange*), drives the accumulation of neurotransmitter (*blue dots*) via the vesicular acetylcholine transporter (*light blue*). The protonation of BoNT leads to the membrane translocation of the L chain into the cytosol (3), which is assisted by the HN domain (*yellow*). The L chain (*red*) is released from the HN domain by the action of the thioredoxin reductase–thioredoxin system (TrxR–Trx, *green*) and Hsp90 (*mud color*), which reduces the inter-chain disulfide bond (*dark yellow*) and assists the refolding of the protease respectively (4). In the cytosol, the L chain displays its metalloprotease activity: BoNT/B, /D, /F, /G cleave VAMP (*blue*), BoNT/A and BoNT/E cleave SNAP-25 (*green*), and BoNT/C cleaves both SNAP-25 and syntaxin (Stx, *dark red*) (5). Each of these proteolytic events is sufficient to cause a prolonged inhibition of neurotransmitter release with consequent neuroparalysis

[1, 19, 20]. HC-C is responsible for the neurospecific binding to a polysialoganglioside and to the luminal domain of a synaptic vesicle protein [19, 21]. The latter has been defined in molecular details for BoNT/B1, BoNT/G, and the hybrid BoNT/DC which bind segment 40–60 of the luminal domain of the synaptic vesicle protein synaptotagmin (Syt) and for BoNT/A1 and BoNT/E1, which in contrast bind specifically to two different segments of the fourth luminal loop of the synaptic vesicle glycoprotein SV2 (for a complete list of references see [1, 21]). It has been also recently shown that BoNT/A1 binding to neuronal glycosylated SV2C involves a protein–protein and a protein-N-glycan interaction [22]. Biophysical, cellular, and functional studies demonstrated that SV2 glycans are essential for BoNT/A1 binding to neurons and its extreme toxicity at the motor nerve terminals. The knowledge of the molecular details of BoNT/A-SV2 drives the development of high-affinity peptides to interfere with toxin binding and therefore to counteract BoNT/A intoxications [22].

Such a dual receptor binding to polysialogangliosides and to a protein receptor ensures a higher binding affinity and is required for the ensuing internalization and trafficking of the toxin within endocytic compartments, which is initiated by synaptic vesicles (SV) retrieval after the release of their neurotransmitter content [19, 21].

Internalization and Trafficking

The BoNT binding to the luminal domain of SV membrane proteins and their synaptic activity-dependent uptake strongly suggest that most of them are endocytosed at nerve terminals inside these organelles. Indeed, after intramuscular injection, BoNT/A1 is rapidly internalized and found in the average number of one–two molecules of toxin inside the lumen of SV within the neuromuscular junction [23]. Therefore, BoNT/A, and probably also the other toxin serotypes, use SV as "Trojan horses" to enter motor neuron terminals in vivo. In fact, during neurotransmitter (NT) release, the lumen of the SV is transiently opened (exposing the luminal domains of the BoNT protein receptors to the outside) and a complex cascade of protein–protein and protein–lipid interactions trigger the recruitment of clathrin and adaptor proteins to the inner leaflet of the plasma membrane, which marks the onset of the endocytic process and thus the SV retrieval [24]. After internalization and uncoating, SV is refilled with NT, a process driven by the electrochemical proton gradient that is generated by the vesicular ATPase proton pump, and the next cycle of neurotransmission begins. Although BoNT activity is mainly restricted to distal synapses and the role of the synaptic vesicle cycle in BoNT/A1 internalization is unquestionable, many recent lines of evidence suggest that synaptic activity-independent, "alternative" pathways also contribute to BoNT/A1 internalization and direct the neurotoxin through retroaxonal transport mechanisms to the central nervous system (CNS). Recently, internalization of BoNT/A1 in a subpopulation of non-recyclable synaptic vesicles whose fate could be to generate retrograde carriers has also been proposed [25]. A more detailed understanding of these direct effects of BoNTs on central circuits will provide valuable information for present and future uses of these neurotoxins in clinical practice [26].

Toxin Translocation

In order to reach their intracellular targets in the cytosol of nerve cells, the catalytically active L domain must be translocated from the SV lumen into the cytosol. The low pH inside the SV lumen induces a structural change of the HN domain leading to its insertion into the membrane and thus an ion translocation channel is formed that assists the passage of the partially unfolded L from the lumenal to the cytosolic side of the SV membrane [1, 27, 28]. The disulfide bridge that links the heavy and light chain must remain intact on the luminal side of the vesicle until the last stage of L translocation [29]. Once it has reached the cytosolic face of SV membrane, the L chain has to reacquire the native structure in order to cleave its substrate and it has been recently shown that the host chaperone heat shock protein 90 (Hsp90) assists the refolding of the L chain after vesicle membrane translocation as already demonstrated for other bacterial toxins such as diphtheria toxin [30, 31]. L remains attached to the SV until the interchain disulfide bond is reduced in the reducing environment of the cytosol, a crucial step for productive release of the L catalytic subunit, which is common to all the BoNT variants [32].

Disulfide Bond Reduction

Host cells possess several redox systems and it was recently found that thioredoxin reductase-thioredoxin (TrxR-Trx) system is responsible for the reduction of disulfide bond of all BoNTs and that it physically interacts with the Hsp90 chaperone on the cytosolic surface of SV, which is the site of toxin translocation [30, 32]. Indeed, inhibitors of the TrxR-Trx redox system prevent the intoxication by BoNTs of neurons in culture and more importantly, largely prevent the BoNT-induced paralysis in mice in vivo, regardless of the serotype involved [32–34]. Moreover, the synergistic effect of Hsp90-specific inhibitor geldanamycin with PX-12, an inhibitor of thioredoxin, indicates that this TrxR-Trx-Hsp90 chaperone-redox machinery, which is exploited by all BoNTs to deliver their catalytic domain into the cytosol, can be considered as a target for drug discovery to prevent and treat botulism, regardless of the serotype (or the subtype) causing the intoxication [30].

Proteolysis of SNARE Proteins

The L chains of BoNTs are metalloproteases with an atom of Zn^{2+} bound to the motif HExxH at the center of the molecule that once released in the cytosol of the nerve terminal, cleave one of the three SNARE proteins: the vesicle-associated membrane protein VAMP, or the presynaptic membrane proteins SNAP-25 or Syntaxin (for a review see [1]). These three proteins form a heterotrimeric coil-coiled SNARE complex, which represents the core of the neuroexocytosis apparatus [35]. The BoNT proteolytic activity is highly specific and directed toward unique peptide bonds within the sequence of their respective SNARE protein targets. BoNT/B, /D, /F, /G cleave VAMP, BoNT/A and BoNT/E cleave SNAP-25, and BoNT/C cleaves both SNAP-25 and syntaxin. In most cases, BoNT cleavage results in the loss of a large part of the cytosolic portion of SNARE proteins, thus preventing the formation of the SNARE complex. In contrast, in the case of BoNT/A and

BoNT/C, the truncated SNAP25 proteins retain most of their sequences (197 and 198 of 206 amino acid residues, respectively) and are capable of forming stable, though non-functional, SNARE complexes. In any cases, the proteolysis of one SNARE protein prevents the formation of a functional SNARE complex and, consequently, the release of neurotransmitter with ensuing neuroparalysis [36, 37]. All subtypes characterized so far share the same cleavage site of the parent serotype with the exception of BoNT/F5 and a chimeric toxin BoNT/FA, which cleave a different peptide bond of VAMP with respect to BoNT/F1 [38, 39]. However, the available evidence suggests that BoNT/A subtypes have different enzymatic rate [40, 41] and it is, therefore, possible that individual subtypes are highly variable in their potency, onset, and duration of action. The exquisite target specificity of botulinum neurotoxins is due to the unique mode of recognition of VAMP, SNAP-25, or syntaxin by the L chain, which involves multiple interactions of the metalloprotease with its substrate including the cleavage site as well as exosites located along the sequence both before and after the hydrolyzed peptide bond [42, 43]. Different SNARE isoforms coexist within the same cell [44], but only some of them are susceptible to proteolysis by the BoNTs and it has been shown that resistance is associated with mutations in the cleavage site or/and at substrate/enzyme binding exosites [45]. The substrate/enzyme co-crystal structures revealed an extensive interface between protease and the SNARE protein and indicate that the multiple interactions sites remote from the L chain active site bring the cleavage region of the substrate close to the L active site [46, 47]. Structural studies using different length substrates or peptidomimetic inhibitors have demonstrated that the BoNT active site has a high degree of plasticity and will adopt different conformations in response to different substrates or to diverse peptide-based inhibitors [48, 49]. The dynamic nature of BoNT active site and the peculiar mode of binding with extensive enzyme–substrate interface explain why long peptide substrates are needed to test the proteolytic activity of the L chain in vitro and also the current lack of specific and high-affinity inhibitors of their metalloprotease activity [43].

Reversibility of Neuroparalysis Induced by BoNTs and Neuromuscular Junction Plasticity

An important feature of BoNT intoxication is its reversibility in vivo. Indeed, the toxin cleaves a SNARE protein as long as it remains intact in the nerve cytosol, but this activity causes neither neuronal cell death nor axonal degeneration in the intoxicated animal, though the animal may die of respiratory failure. Indeed if a botulism patient is kept under mechanical ventilation and appropriate pharmacological treatments, eventually he/she recovers completely, following the inactivation of the toxin and the replacement of the cleaved SNARE [50]. The duration of the BoNT inhibitory effect varies with serotypes [51] and it contributes to determining the severity of human botulism (type A $>$ type B $\gg$ type E) [50, 52].

The main determinant of the duration of neuroparalysis is the L chain lifetime within the terminal and it appears that BoNT/A1 L chain, which has a very remarkable persistence, has a longer lifetime than that of BoNT/E1 because BoNT/E1 L chain is ubiquitinated and targeted to the ubiquitin-proteasome system, whilst BoNT/A1 L chain escapes the action of the cell degradation system by recruiting de-ubiquitinases, i.e. specialized enzymes that remove polyubiquitin chains [53, 54]. In addition to the protease persistence in the cytosol, other factors come into play to determine the duration of action, including the maintenance of truncated SNARE proteins within motor neurons. In fact, the longer duration of the effects of BoNT/A1 and /C1 is also explained, as anticipated above, by the inhibitory action of the truncated SNAP-25 which persist for long time periods at the synapse [36, 55] and the shorter duration of BoNT/E1 is likely determined by the rapid turnover of its truncated SNAP25 [56–58]. New understanding of the mechanisms by which these remarkable toxins or their proteolytic products persist within their motor neuron targets will help to develop, on one hand, BoNT-based therapeutics with improved persistence properties and therefore produce a longer clinical benefit, and on the other hand, BoNT-antidotes which accelerate the toxin degradation and therefore reverse BoNT intoxication.

In addition to the type of BoNT and to the product of SNARE proteolysis, the duration of the paralysis depends also on the dose, the animal species, the mode of administration, and the type of nerve terminal. Regarding the latter, it is known that the local injection of BoNT/A1 and BoNT/B1 at the human autonomic cholinergic nerve terminals induced a longer duration of neuroparalysis (even more than a year) with respect to the shorter duration of action in skeletal nerve terminals (3/4 months in humans) [9]. Since the BoNT poisoned NMJ undergoes a profound remodeling in which Schwann cells play a crucial and active role, the duration of paralysis is also determined by the response of peripheral Schwann cells (which are not present at the autonomic nerve terminals) to the blockade of neuroexocytosis. Indeed, under the effect of growth factors released by Schwann cells and muscles, the motor end plate enlarges and sprouts develop from the unmyelinated motor axon terminal and from the first node of Ranvier [59, 60]. These nerve sprouts follow projections that emerge from perisynaptic Schwann cells, which multiply and migrate from the original NMJ to other sites of the sarcolemma soon after inactivation of the motor axon terminal. New contacts with the muscle fiber are formed. The number of motor end plates on single muscle fibers increases as well as the number of fibers innervated by a single motor axon. Moreover, in the muscle, BoNTs induce alterations similar to those documented in other forms of denervation with fiber atrophy appreciable already in the first 2 weeks after BoNT injection. The new synapses, though immature, can sustain vesicle recycling [60, 61], but are poorly efficient in ACh release [62], providing a limited contribution to the recovery of the neurotransmission from nerve to the muscle fiber. Once a certain level of functionality is re-established at the original site, terminal and nodal sprouts are pruned, and the newly formed synaptic specializations are eliminated [50].

Concluding Remarks and Future Perspective

Botulinum neurotoxins combine potency and specificity with full reversibility at the cellular level, and these unique properties are on the basis of their clinical use. The recent understanding of their detailed modular structure and of their multi-step molecular mechanism of neuron intoxication together with advances in the techniques for production of recombinant proteins, have opened up the opportunity to modify the binding specificity, affinity, and nerve terminal persistence in order to improve their properties in terms of cell targeting and duration of action [63–65]. The duration of BoNTs activity assumes a paramount significance with respect to their therapeutic use because long-lasting BoNTs require fewer injections and lower doses, limiting the possibility of immunization. Moreover, the recent identification of many new toxin variants foster researchers to characterize their biological activity and it is likely that novel BoNTs with improved and/or different therapeutic targets/properties in terms of potency and duration of action will be discovered in the near future and will constitute potential goldmine to be exploited for new clinical applications.

Eventually, the recent identification of inhibitory molecules, which block common steps of nerve intoxication mechanism such as translocation or the reduction of the interchain disulfide bond can be considered as lead compounds for the development of pan-inhibitors of BoNTs regardless of the toxin variant causing intoxication [30, 32, 34].

Acknowledgments Work in the author's laboratory is supported by grants from the University of Padova.

References

1. Rossetto O, Pirazzini M, Montecucco C. Botulinum neurotoxins: genetic, structural and mechanistic insights. Nat Rev Microbiol. 2014;12:535–49.
2. Montecucco C, Rasotto MB. On botulinum neurotoxin variability. MBio. 2015;6:e02131–14.
3. Smith TJ, Hill KK, Raphael BH. Historical and current perspectives on Clostridium botulinum diversity. Res Microbiol. 2015;166:290–302.
4. Blitzer A, Binder WJ. Cosmetic uses of botulinum neurotoxin type A: an overview. Arch Facial Plast Surg. 2002;4:214–20.
5. Dressler D. Clinical applications of botulinum toxin. Curr Opin Microbiol. 2012;15:325–36.
6. Hallett M, Albanese A, Dressler D, Segal KR, Simpson DM, Truong D, et al. Evidence-based review and assessment of botulinum neurotoxin for the treatment of movement disorders. Toxicon. 2013;67:94–114.
7. Scott AB. Botulinum toxin injection into extraocular muscles as an alternative to strabismus surgery. Ophthalmology. 1980;87:1044–9.
8. Wise JB, Greco T. Injectable treatments for the aging face. Facial Plast Surg. 2006;22:140–6.
9. Naumann M, Dressler D, Hallett M, Jankovic J, Schiavo G, Segal KR, et al. Evidence-based review and assessment of botulinum neurotoxin for the treatment of secretory disorders. Toxicon. 2013;67:141–52.

10. Jabbari B. Botulinum toxin treatment of pain disorders. New York: Springer; 2015.
11. Hasegawa K, Watanabe T, Suzuki T, Yamano A, Oikawa T, Sato Y, et al. A novel subunit structure of Clostridium botulinum serotype D toxin complex with three extended arms. J Biol Chem. 2007;282:24777–83.
12. Benefield DA, Dessain SK, Shine N, Ohi MD, Lacy DB. Molecular assembly of botulinum neurotoxin progenitor complexes. Proc Natl Acad Sci USA. 2013;110:5630–5.
13. Lee K, Gu S, Jin L, Le TT, Cheng LW, Strotmeier J, Kruel AM, Yao G, Perry K, Rummel A, Jin R. Structure of a bimodular botulinum neurotoxin complex provides insights into its oral toxicity. PLoS Pathog. 2013;9:e1003690.
14. Fujinaga Y, Sugawara Y, Matsumura T. Uptake of botulinum neurotoxin in the intestine. Curr Top Microbiol Immunol. 2013;364:45–59.
15. Simpson LL. The life history of a botulinum toxin molecule. Toxicon. 2013;68:40–59.
16. Lacy DB, Tepp W, Cohen AC, DasGupta BR, Stevens RC. Crystal structure of botulinum neurotoxin type A and implications for toxicity. Nat Struct Biol. 1998;5:898–902.
17. Kumaran D, Eswaramoorthy S, Furey W, Navaza J, Sax M, Swaminathan S. Domain organization in Clostridium botulinum neurotoxin type E is unique: its implication in faster translocation. J Mol Biol. 2009;386:233–45.
18. Swaminathan S, Eswaramoorthy S. Structural analysis of the catalytic and binding sites of Clostridium botulinum neurotoxin B. Nat Struct Biol. 2000;7:693–9.
19. Binz T, Rummel A. Cell entry strategy of clostridial neurotoxins. J Neurochem. 2009;109:1584–95.
20. Dolly JO, Black J, Williams RS, Melling J. Acceptors for botulinum neurotoxin reside on motor nerve terminals and mediate its internalization. Nature. 1984;307:457–60.
21. Rummel A. Double receptor anchorage of botulinum neurotoxins accounts for their exquisite neurospecificity. Curr Top Microbiol Immunol. 2013;364:61–90.
22. Yao G, Zhang S, Mahrhold S, Lam KH, Stern D, Bagramyan K, et al. N-linked glycosylation of SV2 is required for binding and uptake of botulinum neurotoxin A. Nat Struct Mol Biol. 2016;23:656–62.
23. Colasante C, Rossetto O, Morbiato L, Pirazzini M, Molgo J, Montecucco C. Botulinum neurotoxin type A is internalized and translocated from small synaptic vesicles at the neuromuscular junction. Mol Neurobiol. 2013;48:120–7.
24. Haucke V, Neher E, Sigrist SJ. Protein scaffolds in the coupling of synaptic exocytosis and endocytosis. Nat Rev Neurosci. 2011;12:127–38.
25. Harper CB, Papadopulos A, Martin S, Matthews DR, Morgan GP, Nguyen TH, et al. Botulinum neurotoxin type-A enters a non-recycling pool of synaptic vesicles. Sci Rep. 2016;6:19654.
26. Mazzocchio R, Caleo M. More than at the neuromuscular synapse: actions of botulinum neurotoxin A in the central nervous system. Neuroscientist. 2015;21:44–61.
27. Montal M. Botulinum neurotoxin: a marvel of protein design. Annu Rev Biochem. 2010;79:591–617.
28. Pirazzini M, Azarnia Tehran D, Leka O, Zanetti G, Rossetto O, Montecucco C. On the translocation of botulinum and tetanus neurotoxins across the membrane of acidic intracellular compartments. Biochem Biophys Acta. 2016;1858:467–74.
29. Fischer A, Montal M. Crucial role of the disulfide bridge between botulinum neurotoxin light and heavy chains in protease translocation across membranes. J Biol Chem. 2007;282:29604–11.
30. Azarnia Tehran D, Pirazzini M, Leka O, Mattarei A, Lista F, Binz T, et al. Hsp90 is involved in the entry of clostridial neurotoxins into the cytosol of nerve terminals. Cell Microbiol. 2016; doi:10.1111/cmi.12647.
31. Ratts R, Zeng H, Berg EA, Blue C, McComb ME, Costello CE, et al. The cytosolic entry of diphtheria toxin catalytic domain requires a host cell cytosolic translocation factor complex. J Cell Biol. 2003;160:1139–50.
32. Pirazzini M, Azarnia Tehran D, Zanetti G, Megighian A, Scorzeto M, Fillo S, et al. Thioredoxin and its reductase are present on synaptic vesicles, and their inhibition prevents the paralysis induced by botulinum neurotoxins. Cell Rep. 2014;8:1870–8.

33. Pirazzini M, Bordin F, Rossetto O, Shone CC, Binz T, Montecucco C. The thioredoxin reductase-thioredoxin system is involved in the entry of tetanus and botulinum neurotoxins in the cytosol of nerve terminals. FEBS Lett. 2013;587:150–5.
34. Zanetti G, Azarnia Tehran D, Pirazzini M, Binz T, Shone CC, Fillo S, et al. Inhibition of botulinum neurotoxins interchain disulfide bond reduction prevents the peripheral neuroparalysis of botulism. Biochem Pharmacol. 2015;98:522–30.
35. Sutton RB, Fasshauer D, Jahn R, Brunger AT. Crystal structure of a SNARE complex involved in synaptic exocytosis at 2.4 A resolution. Nature. 1998;395:347–53.
36. Pantano S, Montecucco C. The blockade of the neurotransmitter release apparatus by botulinum neurotoxins. Cell Mol Life Sci. 2014;71(5):793–811.
37. Sudhof TC. The molecular machinery of neurotransmitter release (Nobel lecture). Angew Chem Int Ed Engl. 2014;53:12696–717.
38. Kalb SR, Baudys J, Raphael BH, Dykes JK, Luquez C, Maslanka SE, et al. Functional characterization of botulinum neurotoxin serotype H as a hybrid of known serotypes F and A (BoNT F/A). Anal Chem. 2015;87(7):3911.
39. Kalb SR, Baudys J, Webb RP, Wright P, Smith TJ, Smith LA, et al. Discovery of a novel enzymatic cleavage site for botulinum neurotoxin F5. FEBS Lett. 2012;586(2):109–15.
40. Pellett S, Tepp WH, Whitemarsh RC, Bradshaw M, Johnson EA. vivo onset and duration of action varies for botulinum neurotoxin A subtypes 1-5. Toxicon. 2015;107:37–42.
41. Whitemarsh RC, Tepp WH, Johnson EA, Pellett S. Persistence of botulinum neurotoxin a subtypes 1-5 in primary rat spinal cord cells. PLoS One. 2013;9:e90252.
42. Binz T. Clostridial neurotoxin light chains: devices for SNARE cleavage mediated blockade of neurotransmission. Curr Top Microbiol Immunol. 2013;364:139–57.
43. Chen S. Clostridial neurotoxins: mode of substrate recognition and novel therapy development. Curr Protein Pept Sci. 2014;15:490–503.
44. Bock JB, Scheller RH. SNARE proteins mediate lipid bilayer fusion. Proc Natl Acad Sci U S A. 1999;96:12227–9.
45. Schiavo G, Matteoli M, Montecucco C. Neurotoxins affecting neuroexocytosis. Physiol Rev. 2000;80:717–66.
46. Agarwal R, Schmidt JJ, Stafford RG, Swaminathan S. Mode of VAMP substrate recognition and inhibition of Clostridium botulinum neurotoxin F. Nat Struct Mol Biol. 2009;16:789–94.
47. Breidenbach MA, Brunger AT. Substrate recognition strategy for botulinum neurotoxin serotype A. Nature. 2004;432:925–9.
48. Kumaran D, Rawat R, Ahmed SA, Swaminathan S. Substrate binding mode and its implication on drug design for botulinum neurotoxin A. PLoS Pathog. 2008;4:e1000165.
49. Zuniga JE, Schmidt JJ, Fenn T, Burnett JC, Arac D, Gussio R, et al. A potent peptidomimetic inhibitor of botulinum neurotoxin serotype A has a very different conformation than SNAP-25 substrate. Structure. 2008;16:1588–97.
50. Johnson EA, Montecucco C. Botulism. Handb Clin Neurol. 2008;91:333–68.
51. Eleopra R, Tugnoli V, Quatrale R, Rossetto O, Montecucco C. Different types of botulinum toxin in humans. Mov Disord. 2004;19:S53–9.
52. Cherington M. Clinical spectrum of botulism. Muscle Nerve. 1998;21:701–10.
53. Shoemaker CB, Oyler GA. Persistence of Botulinum neurotoxin inactivation of nerve function. Curr Top Microbiol Immunol. 2013;364:179–96.
54. Tsai YC, Maditz R, C-l K, Fishman PS, Shoemaker CB, Oyler GA, et al. Targeting botulinum neurotoxin persistence by the ubiquitin-proteasome system. Proc Natl Acad Sci U S A. 2010;107:16554–9.
55. Megighian A, Zordan M, Pantano S, Scorzeto M, Rigoni M, Zanini D, et al. Evidence for a radial SNARE super-complex mediating neurotransmitter release at the Drosophila neuromuscular junction. J Cell Sci. 2013;126:3134–40.
56. Eleopra R, Tugnoli V, Rossetto O, De Grandis D, Montecucco C. Different time courses of recovery after poisoning with botulinum neurotoxin serotypes A and E in humans. Neurosci Lett. 1998;256:135–8.

57. Meunier FA, Lisk G, Sesardic D, Dolly JO. Dynamics of motor nerve terminal remodeling unveiled using SNARE-cleaving botulinum toxins: the extent and duration are dictated by the sites of SNAP-25 truncation. Mol Cell Neurosci. 2003;22:454–66.
58. Raciborska DA, Charlton MP. Retention of cleaved synaptosome-associated protein of 25 kDa (SNAP-25) in neuromuscular junctions: a new hypothesis to explain persistence of botulinum A poisoning. Can J Physiol Pharmacol. 1999;77:679–88.
59. Juzans P, Comella JX, Molgo J, Faille L, Angaut-Petit D. Nerve terminal sprouting in botulinum type-A treated mouse levator auris longus muscle. Neuromuscul Disord. 1996;6:177–85.
60. Meunier FA, Schiavo G, Molgo J. Botulinum neurotoxins: from paralysis to recovery of functional neuromuscular transmission. J Physiol Paris. 2002;96:105–13.
61. de Paiva A, Meunier FA, Molgó J, Aoki KR, Dolly JO. Functional repair of motor endplates after botulinum neurotoxin type A poisoning: Biphasic switch of synaptic activity between nerve sprouts and their parent terminals. Proc Natl Acad Sci U S A. 1999;96:3200–5.
62. Rogozhin AA, Pang KK, Bukharaeva E, Young C, Slater CR. Recovery of mouse neuromuscular junctions from single and repeated injections of botulinum neurotoxin A. J Physiol. 2008;586:3163–82.
63. Chen S, Barbieri JT. Engineering botulinum neurotoxin to extend therapeutic intervention. Proc Natl Acad Sci U S A. 2009;106:9180–4.
64. Masuyer G, Chaddock JA, Foster KA, Acharya KR. Engineered botulinum neurotoxins as new therapeutics. Annu Rev Pharmacol Toxicol. 2014;54:27–51.
65. Sikorra S, Litschko C, Muller C, Thiel N, Galli T, Eichner T, et al. Identification and characterization of botulinum neurotoxin A substrate binding pockets and their re-engineering for human SNAP-23. J Mol Biol. 2015;428:372–84.

Botulinum Toxin Treatment of Primary Dystonia

Avram Fraint and Cynthia Comella

Introduction

Dystonia is a sustained or intermittent muscle contraction that causes abnormal movements and/or postures [1]. Prevalence of dystonia is difficult to accurately ascertain due to misdiagnosis and/or under-diagnosis. Nutt et al. estimated its prevalence to be 3.4–29.5 per 100,000, though it is higher in certain communities [2–4]. For example, it is five times higher in Ashkenazi Jews relative to the general population [5]. The annual prevalence rate for primary dystonia is 152 per million, and focal dystonia has the highest relative rate at 117 per million. Prevalence rates for specific types of dystonia have been estimated at 28–183 per million for cervical dystonia (CD), 36 per million for blepharospasm (BPS), and 14 per million for writer's cramp (WC) [3, 6].

There are multiple treatments for dystonia including oral medications, intrathecal infusions, and deep brain stimulation (DBS). Choice of treatment depends on the etiology of the dystonia and the extent of muscle involvement. Treatment of generalized dystonia often relies on oral medications, intrathecal infusions, and/or DBS surgery. However, focal dystonia is best treated with injection of botulinum toxin (BoNT) [1]. The first double-blind, placebo-controlled trial demonstrating the efficacy of botulinum toxin type A (BoNT-A) in CD was published in 1986, and since then its use has been expanded to hundreds of different neurologic conditions.

A. Fraint, M.D. (✉)
Rush University Medical Center – Section of Movement Disorders,
1725 W Harrison Street, Suite 755, Chicago, IL 60612, USA
e-mail: Avram_fraint@rush.edu

C. Comella, M.D.
Rush University Medical Center - Section of Movement Disorders,
1725 W Harrison, Suite 755, Chicago, IL 60612, USA
e-mail: Cynthia_comella@rush.edu

B. Jabbari (ed.), *Botulinum Toxin Treatment in Clinical Medicine*,
DOI 10.1007/978-3-319-56038-0_2

Multiple subsequent studies have demonstrated that it is an effective and safe treatment for multiple forms of dystonia in addition to CD [7].

Classifying Dystonia

The term "primary" dystonia is historically the most consistently used terminology and usually refers to dystonia occurring without other neurological symptoms or pathologic abnormalities [8]. As dystonia is often associated with other neurologic and psychiatric features, this definition was recently refined [9]. The newest classification of dystonia created a category called "isolated" dystonia in which dystonia is the only motor feature seen, with the exception of tremor [1].

Dystonia can also be classified in terms of its age of onset, body region distribution, and temporal evolution. The exact cutoff between early-onset and late-onset dystonia is debated but in general early-onset dystonia is that which occurs before age 20, and late-onset dystonia occurs in patients older than 20 [10]. Early-onset dystonia usually starts in the lower extremity while late-onset dystonia usually starts in the upper body, particularly the muscles of the neck [2]. Classification by age is important in that early-onset dystonia is more likely to have a discoverable cause and is more likely to generalize [1].

Types of Dystonia

Cervical dystonia (CD) is the most common late-onset focal dystonia. It affects the muscles of the neck and shoulders and can take many different forms including horizontal head turning (torticollis), lateral neck tilting (laterocollis), flexion of the head (anterocollis), extension of the head (retrocollis), and shoulder elevation. About two-thirds of patients will have a combination of these movements. Overlying spasms may cause the head tremor seen in about 14% of CD patients [11]. The average age of onset is in the early 40s and the estimated incidence is 0.8 per 100,000 person-years [12]. Many of these patients also develop focal dystonia elsewhere—16% can have oral dystonia, 12% mandibular dystonia, 10% hand or arm dystonia, and 10% have BPS [11]. Overall, about 23% of patients with CD experience spread of their symptoms to contiguous body regions [13].

BPS is characterized by stereotyped, bilateral, synchronous spasms of the orbicularis oculi muscles. These can be clonic with increased blinking, or tonic with sustained eye closures. The spasms vary in duration, and may include eyelid narrowing or closure [14]. BPS affects approximately 16–133 cases per million [10]. It is more common in women, and has a typical age of onset between the fifth and seventh decades. In almost half (47%) of patients, it spreads to adjacent body areas, often within the first 5 years [13]. It may also be associated with a tremor of the head or upper limbs [14].

Focal limb dystonia starts more commonly in the upper rather than lower extremity in adults. In the sub-category of focal hand dystonia (FHD), writer's cramp (WC) and musician's dystonia are the most common. They are considered task-specific in that the patient experiences the dystonia when performing a specific task, but otherwise has normal use of the involved muscles [15]. It usually appears between age 20 and 50, and affects men and women equally [16]. In WC a pen is often held abnormally and there are multiple abnormal postures of the fingers and wrist that can be seen. One study estimated the rate of spread of FHD into another body site to be 38% [13].

Pathophysiology

There is no neuro-anatomical model described that adequately explains the pathophysiology of dystonia. Secondary dystonia has been seen in tumors, infarcts, hemorrhages, arachnoid cysts, demyelinating lesions, and other lesions in the cerebellum and its associated brainstem outputs as well as in the basal ganglia [17, 18]. Functional MRI studies have noted increased activation in the basal ganglia and cerebellum in dystonia [19]. Within the basal ganglia, putaminal lesions in particular are known to cause dystonia [20]. In one study, the putamen was reported to be about 10% larger in patients with primary dystonia [21].

Argyelan et al. suggested that abnormal connections between the cerebellum and thalamus may predict the penetrance of DYT-1 dystonia [22]. Some studies in genetically dystonic rats have shown higher levels of glutamate decarboxylase messenger RNA in Purkinje cells and decreased levels of the same in the deep cerebellar nuclei [23]. Other animal models have shown that dystonia can be induced with pharmacologic manipulation of the cerebellum [24].

Though its involvement is clear, the precise mechanism by which the basal ganglia is involved in producing dystonia is not known. Given that the most effective pharmacologic therapies for dystonia are anticholinergic and dopaminergic medications, dopamine and acetylcholine systems likely play a role in this disorder [17]. Many patients with Parkinson's disease develop dystonia, further implicating the dopaminergic system. Some recent evidence has shown that impaired reciprocal modulation between striatal dopamine and acetylcholine is an important pathophysiological event in DYT-1 dystonia [25–27].

Hallett et al. proposed a loss of inhibition of motor control, leading to a loss in selectivity and a resultant motor overflow as causing symptoms of dystonia. The clinical features of dystonia are thus related to a failure of surround inhibition, and multiple studies using transcranial magnetic stimulation have demonstrated reduced inhibition and abnormal spread of facilitation at the cortical level [28, 29]. Additionally, abnormal plasticity in sensorimotor circuits has been proposed as causing focal dystonia. The core feature of abnormal plasticity in dystonia is a lack of spatial specificity [29]. This could be secondary to lack of inhibition, but there is also spread of maladaptive plasticity into nearby muscle groups [30, 31].

Treatment

For many years, the treatment of dystonia relied on oral medications that had only modest effect on symptoms. High-dose trihexyphenidyl was found to be effective in the treatment of primary dystonia in the mid-1980s [32]. Other medications are frequently used with modest effect—including baclofen and benzodiazepines [33, 34]. In cases of generalized dystonia which is refractory to oral pharmacologic treatment, intrathecal baclofen has been used, though this seems to be effective primarily in secondary dystonia with associated spasticity or pain [25]. Deep brain stimulation (DBS) is also known to be effective in the treatment of dystonia. Several new mediations, including ampicillin for DYT-1, levetiracetam for myoclonus-dystonia, and perampanel for dystonia are currently being investigated [35, 36].

Botulinum toxin has transformed the landscape of the treatment of dystonia in the past 30 years. It is produced by the bacterium *Clostridium botulinum* and it exerts its effect by inhibiting release of acetylcholine (ACh) from nerve terminals into the neuromuscular junction. It thus prevents neuromuscular transmission, resulting in weakness of the targeted muscles. Under normal circumstances, ACh release into the neuromuscular junction occurs via fusion of vesicles that contain ACh within the pre-synaptic membrane. There is a synaptic fusion complex made of soluble *N*-ethylmaleimide-sensitive factor enhancement protein receptor (SNARE) proteins which facilitates ACh release. SNARE proteins form a complex of three proteins, two of which are specific targets for different serotypes of BoNT. These proteins are syntaxin 1, synaptosomal-associated protein 25 (SNAP-25), and synaptobrevin. These proteins are involved in docking and exocytosis of the ACh-containing vesicles at the presynaptic nerve terminal [37, 38].

There are seven serotypes of BoNT, but only types A and B are commercially available and FDA approved for clinical use [39]. Each serotype has a different complex protein structure and each cleaves specific proteins at specific locations on the SNARE complex. In the US, there are currently three commercially available types of BoNT-A, which targets SNAP-25. These include OnabotulinumtoxinA (Onabot), AbobotulinumtoxinA (Abobot), and IncobotulinumtoxinA (Incobot). The fourth type of BoNT-A, similar to Incobot in that it lacks complexing proteins, has completed phase 3 trials [40]. There is one commercially available type of BoNT-B–RimabotulinumtoxinB (Rimabot)—and it targets Synaptobrevin. Potency varies between serotypes, however, no clear dosing equivalencies between the serotypes have been established [41].

Generalized dystonia requires multiple treatment modalities, and while there is a role for botulinum toxin, it is typically used in addition to oral, intrathecal, or surgical options. In these cases, the most painful or disabling dystonic areas are usually targeted. BoNT is the first-line treatment of BPS, CD, laryngeal dystonia, oromandibular dystonia, and focal limb dystonia [26]. There is level B evidence for use of Onabot and Incobot and level C evidence supporting the use of Abobot in the treatment of BPS. BoNT therapy in BPS produces roughly a 2.5-point improvement on the 4-point Global Clinical Improvement (GCI) scale [42]. The most common side

Table 1 Injection sites and potential side effects of BoNT [38]

Pattern of dystonia	Muscles targeted by injections	Side effects
Blepharospasm	Orbicularis oculi Corrugator supercilii Procerus	Ptosis, dry eye, tearing, diplopia
CD: torticollis	SCM (contralateral) Splenius (ipsilateral) Longissimus (ipsilateral)	Neck weakness, dysphagia
CD: laterocollis	Splenius (ipsilateral) Scalene(ipsilateral) SCM (ipsilateral) Levator Scapulae (ipsilateral) Trapezius (ipsilateral)	Neck weakness, dysphagia
CD: retrocollis	Splenius ± semispinalis (bilateral) Upper trapezius (bilateral)	Neck weakness, dysphagia
CD: Anterocollis	SCM (bilateral) Scalene complex (bilateral)	Neck weakness, dysphagia
CD: shoulder elevation	Trapezius (ipsilateral) Levator scapulae (ipsilateral)	Neck weakness, dysphagia

CD (cervical dystonia)

effects observed are periorbital hematoma in 25%, ptosis in 13–54%, dry eyes in 7.1–13%, and blurry vision in 42% [27] (see Table 1). Recommendations for use of BoNT in BPS are based on two Class II studies supporting use of Onabot and one class I study supporting use of Incobot as "probably safe and effective." Abobot received the designation of "possibly effective" in BPS based on one class II study, and there is insufficient evidence to support the use of Rimabot in this disorder. Incobot and Onabot are considered equally effective in treating BPS based on a class I comparative effectiveness study performed in 2011, and two more recent comparative effectiveness studies (Class I and Class III). Abobot and Onabot are considered "possibly equivalent" in the treatment of BPS [27].

For the treatment of CD, Abobot and Rimabot are supported by Level A evidence and evidence for use of Onabot and Incobot is level B [27]. Incobot improved the Toronto Western Spasmodic Torticollis Rating Scale (TWSTRS) total score by almost ten points 4 weeks following injection in one study, and improved severity, disability and pain scores in a second study [43, 44]. Onabot was found to improve CD severity, associated disability, pain, and degree of head turning at rest compared to placebo, but was more likely to produce dysphagia and rhinitis [45, 46]. Commonly involved muscles and BoNT starting doses are outlined in Table 2.

Multiple randomized, double-blind, placebo-controlled trials have proven the efficacy of BoNT in WC. There is level B evidence for use of Abobot and Onabot in the treatment of focal limb dystonia [47]. A study of Abobot in WC reported significant improvements in handwriting scales, writing speed, and symptom severity. All but one of the patients who received Abobot in this study reported weakness of the injected muscles, but most reported persistent benefit and continued treatment 1 year after the initial injection [48]. Although BoNT injections are regarded as the

Table 2 Recommended botulinum toxin doses in CD [29]

Muscle	Onabot (units)	Incobot (units)	Abobot (units)	Rimabot (units)
Sternocleidomastoid	30–50	30–50	100–200	1000–2500
Splenius	50–60	50–60	200–300	2500–5000
Semispinalis	30–40	30–40	60–150	750–1500
Upper trapezius	40–60	40–60	150–200	1000–2500
Levator scapulae	40–60	40–60	150–200	500–1000
Scalene	30–50	30–50	100–200	500–1000

Onabot: onabotulinumtoxinA, *Incobot:* incobotulinumtoxinA, *Abobot:* abobotulinimtoxA, *Rimabot:* rimabotulinumtoxinB

Table 3 Evidence-based recommendations for efficacy of different botulinum toxin formulations [27]

Indication	Level A	Level B	Level C	Level D
Blepharospasm		Onabot Incobot	Abobot	Rimabot
Cervical dystonia	Abobot Rimabot	Onabot Incobot		
Focal hand dystonia		Abobot Onabot		

Onabot: onabotulinumtoxinA, *Incobot:* incobotulinumtoxinA, *Abobot:* abobotulinimtoxA, *Rimabot:* rimabotulinumtoxinB

treatment of choice for spasmodic dysphonia, there have been no randomized clinical trials to establish a recommendation for its use (Table 3).

Some patients may experience clinical benefit as soon as 2 days after injection with BoNT, but the maximal benefit typically occurs 2–6 weeks after injection. After 6 weeks the benefit begins to wane. The usual duration of benefit is between 10 and 16 weeks, and many patients undergo repeat injections every 3 months [39]. Injections are typically started at the lowest possible dose to avoid unwanted side effects, such as those caused by diffusion of the toxin into adjacent muscle groups. In BPS, many patients report dry eyes, bleeding at the injection site, ptosis, and rarely diplopia from weakness of the extra-ocular muscles [39]. In CD, chemodenervation may cause dry mouth, neck weakness, and most commonly dysphagia [27]. The overall rate of dysphagia is 3.4–19.4%, but is dependent upon the brand of BoNT used. Onabot is associated with dysphagia rates between 8.9% and 10.5%, whereas dysphagia can occur in 26.8% of patients receiving Abobot [49]. When using Incobot, dysphagia occurred in 23.4% of patients who received 240 units of toxin and 10.7% of patients who received a smaller dose of 120 units [27]. Regardless of brand, the dysphagia is usually mild and resolves in 2–4 weeks. Patients with anterocollis are particularly susceptible to post-injection dysphagia given the location of the required injections. Injections for focal limb dystonia can result in weakness of the treated limb [39].

Typically BoNT-A is used first in the treatment of dystonia. The specific formulations of the toxin chosen often have to do with factors such as cost, availability to the physician, and physician experience. Electromyography (EMG) or ultrasound (US) can be used, especially in the limbs and neck, to guide the physician into the involved muscles. There is Level I evidence that EMG and US guidance significantly improves injection outcomes [50]. In addition, there are current studies evaluating whether the mapping of motor endplates, where BoNT enters the neuron, will enhance efficacy and reduce side effects. Using motor endplate injections of BoNT may reduce the dose of BoNT necessary for treatment by 50% in CD [51].

It should be noted that despite significant subjective and objective data from clinical trials indicating that dystonia is successfully treated with BoNT, many patients are lost to follow-up. A recent prospective, observational, multi-center, "real world" registry study investigated the efficacy and safety of Onabot in the treatment of CD. It followed 1046 patients with CD who were treatment-naïve (or had not received injections for at least 16 weeks) over three injection cycles. The mean Toronto Western Spasmodic Torticollis Rating Scale (TWSTRS score) in the 479 subjects who completed the treatment protocol decreased from 39.2 at baseline to 27.1 at the final visit. Furthermore, both physicians and patients reported impressions of improvement were increased by the final treatment visit. Despite these improvements, more than half of the patients initially included in the study were lost to follow-up and did not continue treatment with the injecting physician. This may be in part due to the nature of registry studies which have broader subject populations, are longer in duration, and require patients to pay for the medication received. Most of the subjects who withdrew late in the course of the study did receive the full treatment dose but were lost to follow-up—possibly because they did not have the time nor desire to partake in a non-treatment visit. It may also have been that patients who completed the entire study protocol had the more severe disease [52]. Despite these factors, however, it remains unclear why so many patients discontinue what has proven to be a beneficial and safe treatment.

Non-injected formulations of the toxin are also being investigated. In 2013, Lungu et al. studied 24 patients with BPS, adding topical competitive SNAP-25 inhibitor Acetyl-Hexapeptide (AH8) to their BoNT injections. This was a double-blind, placebo-controlled trial in which the primary outcome was time to return to baseline Jankovic Blepharospasm Rating Scale (JBRS) score after BoNT injection and simultaneous initiation of AH8. The study found the medication to be safe and also that the treatment group had a trend toward a longer time until they returned to their baseline JBRS score compared to the placebo group indicating that addition of this medication to the injection could prolong treatment benefit [7, 53].

Conclusion

BoNT is the current treatment of choice for focal dystonia and may be useful for selected areas in generalized dystonia as well. Use of BoNT is supported by multiple studies and its safety and efficacy have been demonstrated multiple times. The major limitation of BoNT relates to dosing and the occurrence of side effects which are mostly due to spread of the toxin into adjacent muscles. Despite its demonstrated efficacy, there are many patients who discontinue therapy for unknown reasons.

References

1. Albanese A, Bhatia K, Bressman SB, et al. Phenomenology and classification of dystonia: a consensus update. Mov Disord. 2013;28:863–73.
2. Albanese A, Barnes MP, Bhatia KP, et al. A systematic review on the diagnosis and treatment of primary (idiopathic) dystonia and dystonia plus syndromes: report of an EFNS/MDS-ES Task Force. Eur J Neurol. 2006;13:433–44.
3. Balash Y, Giladi N. Efficacy of pharmacological treatment of dystonia: evidence-based review including meta-analysis of the effect of botulinum toxin and other cure options. Eur J Neurol. 2004;11:361–70.
4. Nutt JG, Muenter MD, Aronson A, Kurland LT, Melton LJ III. Epidemiology of focal and generalized dystonia in Rochester, Minnesota. Mov Disord. 1988;3:188–94.
5. Bressman SB. Dystonia update. Clin Neuropharmacol. 2000;23:239–51.
6. Defazio G, Jankovic J, Giel JL, Papapetropoulos S. Descriptive epidemiology of cervical dystonia. Tremor Other Hyperkinet Mov (N Y). 2013;3
7. Ramirez-Castaneda J, Jankovic J. Long-term efficacy, safety, and side effect profile of botulinum toxin in dystonia: a 20-year follow-up. Toxicon. 2014;90:344–8.
8. Fahn S, Bressman SB, Marsden CD. Classification of dystonia. Adv Neurol. 1998;78:1–10.
9. Stamelou M, Edwards MJ, Hallett M, Bhatia KP. The non-motor syndrome of primary dystonia: clinical and pathophysiological implications. Brain. 2012;135:1668–81.
10. Defazio G, Abbruzzese G, Livrea P, Berardelli A. Epidemiology of primary dystonia. Lancet Neurol. 2004;3:673–8.
11. Jankovic J, Leder S, Warner D, Schwartz K. Cervical dystonia: clinical findings and associated movement disorders. Neurology. 1991;41:1088–91.
12. Steeves TD, Day L, Dykeman J, Jette N, Pringsheim T. The prevalence of primary dystonia: a systematic review and meta-analysis. Mov Disord. 2012;27:1789–96.
13. Abbruzzese G, Berardelli A, Girlanda P, et al. Long-term assessment of the risk of spread in primary late-onset focal dystonia. J Neurol Neurosurg Psychiatry. 2008;79:392–6.
14. Valls-Sole J, Defazio G. Blepharospasm: update on epidemiology, clinical aspects, and pathophysiology. Front Neurol. 2016;7:45.
15. Pandey S. A practical approach to management of focal hand dystonia. Ann Indian Acad Neurol. 2015;18:146–53.
16. Jedynak PC, Tranchant C, de Beyl DZ. Prospective clinical study of writer's cramp. Mov Disord. 2001;16:494–9.
17. Eskow Jaunarajs KL, Bonsi P, Chesselet MF, Standaert DG, Pisani A. Striatal cholinergic dysfunction as a unifying theme in the pathophysiology of dystonia. Prog Neurobiol. 2015;127–128:91–107.
18. LeDoux MS, Brady KA. Secondary cervical dystonia associated with structural lesions of the central nervous system. Mov Disord. 2003;18:60–9.
19. Peller M, Zeuner KE, Munchau A, et al. The basal ganglia are hyperactive during the discrimination of tactile stimuli in writer's cramp. Brain. 2006;129:2697–708.
20. Lera G, Bhatia K, Marsden CD. Dystonia as the major manifestation of Leigh's syndrome. Mov Disord. 1994;9:642–9.
21. Bradley D, Whelan R, Walsh R, et al. Temporal discrimination threshold: VBM evidence for an endophenotype in adult onset primary torsion dystonia. Brain. 2009;132:2327–35.

22. Argyelan M, Carbon M, Niethammer M, et al. Cerebellothalamocortical connectivity regulates penetrance in dystonia. J Neurosci. 2009;29:9740–7.
23. Naudon L, Delfs JM, Clavel N, Lorden JF, Chesselet MF. Differential expression of glutamate decarboxylase messenger RNA in cerebellar Purkinje cells and deep cerebellar nuclei of the genetically dystonic rat. Neuroscience. 1998;82:1087–94.
24. Raike RS, Jinnah HA, Hess EJ. Animal models of generalized dystonia. NeuroRx. 2005;2:504–12.
25. Albright AL, Ferson SS. Intraventricular baclofen for dystonia: techniques and outcomes. Clinical article. J Neurosurg Pediatr. 2009;3:11–4.
26. Simpson DM, Blitzer A, Brashear A, et al. Assessment: Botulinum neurotoxin for the treatment of movement disorders (an evidence-based review): report of the Therapeutics and Technology Assessment Subcommittee of the American Academy of Neurology. Neurology. 2008;70:1699–706.
27. Simpson DM, Hallett M, Ashman EJ, et al. Practice guideline update summary: Botulinum neurotoxin for the treatment of blepharospasm, cervical dystonia, adult spasticity, and headache: Report of the Guideline Development Subcommittee of the American Academy of Neurology. Neurology. 2016;86:1818–26.
28. Hallett M. Neurophysiology of dystonia: the role of inhibition. Neurobiol Dis. 2011;42:177–84.
29. Morgante F, Klein C. Dystonia. Continuum (Minneap Minn). 2013;19:1225–41.
30. Quartarone A, Pisani A. Abnormal plasticity in dystonia: disruption of synaptic homeostasis. Neurobiol Dis. 2011;42:162–70.
31. Quartarone A, Hallett M. Emerging concepts in the physiological basis of dystonia. Mov Disord. 2013;28:958–67.
32. Burke RE, Fahn S, Marsden CD. Torsion dystonia: a double-blind, prospective trial of high-dosage trihexyphenidyl. Neurology. 1986;36:160–4.
33. Greene P, Shale H, Fahn S. Analysis of open-label trials in torsion dystonia using high dosages of anticholinergics and other drugs. Mov Disord. 1988;3:46–60.
34. Bressman SB, Greene PE. Treatment of hyperkinetic movement disorders. Neurol Clin. 1990;8:51–75.
35. Cao S, Hewett JW, Yokoi F, et al. Chemical enhancement of torsinA function in cell and animal models of torsion dystonia. Dis Model Mech. 2010;3:386–96.
36. Loscher W, Richter A. Piracetam and levetiracetam, two pyrrolidone derivatives, exert antidystonic activity in a hamster model of paroxysmal dystonia. Eur J Pharmacol. 2000;391:251–4.
37. Aoki KR, Guyer B. Botulinum toxin type A and other botulinum toxin serotypes: a comparative review of biochemical and pharmacological actions. Eur J Neurol. 2001;8(Suppl 5):21–9.
38. Truong D, Dressler D, Hallett M. Manual of botulinum toxin therapy. Cambridge, UK. New York: Cambridge University Press; 2009.
39. Shanker V, Bressman SB. Diagnosis and Management of Dystonia. Continuum (Minneap Minn). 2016;22:1227–45.
40. Walker TJ, Dayan SH. Comparison and overview of currently available neurotoxins. J Clin Aesthet Dermatol. 2014;7:31–9.
41. Fraint A, Vittal P, Comella C. Considerations on patient-related outcomes with the use of botulinum toxins: is switching products safe? Ther Clin Risk Manag. 2016;12:147–54.
42. Kollewe K, Mohammadi B, Kohler S, Pickenbrock H, Dengler R, Dressler D. Blepharospasm: long-term treatment with either Botox(R), Xeomin(R) or Dysport(R). J Neural Transm (Vienna). 2015;122:427–31.
43. Comella CL, Jankovic J, Truong DD, Hanschmann A, Grafe S, Group USXCDS. Efficacy and safety of incobotulinumtoxinA (NT 201, XEOMIN(R), botulinum neurotoxin type A, without accessory proteins) in patients with cervical dystonia. J Neurol Sci. 2011;308:103–9.
44. Evidente VG, Fernandez HH, LeDoux MS, et al. A randomized, double-blind study of repeated incobotulinumtoxinA (Xeomin((R))) in cervical dystonia. J Neural Transm (Vienna). 2013;120:1699–707.

45. Charles D, Brashear A, Hauser RA, et al. Efficacy, tolerability, and immunogenicity of onabotulinumtoxina in a randomized, double-blind, placebo-controlled trial for cervical dystonia. Clin Neuropharmacol. 2012;35:208–14.
46. Greene P, Kang U, Fahn S, Brin M, Moskowitz C, Flaster E. Double-blind, placebo-controlled trial of botulinum toxin injections for the treatment of spasmodic torticollis. Neurology. 1990;40:1213–8.
47. Hallett M, Albanese A, Dressler D, et al. Evidence-based review and assessment of botulinum neurotoxin for the treatment of movement disorders. Toxicon. 2013;67:94–114.
48. Kruisdijk JJ, Koelman JH, Ongerboer de Visser BW, de Haan RJ, Speelman JD. Botulinum toxin for writer's cramp: a randomised, placebo-controlled trial and 1-year follow-up. J Neurol Neurosurg Psychiatry. 2007;78:264–70.
49. Chapman MA, Barron R, Tanis DC, Gill CE, Charles PD. Comparison of botulinum neurotoxin preparations for the treatment of cervical dystonia. Clin Ther. 2007;29:1325–37.
50. Grigoriu AI, Dinomais M, Remy-Neris O, Brochard S. Impact of injection-guiding techniques on the effectiveness of botulinum toxin for the treatment of focal spasticity and dystonia: a systematic review. Arch Phys Med Rehabil. 2015;96:2067–78. e2061
51. Delnooz CC, Veugen LC, Pasman JW, Lapatki BG, van Dijk JP, van de Warrenburg BP. The clinical utility of botulinum toxin injections targeted at the motor endplate zone in cervical dystonia. Eur J Neurol. 2014;21:1486–e98.
52. Jankovic J, Adler CH, Charles D, et al. Primary results from the cervical dystonia patient registry for observation of onabotulinumtoxina efficacy (CD PROBE). J Neurol Sci. 2015;349:84–93.
53. Lungu C, Considine E, Zahir S, Ponsati B, Arrastia S, Hallett M. Pilot study of topical acetyl hexapeptide-8 in the treatment for blepharospasm in patients receiving botulinum toxin therapy. Eur J Neurol. 2013;20:515–8.

Botulinum Toxin Treatment in Parkinson's Disease and Atypical Parkinsonian Disorders

Parul Jindal and Joseph Jankovic

Introduction

Therapeutic applications of botulinum toxin (BoNT) have continued to expand into many clinical fields, since its first therapeutic use in the 1970s for strabismus [1]. BoNT was initially approved by the United States Food and Drug Administration (FDA) in 1989 for the treatment of strabismus, blepharospasm, and other facial spasms including hemifacial spasm. The number and scope of therapeutic and non-therapeutic (cosmetic) applications of BoNT is not matched by any other treatments [2, 3]. Besides cosmetic uses, chiefly in the treatment of wrinkles, BoNT has become the standard of care for the management of conditions like focal dystonia (e.g., blepharospasm, cervical dystonia, oromandibular dystonia, writer's cramp), spasticity, hyperhidrosis, hemifacial spasm, and a variety of ophthalmological and otolaryngeal disorders. It is also increasingly used for various gastroenterological and urological indications and as an analgesic therapy including migraines. In this chapter, we will review the role of BoNT in the treatment of multiple symptoms experienced by patients with Parkinson's disease (PD) and atypical parkinsonism (Table 1).

There are five different BoNT available at this time in Europe and America; four contain BoNT serotype A (onabotulinumtoxinA or Botox®, abobotulinumtoxinA or Dysport® and incobotulinumtoxinA or Xeomin®) and the other contains BoNT serotype B (rimabotulinumtoxinB or Myobloc®/NeuroBloc®). There are several other

P. Jindal, M.D. (✉) J. Jankovic, M.D.
Department of Neurology, Parkinson's Disease Center and Movement Disorders Clinic, Baylor College of Medicine, 7200 Cambridge, Suite 9A, Houston, TX 77030-4202, USA
e-mail: jindalneurology@gmail.com; Josephj@bcm.edu

B. Jabbari (ed.), *Botulinum Toxin Treatment in Clinical Medicine*,
DOI 10.1007/978-3-319-56038-0_3

Table 1 Botulinum toxin in the treatment of symptoms associated with Parkinson's disease and atypical parkinsonism

Tremor
Freezing of gait
Dystonia
Blepharospasm and lid apraxia
Bruxism
Limb dystonia—upper and lower extremities—striatal hand/foot
Axial dystonia
Camptocormia
Cervical dystonia
Sialorrhea
Hyperhidrosis
Dysphagia (achalasia)
Seborrhea
Overactive bladder
Constipation
Levodopa-related dystonia
Myoclonus
Dystonic clenched fist
Myorhythmia

forms of BoNT used in other parts of the world, e.g., Prosigne or CBTX-A in China and Meditoxin in South Korea, or are still in development, e.g., daxibotulinumtoxinA (RT002). Potency and doses of BoNT vary depending on the form of toxin and it is, therefore, absolutely critical that the treating clinician is aware of the source and pharmacology of the particular product used. The doses given for a particular toxin cannot be readily transferred to doses of other products, even if they are of the same toxin serotype. Hence, in this chapter different brand names will be mentioned as they have different properties and dosages that are unique to them.

Parkinson's Disease and Atypical Parkinsonism

Parkinson's disease (PD) is a common neurodegenerative disorder, affecting about 1% of the population over the age of 60 years. The mean age of onset is 55 years and men are slightly more frequently affected. According to the United Kingdom PD Society Brain Bank, the clinical criteria for probable PD require the presence of bradykinesia and at least one of the following features: rigidity, rest tremor of 4–6 Hz, or postural instability. In addition, flexed posture and freezing (motor blocks) have been included among classic features of parkinsonism, with PD as the most common form [4]. PD patients may have masked faces, low volume speech, dysphagia, sialorrhea, and shuffling gait. In addition to motor features, the patient

Table 2 Level of evidence support treatment of different symptoms associated with PD with BoNT

Disorder	Level of evidence
Overactive bladder [9]	Level A for BoNT serotype A and B
Hyperhidrosis [9]	Level A for BoNT serotype A, Level B for onabotulinumtoxinA and abobotulinumtoxinA individually
	Level U—rimabotulinumtoxinB and incobotulinumtoxinA
Sialorrhea [9]	Level B—onabotulinumtoxinA, abobotulinumtoxinA and rimabotulinumtoxinB
	Level U—incobotulinumtoxinA
Tremor, freezing of gait, camptocormia, constipation, seborrhea	Level U recommendation
Cervical dystonia [10]	Level A—abobotulinumtoxinA and rimabotulinumtoxinB
	Level B—onabotulinumtoxinA and incobotulinumtoxinA
Blepharospasm [10]	Level B—onabotulinumtoxinA, incobotulinumtoxinA
	Level B—abobotulinumtoxinA
	Level U—rimabotulinumtoxinB
Oromandibular dystonia [11]	Level C—onabotulinumtoxinA, abobotulinumtoxinA
	Level U—rimabotulinumtoxinB and incobotulinumtoxinA

Level A: established as effective (requires at least two consistent class I studies)
Level B: probably effective (requires at least one class I study or at least two consistent class II studies)
Level C: possibly effective (requires at least one class II study or two consistent class III studies)
Level U: inadequate or conflicting data, treatment is unproven

may notice multiple non-motor symptoms such as shoulder pain, depression, sleep problems, forgetfulness, and autonomic problems including orthostatic hypotension, constipation, urinary frequency, urgency, and incontinence. It is increasingly evident that PD is a heterogeneous disorder with variable clinical-pathologic phenotypes and natural history [5].

In addition to PD, there are many other parkinsonian disorders, such as multiple system atrophy (MSA), progressive supranuclear palsy (PSP), and corticobasal degeneration (CBD) that have symptoms which may be amenable to the treatment with BoNT. It is beyond the scope of this review to discuss these atypical parkinsonian disorders but the reader is referred to a recent review article [6].

While levodopa and other dopaminergic and non-dopaminergic drugs are quite effective in controlling the motor and non-motor symptoms of PD and to a lesser degree in atypical parkinsonism, BoNT has emerged as an effective therapeutic option for treatment of many symptoms associated with PD and atypical parkinsonism [6–8] (Table 2). In a retrospective study of 160 patients with idiopathic PD or atypical parkinsonism who received BoNT treatment, the indications for BoNT treatment were pain (50% cases), dystonia (26.2%), sialorrhea (18.7%), camptocormia (1.2%), and freezing of gait (FOG) (0.6%) [12]. Eighty-one percent of all PD patients reported benefits with BoNT treatment and similar results were seen in atypical parkinsonism group, as well. This review is organized according to the various parkinsonian symptoms and signs treated with BoNT.

Tremor

Rest tremor in hand is one of the common features of PD but postural and kinetic tremor may also be present. Re-emergent tremor, which appears after the hand is held in the postural position for some time, is a more bothersome tremor in PD patients than rest tremor as it often interferes with daily activities like holding a newspaper or a cup [13]. Even though tremor usually responds to conventional anti-PD treatment, other treatments such as BoNT may have to be considered when satisfactory relief is not obtained with conventional therapy and before considering deep brain stimulation (DBS).

Phenomenologically, essential tremor (ET) overlaps with re-emergent tremor in that it is a form of postural tremor [14]. BoNT has been shown to be effective in the treatment of essential tremor (ET) in two well-designed double-blind, placebo-controlled studies [15, 16]. Both these studies used onabotulinumtoxinA and showed reduction in the amplitude of tremor. The main complication in both studies was extensor finger weakness. Both studies used "fixed-dose-fixed muscle" approach rather than individualizing the BoNT dose and muscle selection based on specific needs. As a result, we recommend modified protocol with markedly reduced doses in the forearm extensors or completely eliminating injections in the extensor muscle group. In our center, we have achieved comparable tremor control with this modified technique and less incidence of extensor finger weakness [7, 14, 144].

Some studies have shown benefits of BoNT in other types of tremor including PD-related rest tremor. One open-label study examined the effects of BoNT on disabling tremors, classified as dystonic, essential, combination of dystonic and essential, parkinsonian, peripherally induced and cerebellar-outflow tremor and noted that 67% of 51 patients noticed some improvement in tremors with average duration of benefits lasting for 10.5 weeks [17]. In another open-label study, BoNT was injected into forearm and arm of 26 patients (12 with PD and 14 with ET) [18]. At 6 weeks after injection, 38% of the patients (ten total; five PD and five ET) reported moderate to marked subjective improvement in functional benefits. Only ET patients showed statistically significant improvement when pre- and post-injection scores were compared on the Webster Tremor and Global Disability Scales. In 2 of 12 PD patients (17%) and 3 of 14 ET patients (21%) more than 50% reduction in amplitude, assessed by accelerometry, was found after BoNT injections. An earlier study looking at outcome after BoNT treatment in 187 patients with limb disorders, 2 of 15 patients (13.3%) with PD tremor showed marked subjective improvement and significant decrement in tremor amplitude (more than 50% reduction) using quantitative measures [19]. In a single-blind, placebo-controlled study comparing the effects of 25–50 units of BoNT to placebo at 1 month, 60% of the BoNT group demonstrated benefits >30% above the placebo group; 40% improvement in postural PD-like tremor and 57% improvement in ET-like tremor, but there was no significant change in the rest tremor [20]. In a small open-label study seven patients with upper limb PD tremor were injected with incobotulinumtoxinA, using clinical and kinematic assessments to determine the dose and distribution of BoNT [21]. The study showed significant improvement across time points, represented by a reduction in the clinical scale score, in UPDRS Item 20 (rest tremor) at 1, 2, 3 months with respect to the baseline ($p = 0.005$, $p = 0.003$, $p = 0.007$, respectively), Item 21 (action and postural tremor) at 3 months ($p = 0.016$), and spiral drawing at 4 months with respect to the baseline ($p = 0.028$). In a subsequent, 38-week, open-label study using kinematic and biomechanics of tremor for deciding injection pattern of incobotulinumtoxinA in 28 PD patient showed statistically significant decrease in mean UPDRS item 20 at week 16 ($p = 0.006$) and at week 32 ($p = 0.014$), and in the Fahn-Tolosa-Marin Tremor Severity (FTMTS) scores at week 6 ($p = 0.024$) [22]. Further studies are needed to establish the efficacy of BoNT in patients with PD-related tremor [23]. Also, the findings from the published studies suggest that treatment protocols need to be individualized based on tremor type; for example, patients with prominent pronation-supination type hand tremor may require injection into biceps muscles in addition to wrist and finger flexors (Jankovic 2009b). Additionally, kinematic technology may be helpful in guiding the injection pattern when it is difficult to visually judge and decompose the motion involved during the tremor [24].

PD patients, in addition to hand or leg tremor, may also have chin, lip, jaw, or tongue tremor [25, 26]. Jaw tremor resulting in vertical or horizontal oscillation of the mandible may be difficult to treat with conventional dopaminergic medications or other anti-PD therapies [8]. In a case series of three patients with PD jaw tremor, injection of abobotulinumtoxinA (mean dose 53 units in each muscle) in both masseters was associated with subjective and clinical improvement [27]. The improvement in tremor was also noted on the video recording taken before and 4–9 weeks after injections. There were no serious side effects. There is also a case report of BoNT injections in bilateral digastric and masseters in reducing position-sensitive (tremor absent at rest but present when jaw partially opened) jaw tremor that worsened with speaking [28].

Freezing of Gait (FOG)

FOG refers to a sudden inability to initiate or continue ongoing gait, especially when starting to walk, making turns or walking through narrow passages with the associated perception that the feet are "stuck to the ground" [4]. In PD, FOG is associated with disease severity, although it can be seen in early stages of PD, as well [29, 30]. However, if FOG is the first presenting sign, atypical forms of parkinsonism, especially progressive supranuclear palsy (PSP), should be suspected [31]. FOG episodes that are less responsive or nonresponsive to dopaminergic treatments are the greatest therapeutic challenge. Some believe that FOG may be dystonic, associated with disinhibited foot grasp and others believe that it may be mediated by non-dopaminergic mechanisms, including damage to the brainstem pedunculopontine nucleus [29, 32].

Various treatment approaches exist for FOG, including pharmacological agents, surgical options, as well as physiotherapy, including the use of visual cues (e.g., stepping over an obstacle), auditory cues (e.g., musical rhythm), and other sensory techniques [33, 34]. In the treatment of FOG, it is important to distinguish between "on freezing" and "off freezing." "Off freezing," like other PD symptoms can be treated by preventing the patient from going "off." "On freezing" for unclear reasons tends to worsen by increasing the dosage of levodopa. In patients with dopamine-responsive FOG, in addition to dopaminergic medications (levodopa or dopamine agonists), trial of amantadine, rasagiline, selegiline, droxidopa, cholinergic drugs, CNS stimulants, and DBS may also be considered [35–39].

There have been few clinical trials of BoNT for the treatment of FOG. The use of BoNT into the distal leg muscles was based on the theory that involuntary contractions of these muscles may have a role in FOG. These studies involved injection of BoNT serotype A in gastrocnemius and soleus muscles unilaterally or bilaterally [40, 41]. While one of these studies showed marked improvement in 40% of the patients in 6 weeks, these results could not be reproduced in later studies using either BoNT serotype A or B [42–44]. Hence, the use of BoNT for FOG is now used only very rarely [34, 45].

Dystonia

Dystonia is defined as a movement disorder characterized by sustained or intermittent muscle contractions causing abnormal, often repetitive, movements, postures, or both [46]. Dystonic movements are typically patterned (same muscles keep contracting), twisting, and tremulous. Some forms of dystonia, such as blepharospasm and laryngeal dystonia, are not associated with abnormal postures, but are characterized by focal involuntary contractions that interfere with physiological opening or closing of the eyelids or the larynx. About 60% of PD patients with disease onset before age 40 can have different forms of dystonia and 30% of PD patients overall have dystonia [47]. The majority of the cases with dystonia as the presenting PD symptom had involvement of foot, which often can be painful. "Striatal" foot with unilateral equinovarus dystonia posture of the foot with great toe extension, flexion of the remaining toes and extension of the big toe, or "striatal" hand deformity, with flexion at the metacarpophalangeal joint, flexion of distal interphalangeal joints, and ulnar hand deviation may be seen in up to 40% of untreated PD patients with advanced disease [48]. These may be reversible with therapy but if left untreated, will result in fixed deformity. The cause of these deformities is unknown, but may be due to a combination of dystonia, low striatal dopamine, and fibrosis with alterations in soft-tissue plasticity and visco-elasticity [49]. Since levodopa has a variable effect on these deformities, BoNT has been used to effectively correct the abnormal postures in some patients with striatal hand and striatal foot and toe deformities particularly when not accompanied by fixed contractures [50, 51].

Blepharospasm and Lid Apraxia

Blepharospasm is an involuntary, forceful eye closure, which may be present in some patients with PD, but this form of focal dystonia is more common in patients with atypical parkinsonism. When blepharospasm occurs in the setting of parkinsonism, it is often associated with apraxia of eyelid opening (ALO). Indeed, blepharospasm in combination with ALO should raise the possibility of atypical parkinsonism, such as PSP [52].

The mechanism of ALO is not well understood but it has been thought to represent another form of a focal eyelid dystonia due to abnormal contractions of the pretarsal orbicularis oculi, levator palpebrae inhibition, or eyelid freezing [53].

ALO is often difficult to treat with BoNT and is one of the most common reasons for treatment failures in patients thought to have blepharospasm. There are rare reports of injections into the orbital part of orbicularis oculi that might be helpful [54]. Most reports, however, suggest that pre-tarsal injections of BoNT are usually needed to obtain some benefit in patients with ALO [53]. However, when blepharospasm triggers the ALO, then the conventional treatment with BoNT into pretarsal part of the orbicularis oculi can be very effective in treating both sufficiently to obtain optimum results and there is no need to do additional injections [55]. In addition to significantly higher response rate and longer duration of maximum response, pretarsal injections are associated with lower frequency of major side effects such as ptosis [56]. Avoiding the midline of upper lid, the area where the levator palpebrae muscle is located minimizes the risk of ptosis. Injection into the Riolan's muscle at the medial and lateral portions of the upper and lower pre-tarsal orbicularis oculi seems to yield the best results [57]. BoNT can also be used effectively to correct frowning (the procerus sign) when may be a form of upper facial dystonia, particularly common in patients with PSP [58, 59]. In a cross-sectional study, 114 blepharospasm patients who received ≥2 cycles of BoNT serotype A [onabotulinumtoxinA (n = 78), incobotulinumtoxinA (n = 35), or abobotulinumtoxinA (n = 1)] were interviewed immediately before re-injection to evaluate treatment satisfaction, time course of treatment effects, preferred injection intervals, Jankovic Rating Scale (JRS), and Blepharospasm Disability Index (BSDI) [60]. The most frequent injection interval was 12 weeks (46.5% subjects); 30.7% had an interval >12 weeks. 36.6% reported that treatment effects usually declined within 8 weeks; 69.6% within 10 weeks with BSDI scores indicating re-emergence of symptoms before re-injection. Overall, treatment satisfaction was high, but declined at the end of the cycle. Fifty-two percent of the subjects preferred an injection interval of <12 weeks. Although the standard-of-case 12-week interval is commonly used, in some patients flexible, individualized treatment interval may improve treatment satisfaction.

Botulinum toxin therapy is effective in secondary as well as primary blepharospasm, and toxin therapy can improve the quality of life [61, 62]. According to the 2016 AAN evidence-based review of the currently available clinical data available, it was concluded that onabotulinumtoxinA (based on two class II studies) and incobotulinumtoxinA (based on one Class I study) are probably effective in the treatment of blepharospasm (level B recommendation) and abobotulinumtoxinA (based on one Class II study) is possibly effective (level C recommendation). There are no quality studies to confirm the efficacy of rimabotulinumtoxinB (level U recommendation) [10]. The likely reason for the lack of optimal evidence supporting BoNT use in blepharospasm is robust benefits noted with BoNT in the initial open-label studies and the lack of alternate therapies which discouraged newer controlled clinical trials.

In a study comparing onabotulinumtoxinA and abobotulinumtoxinA in 212 patients with blepharospasm, duration of benefits was found to be similar in both groups. AbobotulinumtoxinA arm had higher rate of side effects like ptosis, dry eyes, tearing, blurred vision, double vision, hematoma, and foreign body sensation [63], which were attributed to higher diffusing properties of this toxin. However, Sampaio et al. found no difference between onabotulinumtoxinA and abobotulinumtoxinA with regard to duration of effect or adverse events in a single-blind, randomized comparison [64]. IncobotulinumtoxinA was found to be non-inferior to onabotulinumtoxinA, when compared in 300 patients with blepharospasm in a randomized, double-blind study [65]. There have been studies comparing onabotulinumtoxinA with other formulations such as Prosigne® (not available in the US) [66] and Meditoxin® (not available in the US) [67], and no significant difference was found between the groups. According to the 2016 AAN evidence-based review, incobotulinumtoxinA and onabotulinumtoxinA are equivalent in efficacy for treating blepharospasm based on two Class I effectiveness studies and one Class II study. AbobotulinumtoxinA and onabotulinumtoxinA are possibly equivalent for treating blepharospasm based on one class II study [10].

Oromandibular Dystonia and Bruxism

Oromandibular dystonia (OMD) in a patient with co-existent parkinsonism often suggests the possibility of MSA or some other atypical form of parkinsonism, but it can also be levodopa-induced in patients with PD. OMD is characterized by involuntary repetitive spasms mainly involving masticatory muscles but often includes lingual and pharyngeal muscles [68, 69]. OMD can be jaw-closing, jaw-opening, lateral jaw deviation, or a combination of these abnormal movements as well as bruxism (jaw clenching and teeth grinding) [70]. It can involve lips and tongue (mostly protrusion). Bruxism can occur while the patient is awake or asleep (nocturnal bruxism). If untreated, this can lead to tooth destruction, temporomandibular joint (TMJ) dysfunction, headaches, and disruption of the bed partner's sleep due to grinding sounds.

Supportive therapy includes the use of night guards and dental appliances. BoNT has been used to treat OMD and is most effective in treating jaw-closing and jaw-deviation dystonia [71]. There is limited literature related to the use of BoNT in the management of bruxism [72]. There are only two randomized controlled trials looking at the effectiveness of BoNT in bruxism [73, 74]. Injections are typically given in masseters and temporalis for jaw closing dystonia. Both the studies revealed a reduction in bruxism with BoNT; however, these studies had the small sample size and relied on questionnaires and portable EMG to establish the diagnosis of bruxism. According to a placebo-controlled, parallel design, polysomnogram study, onabotulinumtoxinA injected into masseter and temporalis improved sleep bruxism as demonstrated by significant improvement in clinical global impression ($p < 0.05$) and visual analogue scales ($p < 0.05$) [75].

For jaw-opening OMD, the most important muscle to be targeted with BoNT is the external pterygoid. Digastric and myohyoid muscles are also involved in some cases of jaw-opening dystonia and the submental muscle complex is often injected in our center in patients with jaw-opening dystonia with or without anterocollis and with or without associated parkinsonism. This form of jaw-opening dystonia, also referred to as "hyoid muscle dystonia," may benefit from BoNT injections into the appropriate muscles in about 71% of cases [76]. For jaw deviation, ipsilateral masseter or contralateral external pterygoid muscles may need to be injected to bring the jaw back to normal alignment. When there is associated jaw protrusion, both external pterygoids may be involved and may require injection [77]. The pterygoid muscle injections may have to be performed with EMG guidance, as these muscles are not easy to palpate.

Treatment of OMD with BoNT can improve speech and chewing [78]. An open-label study evaluated onabotulinumtoxinA for OMD in 62 patients and 73% of the subjects had a favorable response based on a global rating scale. In 115 patients with OMD, 42 (37%) visits were followed by some complications, primarily consisting of dysphagia [79]. In another study, 162 patients with OMD (more than half with jaw-closing dystonia) were injected with BoNT serotype A in masseters and submental muscle complex, or both with a mean follow-up of 4.4 ± 3.8 years. On a scale of 0–4 (4 = complete resolution), the mean global effect of BoNT was 3.1 ± 1.0, with the best response in jaw-closing dystonia. Complications such as dysphagia and dysarthria were reported in 11.1% of all treatment visits [70]. In another study, 18 patients with severe bruxism injected with onabotulinumtoxinA in bilateral masseter with the mean dose of 61.7 ± 11.1 units during 123 treatment visits. On a scale of 0–4 where 4 equals total abolishment of grinding the mean peak effect was 3.4 ± 0.9, mean total duration of response was 19.1 ± 17.0 weeks and only one subject (5.6%) reported experiencing dysphagia [71]. Another open-label study explored genioglossus injections of onabotulinumtoxinA for lingual protrusion dystonia in nine patients, who received a mean dose of 13.3 units into each genioglossus muscle [80]. In this study, five patients (55.6%) had moderate or marked reduction in tongue protrusion. One patient developed severe dysphagia requiring placement of a percutaneous gastrostomy (PEG) tube. An observational prospective study investigated the impact of BoNT treatment on the quality of life

(QoL) in 30 patients with prominent lingual dystonia as measured by oromandibular dystonia questionnaire-25 (OMDQ-25) scores [81]. Genioglossus, lateral and medial pterygoids, anterior digastric, masseter, and temporalis muscles were injected with abotulinumtoxinA in 27 patients and onabotulinumtoxinA in three patients. After BoNT treatment, the total OMDQ-25 score reduced from mean of 46.8 at baseline to 38.2 at 4 weeks ($p = 0.004$) and 39.6 at 8 weeks ($p = 0.008$). OnabotulinumtoxinA and abobotulinumtoxinA have received level C rating (possibly effective) for use in OMD [11]. There are no published studies in which incobotulinumtoxinA or rimabotulinumtoxinB were used for the treatment of OMD or bruxism.

Limb Dystonia

Unlike dystonic writer's cramp, which is probably the most common form of focal dystonia associated with abnormal contraction of the muscles of the fingers, wrist and arm producing abnormal posture, often detected by mirror maneuvers [82], the parkinsonian writer's cramp is characterized by an isometric contraction of the hand muscles resulting in a tight grip on the pen and minor flexion of the arm [83]. The data on the use of BoNT in focal hand dystonia (idiopathic rather than PD-related) are based on one class 1 study [84] and one class 2 study [85] of abobotulinumtoxinA and two class 2 studies on onabotulinumtoxinA [86, 87]. The most common side effect reported was the focal weakness. In an evidence-based review of BoNT in the treatment of focal hand dystonia, both abobotulinumtoxinA and onabotulinumtoxinA were considered to be possibly effective (level B recommendation) [11]. There are no published studies using incobotulinumtoxinA or rimabotulinumtoxinB for focal hand dystonia.

In young onset PD, foot dystonia often present as exercise-induced toe cramping that can progress to inversion of the foot and disability. Striatal deformities of the foot with unilateral equinovarus dystonic posture of the foot and extension of the great toe can present in up to 40% of untreated patients with advanced PD. It can also be a form of wearing off dystonia, or less frequently peak dose dyskinesias, in patients on levodopa therapy. There is no class 1 study confirming the efficacy and safety of BoNT for the treatment of foot dystonia but BoNT is widely used off-label for this indication. In an open-label pilot study, onabotulinumtoxinA was used to treat off painful dystonia induced by levodopa in 30 patients with PD [88]. Tibialis posterior, tibialis anterior, gastrocnemius, flexor digitorum longus, and extensor hallucis longus were injected with a median dose 40 IU for each muscle, distributed in two sites. In all patients, the pain originating from afferent nerve fibers within the dystonic muscle, improved within 10 days and seven patients noted an improvement of foot posture on walking.

BoNT has also been found helpful in symptomatic relief of pain and in preventing skin damage in patients with "dystonic clenched fist," a relatively common condition in advanced stages of CBD and other parkinsonian disorders [89]. In one small study, abobotulinumtoxinA was injected into dystonic clenched fist of three CBD patients [90]. Lumbricals, flexor pollicis brevis, flexor digitorum superficialis, and flexor carpi ulnaris muscles were injected. All three patients had significant improvement in pain and muscle relaxation after the first treatment without any functional improvement because of associated apraxia. There was an improvement in hand posture in one patient and gain in palmar hygiene in the other patient. In an observational study of 26 CBD patients, all 11 who received BoNT for their dystonic limb posturing had symptomatic benefits as reflected by improvement in the Unified Dystonia Rating Scale (UDRS) [91]. These studies suggest that BoNT injections for dystonia in CBD can be used to reduce pain, improve hygiene, prevent secondary contractures, and on occasion, improve limb function when applied early in the disease course [92, 178].

Cervical Dystonia

Cervical dystonia is the most common form of axial dystonia. When it is present in patients with PD or other parkinsonian disorders, it often manifests as neck flexion ("dropped head" or "bent spine") and may be accompanied by truncal flexion (camptocormia), scoliosis, pisa syndrome or tilting of the trunk to one side (also known as pleurothotonus) or a combination of these postures [4].

Cervical dystonia is characterized by involuntary patterned contractions of cervical musculature resulting in abnormal movements or postural changes of the head, neck, and shoulders [93, 94]. Cervical dystonia can lead to clinically heterogeneous directional presentations of the neck, such as torticollis, laterocollis, retrocollis, or anterocollis. The patient may have associated shoulder elevation, head oscillation, neck pain, and a variety of alleviating maneuvers, also referred to as sensory tricks [95].

Anterocollis is more typically associated with parkinsonism, specifically PD and MSA [7] whereas neck extension is more typically present in PSP [47]. The neck extension in PSP may be a form of axial rigidity rather than dystonia [47]. Various theories have been proposed for anterocollis including neck extensor myopathy, imbalanced rigidity of anterior and posterior neck muscles, as well as dystonia [182, 96].

BoNT is considered the most effective treatment for cervical dystonia. According to the American Academy of Neurology Practice Guideline report, abobotulinumtoxinA and rimabotulinumtoxinB have level A evidence, whereas onabotulinumtoxinA and incobotulinumtoxinA have level B evidence for the treatment of cervical dystonia [10]. The reason for lack of evidence to support efficacy and safety of BoNT in the treatment of neck flexion (anterocollis), the most common abnormal neck posture in parkinsonism, is because these patients are excluded from cervical dystonia studies of BoNT due to the belief that anterocollis is difficult to treat with BoNT and bilateral injections of sternocleidomastoid and scalene muscles is associated with dysphagia. However, at our center we have successfully treated some of these patients with anterocollis using BoNT, with minimal or no side adverse effects

[7]. Avoiding the lower portions of sternocleidomastoid muscle can also lower the risk of dysphagia. There are case reports of the use of injections of BoNT in the lower third of the sternocleidomastoid in patients with refractory anterocollis with marked benefit and no complications [97]. Deep prevertebral muscles such as longus colli and longus capitis may also be involved in anterocollis, but these are difficult to reach although the injury to vertebral vessels and other complications may be avoided by use of imaging techniques [98, 99]. Sometimes injections into submental muscle complex may be helpful when anterocollis is accompanied by downward jaw deviation due to contractions of the hyoid muscles [7]. Some have categorized anterocollis into conceptual anterocollis, anterocaput, and forward sagittal shift, and have suggested that electromyography, computed tomography, magnetic resonance imaging, FDG-positron emission tomography, endoscopy, and other techniques may need to be utilized to achieve optimal results with BoNT treatment [100]. Retrocollis is relatively easy to treat by injections into posterior neck muscles such as splenius capitis or splenius cervicis [101].

Levodopa-Induced Dyskinesias

Levodopa-induced dyskinesia (LID) is categorized as "peak-dose dyskinesias," "diphasic dyskinesia," and "off-period dystonia" based on the relationship to levodopa dosing. Off-period dyskinesia, typically in a form of dystonia, often responds to adjustments in dopaminergic drugs, addition of catechol-O-methyltransferase (COMT) inhibitor, monoamine oxidase B (MAO-B) inhibitors, dopamine agonists, baclofen, subcutaneous apomorphine, or BoNT [102]. Off-period dystonia accounts for about 30% of the levodopa-induced dyskinesias. Levodopa-related dystonia typically presents when levels of levodopa are rising or falling, but in most cases levodopa-related dystonia is a wearing-off phenomenon. It may be seen in the morning before the first dose of medication or in-between doses. It typically manifests as painful muscle spasms, toe curling, foot flexion, and inversion. Off-period dystonia occurs when the striatal dopamine concentration is low [103, 104]. Both presynaptic dopamine depletion and postsynaptic mechanisms play an important role in LID [103, 105]. Some groups propose that intermittent dosing of levodopa is more likely to shorten the response to each dose of levodopa as compared to a continuous administration [106, 183]. In some cases, BoNT may alleviate prolonged painful foot dystonia. In one study, eight levodopa-treated PD patients with frequent and bothersome cervical-predominant LID, regardless of any antidyskinetic treatment were randomized to receive EMG-guided onabotulinumtoxinA or placebo with normal saline [107]. Assessments occurred at 0, 1, 3 (crossover visit), 4, and 6 months after enrollment, with blinded injections administered at the 0- and 3-month visits. Primary outcome measure was a change in the Goetz dyskinesia rating scale (GDRS, 0–4, higher is worse), modified for the cervical region, 1 month after each injection (1- and 4-month study visits). Only four patients completed the 6-month study before voluntarily stopping due to excessive neck weakness. OnabotulinumtoxinA improved GDRS scores for the resting but not action-induced dyskinesias. Only one subject requested onabotulinumtoxinA injections for ongoing post-study management of his LID.

Myoclonus and Myorhythmia

BoNT may be helpful in the treatment of limb myoclonus associated with CBD or other parkinsonian disorder. Although no well-controlled trials have been conducted, this treatment, however, has been reported to be effective in the treatment of segmental myoclonus [29, 108].

Myorhythmia is described as a repetitive, rhythmic, jerky movement of slow (1–4 Hz) frequency, affecting mainly cranial and limb muscles, usually at rest but sometimes noted also with sustained posture [109]. It may be associated with parkinsonian signs such as rigidity and bradykinesia. BoNT may be safe and effective in the treatment of limb myorhythmia.

Camptocormia

Skeletal and joint deformities, such as striatal hand and feet, bent spine, camptocormia, and pisa syndrome, are common and often under-recognized features of PD and atypical parkinsonism [48, 110–112]. Although usually caused by axial dystonia, there are many pathophysiologic mechanisms of camptocormia, characterized by marked flexion (usually more than 45°) of thoracolumbar spine [23, 96, 113]. Walking typically exacerbates dystonic camptocormia and maneuvers such as "climbing the wall" and supine position tends to relieve the condition. The prevalence of camptocormia in PD has been reported between 4.1% and 17.6% [114]. Conventional anti-PD and anti-spasticity medications are not very beneficial in the treatment of camptocormia. Hence, BoNT and other strategies like DBS may have to be considered in these patients [115]. In one study, 9 of the 11 patients with camptocormia received onabotulinumtoxinA injections into the rectus abdominus with notable improvement in 4 of the 9 patients [116]. These patients had clinical evidence of contraction of rectus abdominus and received injections of between onabotulinumtoxinA 300 and 600 units per treatment visit. The effect lasted for about 3 months after each injection with a mean duration of maximal response in three patients of 10 ± 6 weeks. There have been few negative trials using BoNT serotype A including onabotulinumtoxinA, abobotulinumtoxinA and incobotulinumtoxinA, with injections into only iliopsoas muscle or both iliopsoas and rectus abdominus muscles, using either blind injection technique, ultrasound or CT guidance [117, 139, 179]. Overall, the efficacy of BoNT for camptocormia is controversial, but when the most involved muscles are selected for injection with appropriate dose and skilled technique, the results can be quite satisfactory.

Sialorrhea

Sialorrhea, present in approximately 75% of the patients, is a common source of embarrassment and social handicap, skin irritation around the mouth, and swallowing problems that can lead to impaired quality of life of patients with PD [4].

In a study, where unstimulated saliva production was measured over 5 min revealed that patients with PD produce less saliva than normal controls [163]. Female PD patients produce less saliva than men with Parkinson's disease and levodopa therapy increases the salivary flow in these patients [177]. This suggests that the cause of sialorrhea in PD is due to impaired reflex deglutition rather than hypersecretion. Even in PD patients with no dysphagia complaints, the oral and pharyngeal parts of the swallow are significantly slower; they required more swallows to clear a small amount of liquid and have fewer swallows followed by expiration [162]. The possible causes of impaired deglutition include involvement of motor nucleus of the vagus, degeneration of the myenteric plexus in the esophagus, and flexed posture. In addition, dysregulation of the salivary function due to the involvement of salivary parasympathetic ganglia has also been postulated.

The treatment options for sialorrhea in PD include anticholinergic drugs like oral glycopyrrolate, sublingual ipratropium bromide spray, sublingual atropine drops, clonidine, and modafinil [133]. Side effects of anticholinergic drugs preclude their use, especially in the elderly. BoNT serotype A has been shown to be effective for sialorrhea [147, 149, 151]. In various studies using onabotulinumtoxinA for sialorrhea, the dose ranged from 5 to 50 and 5 units per parotid and submandibular gland, respectively and it significantly reduced drooling in PD, MSA, and DLB patients for approximately 4 months [173]. The typical dose for abobotulinumtoxinA for sialorrhea in three published studies ranged from 75 to 146.2 units and 78.7 units per parotid and submandibular gland, respectively. BoNT type B injections into the parotid and submandibular glands also appear to be effective in the treatment of PD-related sialorrhea and may have a potential advantage over BoNT type A [132, 158]. BoNT serotype B leads to greater incidence of dry mouth when used in the treatment of cervical dystonia and hence may be considered the treatment of choice for sialorrhea [175, 176]. Ultrasound guidance may be helpful in improving the accuracy of injection into the parotid gland [137]. According to the evidence-based review, rimabotulinumtoxinB, abobotulinumtoxinA, and onabotulinumtoxinA all have level B recommendation for sialorrhea. There are insufficient data on the use of incobotulinumtoxinA (level U) for sialorrhea [9]. The facial nerve is close to parotid gland and caution must be taken when injecting for sialorrhea. The optimal number of injections into the parotid gland is debatable; some institutions distribute the dose within two injection sites but other may choose to give up to nine injections distributed in a grid-like pattern [148].

Hyperhidrosis

Sweating disorder, either hypohidrosis or in particular hyperhidrosis were reported by 64% of PD patients and by 12.5% of controls ($p < 0.005$) [174]. Sweating problems, such as "drenching sweats," predominantly happen in off periods and in on periods with dyskinesia. It is suggestive of evidence of dysautonomia and usually does not correlate with severity of the disease. Patients with PD have less sweating in the palms and therefore axial hyperhidrosis could be a compensatory phenomenon for reduced sympathetic function in the extremities in PD patient [169].

There are no studies specifically examining the use of BoNT in sweating disorders in PD patient [7, 23] but this treatment has been found effective in the treatment of essential hyperhidrosis, which is defined as excessive sweating of the palms, feet or axillae [155]. Previous studies have shown the efficacy of intradermal injections of BoNT for focal hyperhidrosis [156, 172]. According to the evidence-based review by Therapeutic and Technology Assessment Subcommittee of the American Academy of Neurology, BoNT has level A evidence for use in axillary hyperhidrosis [9, 157].

Achalasia

Different reasons for swallowing problems in PD patients include proximal dysphagia due to impaired deglutition or flexed neck posture, and achalasia. In Parkinson's patients, reduced pharyngeal constriction and delay in airway closure relative to the arrival of the bolus at the cricopharyngeal (CP) sphincter are the most common abnormalities causing proximal dysphagia [138]. Other studies have suggested hyoid displacement, CP sphincter opening, vocal fold adduction, epiglottic movements, palatal elevation, laryngeal excursions, and prolonged pharyngeal transit time as other reasons for the proximal dysphagia. This can result in the vallecular and pyriform residue, laryngeal penetration, and aspiration.

Several studies have provided evidence for the safe and effective use of BoNT type A for dysfunction of the CP muscle [119, 121, 128, 153]. Injections in the dorsomedial part and on both sides into the ventrolateral part of the CP with doses between 80 and 120 units of abobotulinumtoxinA have been described [170]. Haapaniemi et al. reported good results with the use of onabotulinumtoxinA in posterolateral part of the CP in patients with proximal dysphagia [142].

Achalasia results in aperistalsis and impaired relaxation of the lower esophageal sphincter (LES). Pathophysiologically, achalasia seems to be due to loss of inhibitory neurons within the esophageal myenteric plexus that uses nitric oxide and vasoactive intestinal polypeptides as neurotransmitters [161]. Lewy bodies have been documented in myenteric plexus in PD patient's with achalasia, primarily in the inhibitory vasoactive polypeptide neurons [118]. Also, loss of neurons in the dorsal motor nucleus of the vagus has been described [145]. The treatment of achalasia is directed at reducing the gradient across the lower esophageal sphincter (LES). Laproscopic myotomy and pneumatic dilatation are the most commonly used treatments with comparable clinical efficacy. LES pressure can be transiently reduced by smooth muscle relaxants like BoNT [143, 164]. BoNT presumably counteracts the unopposed LES stimulation by cholinergic neurons, helping to restore the LES to a lower resting pressure by approximately 50% [143, 153]. The total dose of 100 units of onabotulinumtoxinA may need to be endoscopically injected into the LES in multiple aliquots in a ring around the sphincter, increasing the dose to 200 units has been recommended in some studies [123]. OnabotulinumtoxinA markedly improved symptoms in 75% of achalasia patients, but 50% of patients relapsed within 6 months. Patients above age 60 and those with higher esophageal contractility (pressure waves usually >40 mmHg in the esophageal body) tend to have sustained response, sometimes up to 1.5–2 years after a single onabotulinumtoxinA injection [159].

Seborrhea

Seborrhea is a common dermatological disorder associated with PD. Previous studies have shown that parkinsonian male patients show a higher sebum excretion than parkinsonian females and healthy subjects in all the skin locations, with particular significance on the forehead. Different theories for seborrhea have been proposed including increased sebum excretion rate due to hyperactivity of the parasympathetic system, possible action of androgens, excess melanocyte-stimulating hormone secretion because of PD-related dopamine depletion, and high malassezia yeast density on the skin of patients with PD [126, 152]. BoNT injections into the affected skin area may be helpful [7, 171], as it has been found effective in acne, another hypercholinergic dermatologic condition [136, 184]. It has been proposed that BoNT inhibits comedogenesis by interrupting cholinergic transmission between autonomic nerve terminals and secretary glands or by yet unknown anti-inflammatory effects.

Overactive Bladder

Urinary problems may present as urinary frequency and urgency, nocturia and incontinence in patients with PD [181]. Even though these symptoms occur as a consequence of aging detrusor hyperreflexia, which is frequently responsible for these symptoms, it is a relatively common urological problem in the PD population and ranges from 38% to 71% [167]. Detrusor hyperreflexia is presumably a result of the loss of normal inhibition by the basal ganglia and frontal cortex on the sacral spinal cord bladder contractions as a result of which the bladder capacity is much smaller in patients with PD [125, 127]. Urinary retention with or without neurogenic incontinence in parkinsonian patient suggests a diagnosis of MSA [6]. In these patients, EMG reveals signs of denervation in Onuf's nucleus in the sacral spinal cord; this is not seen in PD.

Even though anticholinergic agents, often considered as first-line treatment for overactive bladder, presumably act through "peripheral" mechanisms they often cause cognitive and other central anticholinergic adverse effects, particularly in the elderly [154]. These antimuscarinic drugs include oxybutynin, tolterodine, solifenacin, and darifenacin. Mirabegron, a new beta 3 adrenoreceptor agonist, promotes relaxation of the detrusor smooth muscle and improves urine storage, presumably with fewer side effects [131]. Alpha adrenergic agonists such as alfuzosin, doxazosin, prazosin, terazosin, and tamsulosin do not have a high level of evidence for controlling overactive bladder [122].

BoNT injections into the bladder wall is an effective strategy to increase bladder capacity, and improving urge and incontinence in patients with overactive bladder associated with neurogenic and idiopathic detrusor overactivity [124, 168]. One and 3 months after injection of 200 units botulinum toxin type A into the detrusor muscle, all six patients with parkinsonism (four patients with PD and two with MSA) reported marked reduction in the urinary frequency with no systemic side effects [141]. In another study, 16 PD patients received 500 units of intradetrusor injections of abobotulinumtoxinA and the mean functional bladder capacity increased from 198.6 ± 33.7 to 319 ± 41.1 ml [146]. Similar results have been reproduced in other studies [140, 160].

Based on the result of two class 1 studies of BoNT in neurogenic detrusor overactivity, the Therapeutic and Technology Assessment Subcommittee of the American Academy of Neurology concluded that there is level A evidence for the recommendation that BoNT should be offered as a treatment option for this urinary disorder [9]. In addition to treating detrusor hyperactivity, BoNT has demonstrated promising results for other lower urinary tract symptoms such as voiding dysfunction due to benign prostatic hypertrophy [134].

Constipation

Anismus due to excessive contractions of the muscles of the rectum has been proposed as a mechanism for constipation as a result of functional obstruction at the pelvic outlet by paradoxical contraction of the striated sphincter muscles while straining during defecation [185]. Excessive straining is present in up to 83% of PD patients [135, 165]. Central defecation centers in the lumbosacral spinal cord and sacral parasympathetic nuclei, including Onuf's nuclei control the propulsive actions of the distal colon and defecation [150, 186]. Deposition of Lewy bodies and synuclein pathology in the caudal spinal cord is the most likely substrate for the slow-transit time and dyssynergic defecation observed in the majority of PD patients [129]. Prolonged colon transit time is in part attributed to paradoxical contraction of the puborectalis and external anal sphincter during straining [180, 185]. BoNT injections have been shown to be helpful in the treatment of patients affected by outlet-obstruction constipation and defecatory dysfunction due to pelvic floor dyssynergia [130, 166]. In one study, 10 of the 18 PD patients with outlet constipation, treated with 100 units of type A botulinum toxin, injected into two sites on either side of the puborectalis muscle under ultrasound guidance, reported symptomatic improvement at 2 months evaluation [130]. Anorectal tone, measured by a manometry during straining decreased from 96.2 ± 17.1 to 45.9 ± 16.2 mmHg at 1 month evaluation, and to 56.1 ± 10.7 mmHg at 2 months. Another study involving 10 PD patients with outlet-type constipation injected with BoNT in the puborectalis muscle, showed reduced anorectal tone during straining [120]. There is a need for further and larger double-blind, placebo-controlled studies to establish the safety and efficacy of BoNT in the treatment of constipation in patients with PD [23].

Conclusion

Parkinson's disease (PD) and other parkinsonian syndromes are chronic, progressive neurodegenerative diseases with the multitude of the motor and non-motor symptoms. BoNT is the useful treatment modality for the management of many of these symptoms and can make a significant impact on the quality of life of these patients. It has proven to be a safe and effective therapy for the management of blepharospasm and lid apraxia, cervical dystonia (anterocollis), focal hand dystonia, bruxism, hyperhidrosis, and detrusor overactivity. It is also helpful in the management of foot dystonia, camptocormia, PD-related tremor, constipation, seborrhea, and achalasia. While many conditions are not approved indications, botulinum toxin may be considered in some of these patients with disabling symptoms, unresponsive to other conventional therapies.

Conflict of Interest Dr. Jankovic has received research and/or training grants from Allergan, Inc.; Dystonia Medical Research Foundation; Merz Pharmaceuticals; Revance Therapeutics, Inc.

Dr. Jankovic has served as a consultant or as an advisory committee member for: Allergan, Inc.; Revance Therapeutics, Inc.

References

1. Dressler D. Botulinum toxin drugs: brief history and outlook. J Neural Transm (Vienna). 2016;123(3):277–9.
2. Jankovic J. Botulinum toxin. In: Kompoliti K, Verhagen Metman L, editors. Encyclopedia of movement disorders, vol. 1. Oxford: Academic Press; 2010a. p. 144–50.
3. Jankovic J. Botulinum toxin: State of the art. Mov Disord. 2017. doi:10.1002/mds.27072. In press.

4. Jankovic J. Parkinson's disease: clinical features and diagnosis. J Neurol Neurosurg Psychiatry. 2008;79:368–76.
5. Thenganatt MA, Jankovic J. Parkinson disease subtypes. JAMA Neurol. 2014;71:499–504.
6. Stamelou M, Bhatia KP. Atypical parkinsonism: diagnosis and Treatment. Neurol Clin. 2015;33:39–56.
7. Jankovic J. Disease-oriented approach to botulinum toxin use. Toxicon. 2009;54:614–23.
8. Lotia M, Jankovic J. New and emerging medical therapies in Parkinson's disease. Expert Opin Pharmacother. 2016a;17(7):895–909.
9. Naumann M, Dressler D, Hallett M, Jankovic J, Schiavo G, Segal KR, et al. Evidence-based review and assessment of botulinum neurotoxin for the treatment of secretory disorders. Toxicon. 2013;67:141–52.
10. Simpson DM, Hallett M, Ashman EJ, Comella CL, Green MW, Gronseth GS, et al. Practice guideline update summary: Botulinum neurotoxin for the treatment of blepharospasm, cervical dystonia, adult spasticity, and headache: report of the guideline development Subcommittee of the American Academy of Neurology. Neurology. 2016;86:1818–26.
11. Hallett M, Albanese A, Dressler D, Segal KR, Simpson DM, Truong D, et al. Evidence-based review and assessment of botulinum neurotoxin for the treatment of movement disorders. Toxicon. 2013;67:94–114.
12. Bruno VA, Fox SH, Mancini D, Miyasaki JM. Botulinum toxin use in refractory pain and other symptoms in parkinsonism. Can J Neurol Sci. 2016;43(5):697–702.
13. Jankovic J. How do I examine for re-emergent tremor? Mov Disord Clin Pract. 2016;3:216–7.
14. Lotia M, Jankovic J. Botulinum toxin for the treatment of tremor and tics. Semin Neurol. 2016b;36:54–63.
15. Brin MF, Lyons KE, Doucette J, Adler CH, Caviness JN, Comella CL, et al. A randomized, double masked, controlled trial of botulinum toxin type A in essential hand tremor. Neurology. 2001;56:1523–8.
16. Jankovic J, Schwartz K, Clemence W, Aswad A, Mordaunt J. A randomized, double-blind, placebo-controlled study to evaluate botulinum toxin type A in essential hand tremor. Mov Disord. 1996;11:250–6.
17. Jankovic J, Schwartz K. Botulinum toxin treatment of tremors. Neurology. 1991;41:1185–8.
18. Trosch RM, Pullman SL. Botulinum toxin A injections for the treatment of hand tremors. Mov Disord. 1994;9:601–9.
19. Pullman SL, Greene P, Fahn S, Pedersen SF. Approach to the treatment of limb disorders with botulinum toxin A. Experience with 187 patients. Arch Neurol. 1996;53:617–24.
20. Henderson JM, Ghika JA, Van Melle G, Haller E, Einstein R. Botulinum toxin A in non-dystonic tremors. Eur Neurol. 1996;36:29–35.
21. Rahimi F, Bee C, Debicki D, Roberts AC, Bapat P, Jog M. Effectiveness of BoNT A in Parkinson's disease upper limb tremor management. Can J Neurol Sci. 2013;40:663–9.
22. Rahimi F, Samotus O, Lee J, Jog M. Effective management of upper limb parkinsonian tremor by incobotulinumtoxinA injections using sensor-based biomechanical patterns. Tremor Other Hyperkin Mov. 2015b;5:348.
23. Mills R, Bahroo L, Pagan F. An update on the use of botulinum toxin therapy in Parkinson's disease. Curr Neurol Neurosci Rep. 2015;15:511.
24. Rahimi F, Debicki D, Roberts-South A, Bee C, Bapat P, Jog M. Dynamic decomposition of motion in essential and parkinsonian tremor. Can J Neurol Sci. 2015a;42:116–24.
25. Erer S, Jankovic J. Hereditary chin tremor in Parkinson's disease. Clin Neurol Neurosurg. 2007;109:784–5.
26. Hunker CJ, Abbs JH. Uniform frequency of parkinsonian resting tremor in the lips, jaw, tongue, and index finger. Mov Disord. 1990;5:71–7.
27. Schneider SA, Edwards MJ, Cordivari C, Macleod WN, Bhatia KP. Botulinum toxin A may be efficacious as treatment for jaw tremor in Parkinson's disease. Mov Disord. 2006;21:1722–4.
28. Tarsy D, Ro SI. Unusual position-sensitive jaw tremor responsive to botulinum toxin. Mov Disord. 2006;21:277–8.
29. Jankovic J. Gait disorders. Neurol Clin. 2015;33(1):249–68.

30. Macht M, Kaussner Y, Moller JC, Stiasny-Kolster K, Eggert KM, Kruger HP, et al. Predictors of freezing in Parkinson's disease: a survey of 6,620 patients. Mov Disord. 2007;22:953–6.
31. Giladi N, McDermott MP, Fahn S, Przedborski S, Jankovic J, Stern M, et al. Freezing of gait in PD: prospective assessment in the DATATOP cohort. Neurology. 2001b;56:1712–21.
32. Kuo SH, Kenney C, Jankovic J. Bilateral pedunculopontine nuclei strokes presenting as freezing of gait. Mov Disord. 2008;23:616–9.
33. Ashoori A, Eagleman DM, Jankovic J. Effects of auditory rhythm and music on gait disturbances in Parkinson's disease. Front Neurol. 2015;6:234.
34. Nonnekes J, Snijders AH, Nutt JG, Deuschl G, Giladi N, Bloem BR. Freezing of gait: a practical approach to management. Lancet Neurol. 2015;14:768–78.
35. Espay AJ, Dwivedi AK, Payne M, Gaines L, Vaughan JE, Maddux BN, et al. Methylphenidate for gait impairment in Parkinson disease: a randomized clinical trial. Neurology. 2011a;76:1256–62.
36. Fukada K, Endo T, Yokoe M, Hamasaki T, Hazama T, Sakoda S. L-threo-3,4-dihydroxyphenylserine (L-DOPS) co-administered with entacapone improves freezing of gait in Parkinson's disease. Med Hypotheses. 2013;80:209–12.
37. Malkani R, Zadikoff C, Melen O, Videnovic A, Borushko E, Simuni T. Amantadine for freezing of gait in patients with Parkinson disease. Clin Neuropharmacol. 2012;35:266–8.
38. Moreau C, Delval A, Defebvre L, Dujardin K, Duhamel A, Petyt G, et al. Methylphenidate for gait hypokinesia and freezing in patients with Parkinson's disease undergoing subthalamic stimulation: a multicentre, parallel, randomised, placebo-controlled trial. Lancet Neurol. 2012;11:589–96.
39. Vercruysse S, Vandenberghe W, Munks L, Nuttin B, Devos H, Nieuwboer A. Effects of deep brain stimulation of the subthalamic nucleus on freezing of gait in Parkinson's disease: a prospective controlled study. J Neurol Neurosurg Psychiatry. 2014;85:871–7.
40. Giladi N, Gurevich T, Shabtai H, Paleacu D, Simon ES. The effect of botulinum toxin injections to the calf muscles on freezing of gait in parkinsonism: a pilot study. J Neurol. 2001a;248:572–6.
41. Giladi N, Honigman S. Botulinum toxin injections to one leg alleviate freezing of gait in a patient with Parkinson's disease. Mov Disord. 1997;12:1085–6.
42. Fernandez HH, Lannon MC, Trieschmann ME, Friedman JH. Botulinum toxin type B for gait freezing in Parkinson's disease. Med Sci Monit. 2004;10:CR282–4.
43. Gurevich T, Peretz C, Moore O, Weizmann N, Giladi N. The effect of injecting botulinum toxin type a into the calf muscles on freezing of gait in Parkinson's disease: a double blind placebo-controlled pilot study. Mov Disord. 2007;22:880–3.
44. Wieler M, Camicioli R, Jones CA, Martin WR. Botulinum toxin injections do not improve freezing of gait in Parkinson disease. Neurology. 2005;65:626–8.
45. Zhang LL, Canning SD, Wang XP. Freezing of gait in parkinsonism and its potential drug treatment. Curr Neuropharmacol. 2016;14:302–6.
46. Albanese A, Bhatia K, Bressman SB, Delong MR, Fahn S, Fung VS, et al. Phenomenology and classification of dystonia: a consensus update. Mov Disord. 2013;28(7):863–73.
47. Jankovic J, Tintner R. Dystonia and parkinsonism. Parkinsonism Relat Disord. 2001;8:109–21.
48. Ashour R, Tintner R, Jankovic J. Striatal deformities of the hand and foot in Parkinson's disease. Lancet Neurol. 2005;4:423–31.
49. Doherty KM, van de Warrenburg BP, Peralta MC, Silveira-Moriyama L, Azulay JP, Gershanik OS, et al. Postural deformities in Parkinson's disease. Lancet Neurol. 2011;10(6):538–49.
50. Giladi N, Meer J, Honigman S. The use of botulinum toxin to treat "striatal" toes. J Neurol Neurosurg Psychiatry. 1994;57(5):659.
51. Jankovic J. Botulinum toxin in clinical practice. J Neurol Neurosurg Psychiatry. 2004;75(7):951–7.
52. Azher SN, Jankovic J. Clinical aspects of progressive supranuclear palsy. Handb Clin Neurol. 2008;89:461–73.

53. Clark D, Eggenberger E. Neuro-ophthalmology of movement disorders. Curr Opin Ophthalmol. 2012 Nov;23(6):491–6.
54. Esposito M, Fasano A, Crisci C, Dubbioso R, Iodice R, Santoro L. The combined treatment with orbital and pretarsal botulinum toxin injections in the management of poorly responsive blepharospasm. Neurol Sci. 2014;35:397–400.
55. Kenney C, Jankovic J. Botulinum toxin in the treatment of blepharospasm and hemifacial spasm. J Neural Transm. 2008;115:585–91.
56. Cakmur R, Ozturk V, Uzunel F, Donmez B, Idiman F. Comparison of preseptal and pretarsal injections of botulinum toxin in the treatment of blepharospasm and hemifacial spasm. J Neurol. 2002;249:64–8.
57. Inoue K, Rogers JD. Botulinum toxin injection into Riolan's muscle: somatosensory 'trick'. Eur Neurol. 2007;58:138–41.
58. Hirota N, Hirota M, Mezaki T. Dystonic frowning without blepharospasm. Parkinsonism Relat Disord. 2008;14:579–80.
59. Romano S, Colosimo C. Procerus sign in progressive supranuclear palsy. Neurology. 2001;57:1928.
60. Fezza J, Burns J, Woodward J, Truong D, Hedges T, Verma A. A cross-sectional structured survey of patients receiving botulinum toxin type A treatment for blepharospasm. J Neurol Sci. 2016;367:56–62.
61. Biuk D, Karin AA, Matić S, Barać J, Benasić T, Stiglmayer N. Quality of life in patients with blepharospasm. Coll Antropol. 2013;37(1):29–33.
62. Martinez-Ramirez D, Giugni JC, Hastings E, et al. Comparable botulinum toxin outcomes between primary and secondary blepharospasm: a retrospective analysis. Tremor Other Hyperkinet Mov (N Y). 2014;4:286.
63. Nussgens Z, Roggenkamper P. Comparison of two botulinum-toxin preparations in the treatment of essential blepharospasm. Graefe's Arch Clin Exp Ophthalmol. 1997;235:197–9.
64. Sampaio C, Ferreira JJ, Simoes F, Rosas MJ, Magalhaes M, Correia AP, et al. DYSBOT: a single-blind, randomized parallel study to determine whether any differences can be detected in the efficacy and tolerability of two formulations of botulinum toxin type A—Dysport and Botox—assuming a ratio of 4:1. Mov Disord. 1997;12:1013–8.
65. Roggenkamper P, Jost WH, Bihari K, Comes G, Grafe S, Team NTBS. Efficacy and safety of a new Botulinum toxin type A free of complexing proteins in the treatment of blepharospasm. J Neural Transm. 2006;113:303–12.
66. Quagliato EM, Carelli EF, Viana MA. Prospective, randomized, double-blind study, comparing botulinum toxins type a botox and prosigne for blepharospasm and hemifacial spasm treatment. Clin Neuropharmacol. 2010;33:27–31.
67. Yoon JS, Kim JC, Lee SY. Double-blind, randomized, comparative study of Meditoxin versus Botox in the treatment of essential blepharospasm. Korean J Ophthalmol. 2009;23:137–41.
68. Karp BI, Alter K. Botulinum toxin treatment of blepharospasm, orofacial/oromandibular dystonia, and hemifacial spasm. Semin Neurol. 2016;36(1):84–91.
69. Sinclair CF, Gurey LE, Blitzer A. Oromandibular dystonia: long-term management with botulinum toxin. Laryngoscope. 2013;123:3078–83.
70. Tan EK, Jankovic J. Botulinum toxin A in patients with oromandibular dystonia: long-term follow-up. Neurology. 1999;53:2102–7.
71. Tan EK, Jankovic J. Treating severe bruxism with botulinum toxin. J Am Dent Assoc. 2000;131:211–6.
72. Tinastepe N, Küçük BB, Oral K. Botulinum toxin for the treatment of bruxism. Cranio. 2015;33(4):291–8.
73. Guarda-Nardini L, Manfredini D, Salamone M, Salmaso L, Tonello S, Ferronato G. Efficacy of botulinum toxin in treating myofascial pain in bruxers: a controlled placebo pilot study. Cranio. 2008;26:126–35.
74. Lee SJ, WD MC Jr, Kim YK, Chung SC, Chung JW. Effect of botulinum toxin injection on nocturnal bruxism: a randomized controlled trial. Am J Phys Med Rehabil. 2010;89:16–23.

75. Ondo WG, Simmons JH, Ondo VH, Hunter C, Jankovic J. Onabotulinum toxin-A injections for sleep bruxism: a double-blind, placebo controlled, parallel design, polysomnographic study. Neurology. 2016;78(1)
76. Norby E, Orbelo D, Strand E, Duffy J, Ekbom D, Bower J, et al. Hyoid muscle dystonia: a distinct focal dystonia syndrome. Parkinsonism Relat Disord. 2015;21(10):1210–3.
77. Hallett M, Benecke R, Blitzer A, Comella CL. Treatment of focal dystonias with botulinum neurotoxin. Toxicon. 2009;54:628–33.
78. Thenganatt MA, Fahn S. Botulinum toxin for the treatment of movement disorders. Curr Neurol Neurosci Rep. 2012;12:399–409.
79. Jankovic J, Schwartz K, Donovan DT. Botulinum toxin treatment of cranial-cervical dystonia, spasmodic dysphonia, other focal dystonias and hemifacial spasm. J Neurol Neurosurg Psychiatry. 1990;53:633–9.
80. Esper CD, Freeman A, Factor SA. Lingual protrusion dystonia: frequency, etiology and botulinum toxin therapy. Parkinsonism Relat Disord. 2010;16:438–41.
81. Nastasi L, Mostile G, et al. Effect of botulinum toxin treatment on quality of life in patients with isolated lingual dystonia and oromandibular dystonia affecting the tongue. J Neurol. 2016;263(9):1702–8.
82. Sitburana O, Wu LJ, Sheffield JK, Davidson A, Jankovic J. Motor overflow and mirror dystonia. Parkinsonism Relat Disord. 2009;15(10):758–61.
83. Tolosa E, Compta Y. Dystonia in Parkinson's disease. J Neurol. 2006;253(Suppl 7):VII7–13.
84. Kruisdijk JJM, Koelman JHTM, de Visser BWO, de Haan RJ, Speelman JD. Botulinum toxin for writer's cramp: a randomised, placebo-controlled trial and 1-year follow-up. J Neurol Neurosurg Psychiatry. 2007;78(3):264–70.
85. Contarino MF, Kruisdijk JJM, Koster L, et al. Sensory integration in writer's cramp: comparison with controls and evaluation of botulinum toxin effect. Clin Neurophysiol. 2007;118(10):2195–206.
86. Tsui JK, Bhatt M, Calne S, Calne DB. Botulinum toxin in the treatment of writer's cramp: a double-blind study. Neurology. 1993;43:183–5.
87. Yoshimura DM, Aminoff MJ, Olney RK. Botulinum toxin therapy for limb dystonias. Neurology. 1992;42:627–30.
88. Pacchetti C, Albani G, Martignoni E, Godi L, Alfonsi E, Nappi G. "Off" painful dystonia in Parkinson's disease treated with botulinum toxin. Mov Disord. 1995;10:333–6.
89. Mahapatra RK, Edwards MJ, Schott JM, Bhatia KP. Corticobasal degeneration. Lancet Neurol. 2004;3:736–43.
90. Cordivari C, Misra VP, Catania S, Lees AJ. Treatment of dystonic clenched fist with botulinum toxin. Mov Disord. 2001;16:907–13.
91. Shehata HS, Shalaby NM, Esmail EH, Fahmy E. Corticobasal degeneration: clinical characteristics and multidisciplinary therapeutic approach in 26 patients. Neurol Sci. 2015;36:1651–7.
92. Armstrong MJ. Diagnosis and treatment of corticobasal degeneration. Curr Treat Options Neurol. 2014;16:282.
93. Defazio G, Jankovic J, Giel JL, Papapetropoulos S. Descriptive epidemiology of cervical dystonia. Tremor Other Hyperkin Mov. 2013;3
94. Jankovic J, Tsui J, Bergeron C. Prevalence of cervical dystonia and spasmodic torticollis in the United States general population. Parkinsonism Relat Disord. 2007;13:411–6.
95. Patel N, Hanfelt J, Marsh L, Jankovic J, Members of the Dystonia Coalition. Alleviating manoeuvres (sensory tricks) in cervical dystonia. J Neurol Neurosurg Psychiatry. 2014;85(8):882–4.
96. Jankovic J. Camptocormia, head drop and other bent spine syndromes: heterogeneous etiology and pathogenesis of Parkinsonian deformities. Mov Disord. 2010;25(5):527–8b.
97. Peng-Chen Z, Thompson A, Rodriguez RL. Bilateral lower sternocleidomastoid Botulinum toxin injections to address refractory Anterocollis. Neurologist. 2016;21:30–1.
98. Allison SK, Odderson IR. Ultrasound and electromyography guidance for injection of the Longus Colli with Botulinum toxin for the treatment of cervical dystonia. Ultrasound Q. 2016;32(3):302–6.

99. Herting B, Wunderlich S, Glockler T, Bendszus M, Mucha D, Reichmann H, et al. Computed tomographically-controlled injection of botulinum toxin into the longus colli muscle in severe anterocollis. Mov Disord. 2004;19:588–90.
100. Finsterer J, Maeztu C, Revuelta GJ, Reichel G, Truong D. Collum-caput (COL-CAP) concept for conceptual anterocollis, anterocaput, and forward sagittal shift. J Neurol Sci. 2015;355:37–43.
101. Papapetropoulos S, Baez S, Zitser J, Sengun C, Singer C. Retrocollis: classification, clinical phenotype, treatment outcomes and risk factors. Eur Neurol. 2008;59:71–5.
102. Vijayakumar D, Jankovic J. Drug-induced dyskinesia, part 1: treatment of levodopa-induced dyskinesia. Drugs. 2016;76:759–77.
103. Bezard E, Brotchie JM, Gross CE. Pathophysiology of levodopa-induced dyskinesia: potential for new therapies. Nat Rev Neurosci. 2001;2:577–88.
104. Huot P, Johnston TH, Koprich JB, Fox SH, Brotchie JM. The pharmacology of L-DOPA-induced dyskinesia in Parkinson's disease. Pharmacol Rev. 2013;65:171–222.
105. Hong JY, JS O, Lee I, Sunwoo MK, Ham JH, Lee JE, et al. Presynaptic dopamine depletion predicts levodopa-induced dyskinesia in de novo Parkinson disease. Neurology. 2014;82:1597–604.
106. Bastide MF, Meissner WG, Picconi B, Fasano S, Fernagut PO, Feyder M, et al. Pathophysiology of L-dopa-induced motor and non-motor complications in Parkinson's disease. Prog Neurobiol. 2015;132:96–168.
107. Espay AJ, Vaughan JE, Shukla R, Gartner M, Sahay A, Revilla FJ, et al. Botulinum toxin type A for levodopa-induced cervical dyskinesias in Parkinson's disease: unfavorable risk-benefit ratio. Mov Disord. 2011b;26:913–4.
108. Mills K, Mari Z. An update and review of the treatment of myoclonus. Curr Neurol Neurosci Rep. 2015;15:512.
109. Baizabal-Carvallo JF, Cardoso F, Jankovic J. Myorhythmia: phenomenology, etiology, and treatment. Mov Disord. 2015;30:171–9.
110. Ashour R, Jankovic J. Joint and skeletal deformities in Parkinson's disease, multiple system atrophy, and progressive supranuclear palsy. Mov Disord. 2006;21:1856–63.
111. Barone P, Santangelo G, Amboni M, Pellecchia MT, Vitale C. Pisa syndrome in Parkinson's disease and parkinsonism: clinical features, pathophysiology, and treatment. Lancet Neurol. 2016;15(10):1063–74.
112. Bertram KL, Stirpe P, et al. Treatment of camptocormia with botulinum toxin. Toxicon. 2015;107(Pt A):148–53.
113. Srivanitchapoom P, Hallett M. Camptocormia in Parkinson's disease: definition, epidemiology, pathogenesis and treatment modalities. J Neurol Neurosurg Psychiatry. 2016;87:75–85.
114. Peeraully T, Tan E-K. Camptocormia in Parkinson's disease: dystonia or myopathy? Basal Ganglia. 2012;2:1–3.
115. Hellmann MA, Djaldetti R, Israel Z, Melamed E. Effect of deep brain subthalamic stimulation on camptocormia and postural abnormalities in idiopathic Parkinson's disease. Mov Disord. 2006;21:2008–10.
116. Azher SN, Jankovic J. Camptocormia: pathogenesis, classification, and response to therapy. Neurology. 2005;65:355–9.
117. Colosimo C, Salvatori FM. Injection of the iliopsoas muscle with botulinum toxin in camptocormia. Mov Disord. 2009;24:316–7.
118. Adler CH, Beach TG. Neuropathological basis of nonmotor manifestations of Parkinson's disease. Mov Disord. 2016;31(8):1114–9.
119. Ahsan SF, Meleca RJ, Dworkin JP. Botulinum toxin injection of the cricopharyngeus muscle for the treatment of dysphagia. Otolaryngology. 2000;122:691–5.
120. Albanese A, Brisinda G, Bentivoglio AR, Maria G. Treatment of outlet obstruction constipation in Parkinson's disease with botulinum neurotoxin A. Am J Gastroenterol. 2003;98:1439–40.
121. Alfonsi E, Merlo IM, Ponzio M, Montomoli C, Tassorelli C, Biancardi C, et al. An electrophysiological approach to the diagnosis of neurogenic dysphagia: implications for botulinum toxin treatment. J Neurol Neurosurg Psychiatry. 2010;81:54–60.

122. Andersson KE, Chapple CR, Cardozo L, Cruz F, Hashim H, Michel MC, et al. Pharmacological treatment of overactive bladder: report from the international consultation on incontinence. Curr Opin Urol. 2009;19:380–94.
123. Annese V, Bassotti G, Coccia G, Dinelli M, D'Onofrio V, Gatto G, et al. A multicentre randomised study of intrasphincteric botulinum toxin in patients with oesophageal achalasia. GISMAD Achalasia Study Group. Gut. 2000;46:597–600.
124. Apostolidis A, Fowler CJ. The use of botulinum neurotoxin type A (BoNTA) in urology. J Neural Transm. 2008;115:593–605.
125. Araki I, Kuno S. Assessment of voiding dysfunction in Parkinson's disease by the international prostate symptom score. J Neurol Neurosurg Psychiatry. 2000;68:429–33.
126. Arsic Arsenijevic VS, Milobratovic D, Barac AM, Vekic B, Marinkovic J, Kostic VS. A laboratory-based study on patients with Parkinson's disease and seborrheic dermatitis: the presence and density of Malassezia yeasts, their different species and enzymes production. BMC Dermatol. 2014;14:5.
127. Blackett H, Walker R, Wood B. Urinary dysfunction in Parkinson's disease: a review. Parkinsonism Relat Disord. 2009;15:81–7.
128. Blitzer A, Sulica L. Botulinum toxin: basic science and clinical uses in otolaryngology. Laryngoscope. 2001;111:218–26.
129. Borghammer P, Knudsen K, Brooks DJ. Imaging systemic dysfunction in Parkinson's disease. Curr Neurol Neurosci Rep. 2016;16:51.
130. Cadeddu F, Bentivoglio AR, Brandara F, Marniga G, Brisinda G, Maria G. Outlet type constipation in Parkinson's disease: results of botulinum toxin treatment. Aliment Pharmacol Ther. 2005;22:997–1003.
131. Chapple CR, Cardozo L, Nitti VW, Siddiqui E, Michel MC. Mirabegron in overactive bladder: a review of efficacy, safety, and tolerability. Neurourol Urodyn. 2014;33:17–30.
132. Chinnapongse R, Gullo K, Nemeth P, Zhang Y, Griggs L. Safety and efficacy of botulinum toxin type B for treatment of sialorrhea in Parkinson's disease: a prospective double-blind trial. Mov Disord. 2012;27:219–26.
133. Chou KL, Evatt M, Hinson V, Kompoliti K. Sialorrhea in Parkinson's disease: a review. Mov Disord. 2007;22:2306–13.
134. Chuang YC, Chancellor MB. The application of botulinum toxin in the prostate. J Urol. 2006;176:2375–82.
135. Damian A, Adler CH, Hentz JG, Shill HA, Caviness JN, Sabbagh MN, et al. Autonomic function, as self-reported on the SCOPA-autonomic questionnaire, is normal in essential tremor but not in Parkinson's disease. Parkinsonism Relat Disord. 2012;18:1089–93.
136. Diamond A, Jankovic J. Botulinum toxin in dermatology—beyond wrinkles and sweat. J Cosmet Dermatol. 2006;5:169.
137. Dogu O, Apaydin D, Sevim S, Talas DU, Aral M. Ultrasound-guided versus 'blind' intraparotid injections of botulinum toxin-A for the treatment of sialorrhoea in patients with Parkinson's disease. Clin Neurol Neurosurg. 2004;106:93–6.
138. Ellerston JK, Heller AC, Houtz DR, Kendall KA. Quantitative measures of swallowing deficits in patients with Parkinson's disease. Ann Otol Rhinol Laryngol. 2016;125:385–92.
139. Fietzek UM, Schroeteler FE, Ceballos-Baumann AO. Goal attainment after treatment of parkinsonian camptocormia with botulinum toxin. Mov Disord. 2009;24:2027–8.
140. Giannantoni A, Conte A, Proietti S, Giovannozzi S, Rossi A, Fabbrini G, et al. Botulinum toxin type A in patients with Parkinson's disease and refractory overactive bladder. J Urol. 2011;186:960–4.
141. Giannantoni A, Rossi A, Mearini E, Del Zingaro M, Porena M, Berardelli A. Botulinum toxin A for overactive bladder and detrusor muscle overactivity in patients with Parkinson's disease and multiple system atrophy. J Urol. 2009;182:1453–7.
142. Haapaniemi JJ, Laurikainen EA, Pulkkinen J, Marttila RJ. Botulinum toxin in the treatment of cricopharyngeal dysphagia. Dysphagia. 2001;16:171–5.
143. Hoogerwerf WA, Pasricha PJ. Pharmacologic therapy in treating achalasia. Gastrointest Endosc Clin N Am. 2001;11:311–24. vii

144. Jankovic J. The use of botulinum toxin in tic disorders and essential hand and head tremor. In: Truong D, Dressler D, Hallett M, editors. Manual of botulinum toxin therapy. Cambridge: Cambridge University Press; 2013. p. 160–7.
145. Johnston BT, Colcher A, Li Q, Gideon RM, Castell JA, Castell DO. Repetitive proximal esophageal contractions: a new manometric finding and a possible further link between Parkinson's disease and achalasia. Dysphagia. 2001;16:186–9.
146. Kulaksizoglu H, Parman Y. Use of botulinim toxin-A for the treatment of overactive bladder symptoms in patients with Parkinsons's disease. Parkinsonism Relat Disord. 2010;16:531–4.
147. Lagalla G, Millevolte M, Capecci M, Provinciali L, Ceravolo MG. Botulinum toxin type A for drooling in Parkinson's disease: a double-blind, randomized, placebo-controlled study. Mov Disord. 2006;21:704–7.
148. Lakraj AA, Moghimi N, Jabbari B. Sialorrhea: anatomy, pathophysiology and treatment with emphasis on the role of botulinum toxins. Toxins (Basel). 2013;5:1010–31.
149. Lipp A, Trottenberg T, Schink T, Kupsch A, Arnold G. A randomized trial of botulinum toxin A for treatment of drooling. Neurology. 2003;61:1279–81.
150. Lynch AC, Frizelle FA. Colorectal motility and defecation after spinal cord injury in humans. Prog Brain Res. 2006;152:335–43.
151. Mancini F, Zangaglia R, Cristina S, Sommaruga MG, Martignoni E, Nappi G, et al. Double-blind, placebo-controlled study to evaluate the efficacy and safety of botulinum toxin type A in the treatment of drooling in parkinsonism. Mov Disord. 2003;18:685–8.
152. Martignoni E, Godi L, Pacchetti C, Berardesca E, Vignoli GP, Albani G, et al. Is seborrhea a sign of autonomic impairment in Parkinson's disease? J Neural Transm. 1997;104:1295–304.
153. Moonen AJ, Boeckxstaens GE. Management of achalasia. Gastroenterol Clin N Am. 2013;42:45–55.
154. Mostile G, Jankovic J. Treatment of dysautonomia associated with Parkinson's disease. Parkinsonism Relat Disord. 2009;15(Suppl 3):S224–32.
155. Murray CA, Cohen JL, Solish N. Treatment of focal hyperhidrosis. J Cutan Med Surg. 2007;11:67–77.
156. Naumann M, Jost W. Botulinum toxin treatment of secretory disorders. Mov Disord. 2004;19(Suppl 8):S137–41.
157. Naumann M, So Y, Argoff CE, et al. Assessment: botulinum neurotoxin in the treatment of autonomic disorders and pain (an evidence-based review): report of the Therapeutics and Technology Assessment Subcommittee of the American Academy of Neurology. Neurology. 2008;70:1707–14.
158. Ondo WG, Hunter C, Moore W. A double-blind placebo-controlled trial of botulinum toxin B for sialorrhea in Parkinson's disease. Neurology. 2004;62:37–40.
159. Pasricha PJ, Rai R, Ravich WJ, Hendrix TR, Kalloo AN. Botulinum toxin for achalasia: long-term outcome and predictors of response. Gastroenterology. 1996;110:1410–5.
160. Patel AK, Patterson JM, Chapple CR. Botulinum toxin injections for neurogenic and idiopathic detrusor overactivity: a critical analysis of results. Eur Urol. 2006;50:684–709. discussion 709-610
161. Pfeiffer RF. Neurologic presentations of gastrointestinal disease. Neurol Clin. 2010;28:75–87.
162. Pinnington LL, Muhiddin KA, Ellis RE, Playford ED (2000) Non-invasive assessment of swallowing and respiration in Parkinson's disease. J Neurol 247:773–777.
163. Proulx M, de Courval FP, Wiseman MA, Panisset M. Salivary production in Parkinson's disease. Mov Disord. 2005;20:204–7.
164. Richter JE, Boeckxstaens GE. Management of achalasia: surgery or pneumatic dilation. Gut. 2011;60:869–76.
165. Rodriguez-Blazquez C, Forjaz MJ, Frades-Payo B, de Pedro-Cuesta J, Martinez-Martin P, Longitudinal Parkinson's Disease Patient Study ELdPcEdPG. Independent validation of the scales for outcomes in Parkinson's disease-autonomic (SCOPA-AUT). Eur J Neurol. 2010;17:194–201.

166. Rossi M, Merello M, et al. Management of constipation in Parkinson's disease. Expert Opin Pharmacother. 2015;16(4):547–57.
167. Sakakibara R, Tateno F, Nagao T, Yamamoto T, Uchiyama T, Yamanishi T, et al. Bladder function of patients with Parkinson's disease. Int J Urol. 2014;21:638–46.
168. Sakakibara R, Panicker J, Finazzi-Agro E, Iacovelli V, Bruschini H, The Parkinson's Disease Subcomittee, The Neurourology Promotion Committee in The International Continence Society. A guideline for the management of bladder dysfunction in Parkinson's disease and other gait disorders. Neurourol Urodyn. 2016;35:551–63.
169. Schestatsky P, Valls-Sole J, Ehlers JA, Rieder CR, Gomes I. Hyperhidrosis in Parkinson's disease. Mov Disord. 2006;21:1744–8.
170. Schneider I, Thumfart WF, Pototschnig C, Eckel HE. Treatment of dysfunction of the cricopharyngeal muscle with botulinum A toxin: introduction of a new, noninvasive method. Ann Otol Rhinol Laryngol. 1994;103:31–5.
171. Sheffield JK, Jankovic J. Botulinum toxin in the treatment of tremors, dystonias, sialorrhea and other symptoms associated with Parkinson's disease. Expert Rev Neurother. 2007;7:637–47.
172. Solish N, Bertucci V, Dansereau A, Hong HC, Lynde C, Lupin M, et al. A comprehensive approach to the recognition, diagnosis, and severity-based treatment of focal hyperhidrosis: recommendations of the Canadian Hyperhidrosis Advisory Committee. Dermatol Surg. 2007;33:908–23.
173. Srivanitchapoom P, Pandey S, Hallett M. Drooling in Parkinson's disease: a review. Parkinsonism Relat Disord. 2014;20(11):1109–18.
174. Swinn L, Schrag A, Viswanathan R, Bloem BR, Lees A, Quinn N. Sweating dysfunction in Parkinson's disease. Mov Disord. 2003;18:1459–63.
175. Tintner R, Gross R, Winzer UF, Smalky KA, Jankovic J. Autonomic function after botulinum toxin type A or B: a double-blind, randomized trial. Neurology. 2005;65:765–7.
176. Tison F, Yekhlef F, Chrysostome V, Sourgen C. Prevalence of multiple system atrophy. Lancet. 2000;355:495–6.
177. Tumilasci OR, Cersosimo MG, Belforte JE, Micheli FE, Benarroch EE, Pazo JH. Quantitative study of salivary secretion in Parkinson's disease. Mov Disord. 2006;21:660–7.
178. Vanek ZF, Jankovic J. Dystonia in corticobasal degeneration. Adv Neurol. 2000;82:61–7.
179. von Coelln R, Raible A, Gasser T, Asmus F. Ultrasound-guided injection of the iliopsoas muscle with botulinum toxin in camptocormia. Mov Disord. 2008;23:889–92.
180. Wang CP, Sung WH, Wang CC, Tsai PY. Early recognition of pelvic floor dyssynergia and colorectal assessment in Parkinson's disease associated with bowel dysfunction. Colorectal Dis. 2013;15:e130–7.
181. Winge K, Fowler CJ. Bladder dysfunction in parkinsonism: mechanisms, prevalence, symptoms, and management. Mov Disord. 2006;21:737–45.
182. van de Warrenburg BP, Cordivari C, Ryan AM, Phadke R, Holton JL, Bhatia KP, Hanna MG, Quinn NP. The phenomenon of disproportionate antecollis in Parkinson's disease and multiple system atrophy. Mov Disord. 2007;22(16):2325–31.
183. Tarakad A, Jankovic J. Diagnosis and management of Parkinson's disease. Semin Neurol. 2017;37(2):118–26.
184. Wollina U, Konrad H, Petersen S. Botulinum toxin in dermatology—beyond wrinkles and sweat. J Cosmet Dermatol. 2005;4(4):223–7.
185. Mathers SE, Kempster PA, Law PJ, Frankel JP, Bartram CI, Lees AJ, Stern GM, Swash M. Anal sphincter dysfunction in Parkinson's disease. Arch Neurol. 1989;46(10):1061–4.
186. de Groat WC, Nadelhaft I, Milne RJ, Booth AM, Morgan C, Thor K. Organization of the sacral parasympathetic reflex pathways to the urinary bladder and large intestine. J Auton Nerv Syst. 1981;3(2-4):135–60.

Applications of Botulinum Toxin in the Urinary Tract

Saman Shafaat Talab, Hossein Sadeghi-Nejad, and Patricia E. Gilhooly

Introduction

Lower urinary tract appears to have a simple mission—to store and empty urine. To accomplish this mission, however, a well-orchestrated and complex sequence of neuromuscular events is required. The bladder has to painlessly store urine at a low pressure, to sense when the bladder is reaching its capacity, and then at appropriate intervals, empty to completion under low pressure and volitional control. The smooth muscle of the bladder, i.e., the detrusor muscle, the bladder outlet composed of the intrinsic smooth muscle of the bladder neck, trigone, and posterior urethra surrounded by extrinsic striated muscle, and the pelvic floor striated musculature work in a coordinated fashion as governed by complex networking of both the central and peripheral nervous systems. Although all the various pre- and post-synaptic receptor subtypes have not as yet been defined in voiding function/dysfunction, most pharmacologic intervention has been aimed at muscarinic receptors, and more recently, beta 3 adrenergic receptors, of the bladder, and alpha adrenergic receptors at the bladder outlet.

Antimuscarinic drug therapies can have significant side effects common with anticholinergic medications such as dry mouth, constipation, dry eyes, blurred vision, headaches, and potential risk for serious cardiac and CNS adverse events. Such events limit the tolerability of these therapies and even if manageable, some patients' symptoms are refractory to their use.

In this chapter, the authors review applications of botulinum toxin A (BoNTA) in urology that mainly include the management of patients with lower urinary tract disorders that have not responded to traditional first-line therapies.

S.S. Talab, M.D. (✉)
Division of Urology, Department of Surgery, Rutgers New Jersey Medical School, Newark, NJ, USA
e-mail: ss2496@njms.rutgers.edu

H. Sadeghi-Nejad, M.D., F.A.C.S • P.E. Gilhooly, M.D., F.A.C.S
Division of Urology, Department of Surgery, Rutgers New Jersey Medical School, Newark, NJ, USA

VA New Jersey Health Care System, East Orange, NJ, USA
e-mail: hossein@ix.netcom.com ; Patricia.Gilhooly@va.gov

B. Jabbari (ed.), *Botulinum Toxin Treatment in Clinical Medicine*,
DOI 10.1007/978-3-319-56038-0_4

Mechanism of Action: Botulinum Toxin A in the Lower Urinary Tract

Two types of cell surface receptors for botulinum toxin A (BoNTA) have been identified: gangliosides and the synaptic vesicle-associated protein2 (SV2) family. The heavy chain of BoNTA binds to SV2 receptor of the presynaptic neuron. Following endocytic internalization, BoNTA exerts its effects via cleavage of synaptosome-associated protein (SNAP25) within the synaptic fusion complex in presynaptic neurons and subsequently inhibits fusion of neurotransmitter-containing vesicles with the neuronal cell membrane. The end result of this process is disruption of acetylcholine release into the neuromuscular junction that leads to temporary muscle denervation and paralysis [1, 2].

Immunohistochemical evaluation has demonstrated that BoNTA predominantly accumulates in parasympathetic nerve endings at the neuromuscular junction [3]. It has been shown, however, that bladder urothelium also contains muscarinic receptors [4] and, in addition to cholinergic efferent innervation, human urothelium releases neurotransmitters including acetylcholine that can act on nearby urothelium as well as on afferent fibers [5]. More recently, SV2 receptor and SNAP25 protein have also been mapped to the human bladder urothelium [6]. These findings suggest that, in addition to the neuromuscular junction, BoNTA may also act through the urothelial layer by affecting bladder sensory input. Furthermore, it has been shown that BoNTA modulates bladder sensory neurotransmission by inhibition of adenosine triphosphate and substance P release, as well as through a reduction of the axonal expression of capsaicin and purinergic receptors [7]. These findings suggest that alteration of both afferent and efferent fibers may play a role in the therapeutic effects of BoNTA in lower urinary tract disorders.

Botulinum Toxin for Management of Lower Urinary Tract Disorders

Application of BoNTA in the urinary tract was first reported by Dykstra et al. in 1988 when they injected botulinum A toxin into the rhabdosphincter of 11 men with spinal cord injury (SCI) and detrusor-sphincter dyssynergia (DSD) [8]. Schurch et al. in 2000, for the first time, reported intra-detrusor injection of BoNTA for the treatment of neurogenic bladder detrusor overactivity in spinal cord injury patients [9]. Following several placebo-controlled RCTs [10–13] with promising outcomes, the US Food and Drug Administration (FDA) approved the application of onabotulinumtoxin A for the treatment of urge urinary incontinence due to neurogenic detrusor overactivity (NDO) in 2011 and for overactive bladder in 2013. Following FDA approval, use of BoNTA has been gaining popularity among urologists as third-line treatment of refractory neurogenic bladder overactivity and overactive bladder symptoms according to the most recent American Urological Association guidelines [14]. Several other urologic indications have been reported in the literature that we will review later in this chapter (Table 1).

Table 1 Urological application of botulinum toxin A

Diagnosis	Injection site	Recommended doses	AUA/EAU recommendations/ guidelines
Neurogenic detrusor overactivity	Intradetrusor	200–300 U	FDA approved 2011 for adults EAU: LE 1a/ GR A
Idiopathic detrusor overactivity/refractory overactive bladder	Intradetrusor	100–300 U	FDA approved 2013 for adults AUA: 3rd line treatment (100 U) EAU: GR A (100 U)
Interstitial cystitis/ bladder pain syndrome	Intradetrusor	100–200 U	AUA: 4th line treatment EAU: GR A (submucosal injection + hydrodistension) GR C (intradetrusor and trigonal injection)
Detrusor sphincter dyssynergia	Intrasphincteric	100 U	Data are inconclusive
Obstructive voiding symptoms/benign prostatic hypertrophy	Intraprostatic	100–300 U	Data are inconclusive

FDA Food and Drug Administration, *AUA* American Urological Association, *EAU* European Association of Urology, *LE* level of evidence, *GR* grade of recommendation

Botulinum Toxin for Neurogenic Detrusor Overactivity (NDO)

Voiding dysfunction in patients with neurogenic lesions such as patients with SCI above the sacral spinal cord or multiple sclerosis (MS) commonly presents with mixed storage symptoms (urinary frequency and urgency, decreased bladder capacity and incontinence caused by involuntary contractions of the detrusor muscle of the bladder) and voiding symptoms (urinary hesitancy, slow or interrupted flow, and incomplete bladder emptying frequently caused by DSD). In this section, we will discuss the role of bladder chemo-denervation in the management of neurogenic bladder overactivity, officially known as neurogenic detrusor overactivity [15]. The use of BoNTA for the treatment of NDO was first reported by Schurch et al. in 2000 [16]. In this pioneering study, 200–300 U of BoNTA was injected into the detrusor muscle of 21 patients with NDO and urinary urge incontinence secondary to SCI. The results showed complete urinary continence in 17 of 19 cases and significant increase in bladder capacity (296–480 ml, $p < 0.016$), as well as decrease in mean maximum detrusor voiding pressure (65–35 cmH_2O, $p < 0.016$) at 6 weeks follow-up. Among 11 patients available for follow-up at 16 and 36 weeks, ongoing improvement in bladder function was evident in all patients.

Following this initial report, in 2005 Schurch et al. published a randomized double-blind placebo-controlled trial in 59 patients with urinary incontinence caused by neurogenic detrusor overactivity (300 U in 19 patients, 200 U in 19 patients, and placebo in 21 patients) [17]. The results confirmed the efficacy of 200 or 300 units of BoNTA compared with placebo in these patients. Benefits were generally maintained for the duration of the 24-week study.

In 2007, Ehren et al. also reported the effect of abobotulinum toxin type A (Dysport®) in a randomized, placebo-controlled, double-blind study in patients with urge incontinence due to neurogenic detrusor overactivity [18]. Thirty-one patients underwent intra-detrusor injection of 500 U BoNTA or placebo. Patients were followed for 26 weeks and cystometric evaluation revealed significantly higher bladder capacity along with a decrease in maximum detrusor pressure. They also reported significant improvement in urinary frequency, as well as the quality of life parameters.

Following initial reports regarding the effectiveness of intradetrusor injection of BoNTA in neurogenic bladder overactivity in small RCTs, several large multicenter randomized and placebo-controlled phase III studies were published. Cruz et al. reported a multicenter RCT that included 275 patients (SCI; $n = 121$, MS; $n = 154$) randomized into three groups of placebo, BoNTA 200 U and 300 U [11]. The results showed that both doses of BoNTA significantly reduced incontinence episodes and improved urodynamic parameters, as well as, quality of life in the study population. Both doses were well tolerated with comparable clinical effectiveness and duration of effect. Similar findings were reported by Ginsberg et al. where 416 patients with neurogenic bladder overactivity secondary to MS ($n = 227$) and SCI ($n = 189$) were randomized into three groups of placebo, BoNTA 200 U and 300 U [10]. BoNTA 200 U and 300 U significantly decreased mean urinary incontinence episodes per week at the 6 weeks follow-up by 21 and 23 episodes per week respectively, compared to nine episodes in the placebo group. Similarly, significant improvement of urodynamic indices and quality of life scores were also reported. Both doses demonstrated similar effectiveness. Data from numerous studies confirmed the therapeutic effects of intradetrusor BoNTA injection in patients with neurogenic lesions and overactive bladder, with consensus that repeated injections are necessary to maintain the outcomes. Giannantoni et al. reported the effect of repeated injections of 300 U of BoNTA into the detrusor in 17 patients with SCI and detrusor overactivity who were followed for 6 years [19]. Repeat injections were performed whenever patients had worsening of clinical symptoms. The mean number of injections for each patient and mean interval between two consecutive injections were 7.2 ± 1.3 and 11.0 ± 2.4 months, respectively. The results showed that repeated injections of BoNTA provide sustained symptomatic improvement over the entire duration of follow-up and even amelioration of upper-tract function without inducing any systemic side effects allowing patients to minimize anticholinergic drug use.

More recently, Kennelly et al. published a 3-year, prospective multicenter extension study [20] to assess the long-term safety and maintenance of efficacy of intradetrusor BoNTA injection in 396 patients who initially were enrolled in the phase III trials [10, 11]. They reported that 200 U of BoNTA continued to reduce urinary incontinence episodes/day (range −3.2 to −4.1 from baseline), with the sustained improvement of volume per void, as well as the quality of life. Results from 200 U and 300 U injections were comparable and overall median duration of effect was 9 months for patients who received 200 U of intradetrusor BoNTA. With UTI and urinary retention being the most common adverse effects, the findings demonstrated that long-term safety of BoNTA following multiple treatments is consistent with its reported safety profile from phase III studies, suggesting that BoNTA does not have a cumulative dose or duration toxicity.

Application of BoNTA in children with neurogenic bladder hyperactivity was reported for the first time by Schulte-Baukloh et al. in 2002 [21]. They reported significant improvement of urodynamic parameters in 17 children with detrusor hyperreflexia secondary to myelomeningocele following injection of 85–300 U of BoNTA. In a systematic review of six published articles, intradetrusor injection of 10–12 U/kg of BoNTA in children with neurogenic detrusor overactivity has been shown to significantly improve clinical and urodynamic variables (65–87% became completely dry) without major adverse effects [22]. In a prospective study of 17 patients with 4 years of follow-up, similar findings were reported by Figueroa et al. [23]. In addition to 70.6% patient/parental satisfaction, 14/17 children (87.5%) who underwent BoNTA injection were spared reconstruction surgery (i.e., bladder augmentation).

These data demonstrated that BoNTA intra-detrusor injection is a safe, therapeutic option in NDO and an acceptable alternative to invasive reconstructive surgical approaches. Many patients with NDO may already be catheterizing themselves. For patients who are not doing clean intermittent catheterization (CIC), however, they may need to start CIC after BoNTA injections into the bladder if they have subsequent difficulty adequately emptying their bladder. This is a matter of serious concern for neurologic patients with poor upper extremity coordination and strength.

Botulinum Toxin for Idiopathic Detrusor Overactivity (IDO)/ Refractory Overactive Bladder (OAB)

Overactive bladder is characterized by a sudden and unexpected urge to urinate that patients cannot control and, in some patients, may result in urinary incontinence. The condition is also associated with increased daytime frequency and nocturia. IDO/OAB can have a significantly negative impact on patient's quality of life, work productivity, and sleep quality.

In the National Overactive Bladder Evaluation (NOBEL) study, the overall prevalence of overactive bladder was reported in up to 16.9% of the US population ≥18 years of age. The prevalence of overactive bladder increases with age and has been reported in up to 30% of those aged 75 years or older [24]. Considering the high prevalence of overactive bladder, the introduction of new treatment modalities with the promising clinical outcome and the acceptable safety profile was a huge step-forward in the management of this group of patients.

Following numerous reports regarding promising outcomes of intradetrusor injection of BoNTA in patients with neurogenic detrusor overactivity, its application has been extended to patients with non-neurogenic bladder overactivity refractory to anticholinergic medications. The first study in this regard was published by Dykstra et al. in 2003 [25]. They reported significant improvement of urinary frequency in 15 females with idiopathic overactive bladder following intra-detrusor injection of botulinum toxin type B (2500–15,000 U). The clinical response was comparable among all doses. However, the correlation between the dosage used and the duration of effect was very significant (correlation coefficient = 0.96, $p < 0.001$).

Dmochowski et al. published a multicenter double-blind RCT in 2010, involving 313 patients with idiopathic overactive bladder and urinary urgency incontinence experiencing eight or more urinary urgency incontinence episodes a week and eight or more micturitions daily at baseline [26]. Patients were randomized into six groups of 50, 100, 150, 200, or 300 U intradetrusor BoNTA, vs. placebo. The outcome was evaluated by using a 7-day bladder diary and the patients were followed up to 36 weeks. The durable clinical response was observed in all patients who received BoNTA 100–300 U. Doses greater than 150 U showed minimal additional or clinically relevant improvement in patients' symptoms along with the dose-dependent increase in PVR and need for clean intermittent catheterization (CIC). Authors suggested 100 U BoNTA as the appropriate dose for a balanced clinical response and safety profile. Similar findings were subsequently reported by Denys et al. in another randomized double-blind RCT that enrolled 99 patients with idiopathic overactive bladder who received 50, 100, and 150 U of BoNTA vs. placebo [27].

A clinical phase III study investigating the efficacy of intradetrusor BoNTA in patients with OAB and urinary incontinence inadequately managed with anticholinergics was published in 2013 [12]. In this study, 557 patients were randomly assigned into two groups of BoNTA 100 U vs. placebo and followed for 24 weeks. The authors reported that 100 U of BoNTA injection significantly decreased urinary incontinence episodes vs placebo (−2.65 vs −0.87, $p < 0.001$) and 22.9% vs 6.5% of patients became completely continent. Significant improvement of health-related quality of life was also seen in the BoNTA group. Another phase III study also reported similar findings with significant and clinically relevant improvements in OAB symptoms following injection of 100 U BoNTA [13]. Analysis of pooled data from 2 phase III studies showed that 100 U of BoNTA injection significantly reduces episodes of daily urinary incontinence from baseline at week 12 compared to placebo (2.80 vs. 0.95 episodes/day; $p < 0.001$) [28]. Moreover, it was shown that 27.1% of the BoNTA patients became completely continent as compared to 8.4% of patients in the placebo group ($p < 0.001$). Adverse effects were well tolerated, with a comparable incidence in all groups.

One double-blind, double-placebo–controlled trial by Visco et al. investigated the difference in efficacy and safety of oral anticholinergic therapy vs. 100 U BoNTA injection in 241 women with OAB with urgency urinary incontinence [29]. Treatment with either anticholinergics or BoNTA was associated with a comparable mean reduction in the frequency of daily episodes of incontinence (−3.4 versus −3.3; $p = 0.81$). Furthermore, patients receiving BoNTA were less likely to have dry mouth and more likely to have complete resolution of urinary incontinence. In view of the higher rates of transient urinary retention and urinary tract infections, the authors suggested that considering comparable clinical outcomes for these two treatment approaches, the side effect profile, as well as the route of administration should be discussed with patients before final treatment decisions are made.

These, plus other supporting studies, confirm the efficacy of BoNTA in the treatment of refractory IDO with an acceptable safety profile. Patients who opt to pursue the option of BoNTA must accept the risk, albeit low at the 100 U dose, that they may need to start CIC if their postvoid residual urine measurement (PVR) rises to an unacceptable level.

Botulinum Toxin for Detrusor Sphincter Dyssynergia (DSD)

Detrusor sphincter dyssynergia is an involuntary contraction of the external sphincter during detrusor contraction. DSD can cause a functional obstruction with high-pressure voiding and incomplete emptying. It is a common cause of voiding dysfunction in patients with upper motor neuron disease including patients with spinal cord injury above the sacral spinal cord and multiple sclerosis [30]. Various therapeutic strategies have been proposed including medical treatment (spasmolytic agents, alpha blockers) and surgery (sphincterotomy) with suboptimal outcome and significant side effects.

BoNTA was originally used for the treatment of DSD in spinal cord injury (SCI) patients [8]. In 1996, Schurch et al. reported a prospective study in 24 patients with DSD secondary to SCI who underwent injection of BoNTA into the external sphincter with promising results. They reported a significant improvement of PVR postoperatively and the effects lasted 3–9 months [31]. Similar findings were published in 2002 in a randomized double-blind lidocaine-controlled study on 13 patients with DSD/SCI that showed a significant reduction in PVR and maximal urethral pressure up to 1 month after injection [32]. We found only one published RCT with a true control group studying intra-sphincter injection of BoNTA in patients with the history of multiple sclerosis (MS) and DSD [33]. This study included 86 patients (placebo: 41; 100 U of BoNTA: 45) who were followed up to 4 months. The results showed that in the study population a single injection of 100 U of BoNTA does not decrease post-voiding residual urine volume after 1 month. Compared to the placebo group, however, patients in the BoNTA group showed an increase in voided volume by 54% ($p = 0.02$), a decrease in pre-micturition pressure by 29% ($p = 0.02$), and in maximal detrusor pressures by 21% ($p = 0.02$). At the end of 4 months follow-up, International Prostate Symptom Score (IPSS) improved significantly in both groups despite some of the better urodynamic parameters seen after BoNTA.

Accordingly, larger placebo-controlled studies with more quantitative measures, as well as patient-reported outcomes with longer follow-up to assess duration of effect are required before any definitive conclusion regarding the effectiveness of BoNTA injection into the rhabdosphincter in patients with DSD can be made. Nonetheless, considering the promising outcomes of BoNTA injection into the sphincter in some studies (i.e., decrease in PVR) [31, 32], intra-sphincteric injection of BoNTA can be tried in a patient who has failed alpha blockers in an attempt to avoid chronic catheterization.

Botulinum Toxin for Obstructive Voiding Symptoms/Benign Prostatic Hypertrophy (BPH)

Benign prostatic hyperplasia is one of the most common disorders in aging men, resulting in a significant burden on patients' general quality of life. Patients usually present with lower urinary tract symptoms (LUTS) that stem from urethral and bladder outlet obstruction. These symptoms include frequency, urgency, slow urine stream, incomplete bladder emptying, hesitancy, straining, and nocturia.

Maria et al. reported the first off-label use of BoNTA in BPH patients [34]. In this study, 30 patients with an average prostate volume of 52 cc were randomly assigned to receive intraprostatic injection of 200 U of BoNTA vs saline. They reported significant improvement of subjective symptoms in 13/15 patients in the treatment group and 3/15 in the control group ($p = 0.0007$). Moreover, symptom scores were reduced by 65% compared to baseline in the BoNTA group vs minimal change in control patients. More interestingly, the authors reported 51% decrease in PSA and significant reduction of prostate size up to 12 months after intraprostatic BoNTA injection (52.6 ± 10.6 cc vs. 20.5± 8 cc).

Subsequently, Chuang et al. published two studies investigating the effectiveness of intraprostatic injection of BoNTA in prostates <30 cc (21 patients, 100 U injection) and >30 cc (20 patients, 200 U injection) [35, 36]. The results showed that lower urinary tract symptoms and quality of life indices improved by >30% in 76% of the men, and four of five men with urinary retention for >1 month could void spontaneously at 1 week to 1 month after the BoNTA injection. However, in contradiction to the findings of Maria et al., they reported minimal change in prostate volume following BoNTA injection, suggesting that inhibitory effects of the toxin on smooth muscle cell tone and modulation of afferent neural function may play an important role in the therapeutic effects of BoNTA in BPH patients.

More recently, McVary et al. published a phase II multicenter, placebo-controlled, RCT using BoNTA 200 U to treat men with moderate LUTS due to BPH where 315 patients were randomized into BoNTA ($n = 158$) or placebo ($n = 157$) groups [37]. In contrast to the previous reports, this study showed improvement of International Prostate Symptom Score (IPSS) from baseline in both BoNTA and placebo groups (−6.3 vs −5.6 points, $p < 0.001$) with no difference between the groups. However, the improvement was observed in the peak urinary flow rate, which was significant only at week 6 compared to placebo. Similar findings were reported by Marberger et al. in another multicenter double-blind randomized, placebo-controlled study ($n = 380$) that showed significant improvement of IPSS and Qmax following intraprostatic injection of BoNTA (100 U, 200 U, and 300 U) and saline with no significant difference between all groups including the placebo [38].

Overall, there is not enough current data to support the use of BoNTA as first-line therapy for BPH with LUTS. In view of some of the promising findings, however, there may be an indication for a trial of this therapy in a select group of challenging patients who have failed optimum medical therapy and are not deemed good surgical candidates.

Botulinum Toxin for Interstitial Cystitis/Bladder Pain Syndrome (IC/BPS)

Interstitial Cystitis/Bladder Pain Syndrome is a chronic and debilitating syndrome defined as pelvic pain, pressure, or discomfort that is related to the urinary bladder and associated with at least one other urinary symptom such as urgency, frequency, or nocturia [39]. The term "interstitial cystitis" should probably be used in cases with typical cystoscopic and pathologic features. However, in recent years the term IC/PBS includes all cases of urinary pain that cannot be attributed to other causes, such as infection or urinary stone. The etiology of IC/BPS is unknown and, accordingly, the management of these patients is usually challenging and multi-pronged.

In a pilot study of 13 females, Smith et al. showed that intradetrusor injection of 100–200 U BoNTA decreased interstitial cystitis symptoms and mean Interstitial Cystitis Problem Index (ISPI) scores by 71% and 69%, respectively. They also reported that daytime frequency, nocturia, and pain by Visual Analog Scale (VAS) decreased by 44%, 45%, and 79%, respectively ($p < 0.01$) [40]. Following this initial report, beneficial effects of BoNTA injection in IC/BPS were reported in other small case series [41, 42].

The first prospective RCT in this area was published in 2009 by Kuo and Chancellor [43] in which they compared hydrodistention of the bladder, i.e., a filled bladder under pressure for a determined amount of time which in this study was 80 cmH_2O for 15 min ± BoNTA. Sixty-seven patients were randomized to three groups of: 200 U + hydrodistention ($n = 15$), 100 U + hydrodistention ($n = 29$), and hydrodistention alone ($n = 23$) [43]. The findings revealed that IC/BMP symptom score significantly improved in all groups. However, at 3-month follow-up, pain visual analog scale, cystometric bladder capacity, and global response assessment improved only in the BoNTA group. Moreover, they showed that 200 U injection has no significant therapeutic superiority to 100 U while injection of 100 U has a better safety profile.

Another study of patients with a diagnosis of IC/BPS showed that injection of 100 U BoNTA in the trigone significantly improved pain, frequency, and quality of life [44]. Furthermore, the authors demonstrated that beneficial effects of a single treatment were retained up to 9 months in greater than 50% of the patients.

More recently, a multicenter, double-blind, placebo-controlled trial showed that injections of 100 U of BoNTA effectively reduced bladder pain symptoms in patients with IC/BPS. In this study, 60 patients underwent injection of 100 U BoNTA and hydrodistention or normal saline injection and hydrodistention [45]. At 8 weeks follow-up, a significantly greater reduction of pain score was seen in the BoNTA group compared to the control group (-2.6 ± 2.8 versus -0.9 ± 2.2; $p = 0.02$). Cystometric bladder capacity was also significantly increased in the BoNTA group while other variables including frequency, voided volume, and PVR were similar between two groups.

Two main mechanisms were suggested by the authors for an explanation of BoNTA effectiveness in IC/BPS patients: modulation of sensory nerve transmission affecting pain perception, as well as inhibition of acetylcholine release in the neuromuscular junction leading to increased bladder capacity [45].

Although larger placebo-controlled trials are needed before FDA approval for this application, the results with 100 U thus far are encouraging enough that the American Urologic Association Guidelines include 100 U BoNTA as a fourth line treatment option for this very diverse and often very desperate patient cadre.

Other Potential Applications of Botulinum Toxin

Patients with chronic prostatitis/chronic pelvic pain syndrome (CP/CPPS) most commonly present with pain that is usually localized to the perineum, suprapubic area, and penis but can also occur in the testes, groin, or low back. Pain during and after ejaculation, as well as storage and voiding urinary symptoms are associated with this syndrome in the majority of the patients. CP/CPPS has a significant negative impact on patient's quality of life with very high socioeconomic burden [46]. In a study of 11 patients with CPPS, transurethral perisphincteric injections of 200 U of BoNTA showed improvement in pelvic pain [47]. Another trial of 13 patients diagnosed with CPPS showed the beneficial effect of injections of 100 U of BoNTA into the perineal body and bulbospongiosus muscle with the treatment response rate of 30% compared to 13% in the control patients [48]. In a recent prospective double-blind and randomized placebo-controlled study, 60 patients with CPPS underwent transurethral intraprostatic injection of 100–200 U of BoNTA (based on prostate size) or placebo. The results showed significant improvement of pain, reflected by a decrease in the VAS by 62.3%, 72.4%, and 82.1% compared to baseline at 1, 3, and 6 months after injection ($p < 0.001$).

In a case report, intradetrusor injection of BoNTA was reported to facilitate intravesical BCG treatment in a patient with bladder cancer with refractory urge incontinence after BCG instillation [49]. In another case, the effectiveness of intradetrusor BoNTA for the management of refractory autonomic dysreflexia and severe hypertension in an 11-year-old with neurogenic bladder secondary to T4 paraplegia has been reported [50]. Moreover, potential clinical benefits of periureteral BoNTA injection to improve ureteral stent tolerability and stent-related pain have been demonstrated [51].

Although large randomized control trials are necessary before any definite conclusions regarding indications for BoNTA injections in this group of patients may be reached, modulation of sensory neural pathway affecting pain perception may play a role in its effectiveness.

Injection Techniques

Bladder

Variables involved in intradetrusor BoNTA administration include the amount and dose of toxin, the concentration of the solution, injection technique, and the number/location of injections, as well as the type of scope, needle, and anesthesia.

The dose of toxin for each treatment session mainly depends on the initial indication as has been discussed previously in this chapter. A wide range of concentrations for the preparation of the solution has also been reported by various authors that range from 10 U to 100 U per ml of preservative-free normal saline with total injected volume of up to 30 cc [49, 52–54]. The total number of injections per treatment session has also been reported to vary from 10 to 50 sites, with 20–30 sites as the most commonly used protocol. Despite the wide range of variability regarding concentration and injected volume, we could not find any study representing the optimum treatment protocol and it seems that surgeon preference and experience are the determining factors.

Distribution of the injection sites is also a matter of debate among urologists. Some urologists distribute the injections over the lateral and posterior bladder walls sparing the trigone area [52, 55]. The idea behind sparing the trigone is potential distal ureteral paralysis and subsequent vesicoureteral reflux, though this has never been shown in clinical studies. On the other hand, due to the high density of nerve endings in the trigone area, others suggest that trigonal injection may offer additional clinical benefits. At the time of this writing, there is still no consensus regarding the efficacy of trigonal versus bladder body injections [56] (Fig. 1).

Similar controversy also exists regarding the depth of injection. In the majority of studies, BoNTA has been injected directly into the detrusor muscle. However, submucosal injection of toxin was later described with the idea that there would be more effect on the afferent nerve fibers and subsequent improvement in outcome, but this has not been confirmed by clinical studies [43, 57].

The injection process using a long, flexible needle has been performed under general and spinal anesthesia, as well as intravenous sedation in a same day surgery settings. Others have reported that patients tolerate the procedure well under local anesthesia (using intravesical lidocaine) in office-based settings [58]. Both flexible and rigid cystoscopes have been used for intradetrusor injection [52, 59]. However, rigid cystoscopy in an operating room setting seems to be the most commonly used approach.

Urethral Sphincter

Administration of BoNTA into the external sphincter has been reported both under direct cystoscopic vision and by transperineal injection [33, 47]. Using cystoscopy, the external sphincter needs to be localized first followed by injection of BoNTA at 12, 3, 6, and 9 o'clock positions. In our experience, spinal anesthesia is the preferred anesthesia technique in these cases since it reliably results in a relaxed sphincter with optimal visualization and ease of injection. Transperineal injection is feasible in both males and females via a single injection using striated sphincter electromyography for localization [32].

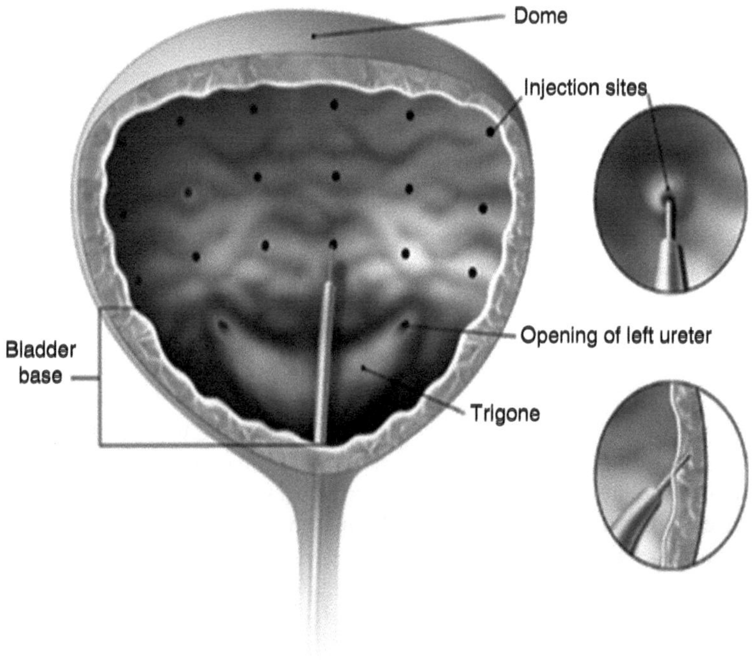

Fig. 1 Injection pattern for intradetrusor injections for the treatment of neurogenic detrusor overactivity and overactive bladder [68]

Adverse Effects and Contraindications

Administration of BoNTA into the lower urinary tract is a generally safe and well-tolerated procedure. Moreover, repeated intradetrusor injection of BoNTA has been shown to be a safe therapeutic approach [60, 61]. Most common reported side effects are urinary tract infection and urinary retention. Post procedure urinary tract infection has been reported in more than 50% of the patients with neurogenic detrusor overactivity [62, 63] and in up to 25% of patients with idiopathic overactive bladder [12, 13, 28]. However, the incidence of UTI complicated by urosepsis is rare. The neurogenic bladder population generally has a high rate of bacteriuria which has prompted us to routinely use peri-procedural antibiotic prophylaxis (but not aminoglycosides). Some studies have shown post-procedure urinary retention in 21–23% of the patients with neurogenic detrusor overactivity and in 5.8% of patients with idiopathic bladder overactivity. The need to initiate de novo CIC after BoNTA injection has also been reported in 6–88% of the patients [21, 59, 64, 65]. However, the presence of retention is usually unrelated to the treatment outcome. In a multivariate analysis of 217 patients with idiopathic bladder overactivity, it has been shown that male gender and baseline PVR >100 ml are independent predictors of post-procedure urinary retention [66]. Dysuria, hematuria, and epididymitis have also been reported [13, 67].

Of note, the safety and efficacy of the use of BoNTA in patients under 18 years of age for the treatment of OAB, and detrusor overactivity associated with a neurologic condition are not established as of January 2016 [68].

Systemic effects of BoNTA such as generalized weakness, blurred vision, or diplopia secondary to intradetrusor application are extremely rare [69]. This is most likely due to minimal systemic absorption, as well as low injection doses which is well below the fatal dose of botulinum toxin [70].

The main contraindications for BoNTA injection into the urinary tract include myasthenia gravis, Eaton-Lambert syndrome, breastfeeding, pregnancy, intake of any medication that may interfere with neuromuscular transmission (such as aminoglycosides), active urinary tract infection, and history of allergy to botulinum toxin [71].

Costs

Visco et al. recently published a study comparing the cost-effectiveness of intravesical BoNTA (100 U) injection with anticholinergic medications for the treatment of idiopathic overactive bladder [72]. The results showed that intravesical BoNTA and anticholinergic medications have similar costs and efficacy in the first 6 months of treatment ($1266 vs $1339, respectively). However, in a 9-month period, BoNTA may have significantly lower costs with comparable clinical outcomes ($207 vs $305 per month, respectively).

Previously, Wu et al. had reported similar findings demonstrating that, as compared to anticholinergic medications, BoNTA injection was cost-effective for the treatment of refractory urge incontinence [73]. The incremental cost-effectiveness ratio was calculated as $14,377 per quality adjusted life-year. A treatment modality is often considered cost-effective when the incremental cost-effectiveness ratio is less than $50,000 per quality adjusted life-year. The authors also reported that anticholinergics may become cost-effective if patients are highly compliant with the treatment protocol or if the costs of BoNTA injection procedure increase substantially.

Conclusions

Injection of BoNTA in the lower urinary tract is a minimally invasive therapeutic option for patients with refractory and debilitating urologic diseases such as neurogenic detrusor overactivity, idiopathic overactive bladder, and interstitial cystitis/painful bladder syndrome. The injection procedure is fairly simple, feasible in office-based or same day surgery settings, widely available with generally acceptable safety profile making multiple procedures a valid option. Importantly, BoNTA administration in the lower urinary tract offers a valuable long term, temporary alternative to failed conservative medical treatments and has the potential to postpone invasive and irrevocable surgical reconstruction.

References

1. Benoit RM, et al. Structural basis for recognition of synaptic vesicle protein 2C by botulinum neurotoxin A. Nature. 2014;505(7481):108–11.
2. Dong M, et al. SV2 is the protein receptor for botulinum neurotoxin A. Science. 2006;312(5773):592–6.
3. Coelho A, et al. Distribution of the high-affinity binding site and intracellular target of botulinum toxin type A in the human bladder. Eur Urol. 2010;57(5):884–90.
4. Hawthorn MH, et al. Urothelium-derived inhibitory factor(s) influences on detrusor muscle contractility in vitro. Br J Pharmacol. 2000;129(3):416–9.
5. Andersson KE, Yoshida M. Antimuscarinics and the overactive detrusor—which is the main mechanism of action? Eur Urol. 2003;43(1):1–5.
6. Hanna-Mitchell AT, et al. Effect of botulinum toxin A on urothelial-release of ATP and expression of SNARE targets within the urothelium. Neurourol Urodyn. 2015;34(1):79–84.
7. Apostolidis A, Dasgupta P, Fowler CJ. Proposed mechanism for the efficacy of injected botulinum toxin in the treatment of human detrusor overactivity. Eur Urol. 2006;49(4):644–50.
8. Dykstra DD, et al. Effects of botulinum A toxin on detrusor-sphincter dyssynergia in spinal cord injury patients. J Urol. 1988;139(5):919–22.
9. Schurch B, Schmid DM, Stohrer M. Treatment of neurogenic incontinence with botulinum toxin A. N Engl J Med. 2000;342(9):665.
10. Ginsberg D, et al. Phase 3 efficacy and tolerability study of onabotulinumtoxinA for urinary incontinence from neurogenic detrusor overactivity. J Urol. 2012;187(6):2131–9.
11. Cruz F, et al. Efficacy and safety of onabotulinumtoxinA in patients with urinary incontinence due to neurogenic detrusor overactivity: a randomised, double-blind, placebo-controlled trial. Eur Urol. 2011;60(4):742–50.
12. Nitti VW, et al. OnabotulinumtoxinA for the treatment of patients with overactive bladder and urinary incontinence: results of a phase 3, randomized, placebo controlled trial. J Urol. 2013;189(6):2186–93.
13. Chapple C, et al. OnabotulinumtoxinA 100 U significantly improves all idiopathic overactive bladder symptoms and quality of life in patients with overactive bladder and urinary incontinence: a randomised, double-blind, placebo-controlled trial. Eur Urol. 2013;64(2):249–56.
14. Gormley EA, et al. Diagnosis and treatment of overactive bladder (non-neurogenic) in adults: AUA/SUFU guideline amendment. J Urol. 2015;193(5):1572–80.
15. Fowler CJ, Griffiths D, de Groat WC. The neural control of micturition. Nat Rev Neurosci. 2008;9(6):453–66.
16. Schurch B, et al. Botulinum-a toxin for treating detrusor hyperreflexia in spinal cord injured patients: a new alternative to anticholinergic drugs? Preliminary results. J Urol. 2000;164(3 Pt 1):692–7.
17. Schurch B, et al. Botulinum toxin type a is a safe and effective treatment for neurogenic urinary incontinence: results of a single treatment, randomized, placebo controlled 6-month study. J Urol. 2005;174(1):196–200.
18. Ehren I, et al. Efficacy and impact of botulinum toxin A on quality of life in patients with neurogenic detrusor overactivity: a randomised, placebo-controlled, double-blind study. Scand J Urol Nephrol. 2007;41(4):335–40.
19. Giannantoni A, et al. Six-year follow-up of botulinum toxin A intradetrusorial injections in patients with refractory neurogenic detrusor overactivity: clinical and urodynamic results. Eur Urol. 2009;55(3):705–11.
20. Kennelly M, et al. Efficacy and safety of onabotulinumtoxinA therapy are sustained over 4 years of treatment in patients with neurogenic detrusor overactivity: final results of a long-term extension study. Neurourol Urodyn. 2015;36(2):368–75.
21. Schulte-Baukloh H, et al. Efficacy of botulinum-a toxin in children with detrusor hyperreflexia due to myelomeningocele: preliminary results. Urology. 2002;59(3):325–7. discussion 327–8

22. Game X, et al. Botulinum toxin-A (Botox) intradetrusor injections in children with neurogenic detrusor overactivity/neurogenic overactive bladder: a systematic literature review. J Pediatr Urol. 2009;5(3):156–64.
23. Figueroa V, et al. Single-center experience with botulinum toxin endoscopic detrusor injection for the treatment of congenital neuropathic bladder in children: effect of dose adjustment, multiple injections, and avoidance of reconstructive procedures. J Pediatr Urol. 2014;10(2):368–73.
24. Stewart WF, et al. Prevalence and burden of overactive bladder in the United States. World J Urol. 2003;20(6):327–36.
25. Dykstra D, Enriquez A, Valley M. Treatment of overactive bladder with botulinum toxin type B: a pilot study. Int Urogynecol J Pelvic Floor Dysfunct. 2003;14(6):424–6.
26. Dmochowski R, et al. Efficacy and safety of onabotulinumtoxinA for idiopathic overactive bladder: a double-blind, placebo controlled, randomized, dose ranging trial. J Urol. 2010;184(6):2416–22.
27. Denys P, et al. Efficacy and safety of low doses of onabotulinumtoxinA for the treatment of refractory idiopathic overactive bladder: a multicentre, double-blind, randomised, placebo-controlled dose-ranging study. Eur Urol. 2012;61(3):520–9.
28. Sievert KD, et al. OnabotulinumtoxinA 100U provides significant improvements in overactive bladder symptoms in patients with urinary incontinence regardless of the number of anticholinergic therapies used or reason for inadequate management of overactive bladder. Int J Clin Pract. 2014;68(10):1246–56.
29. Visco AG, et al. Anticholinergic therapy vs. onabotulinumtoxina for urgency urinary incontinence. N Engl J Med. 2012;367(19):1803–13.
30. Andersen JT, Bradley WE. The syndrome of detrusor-sphincter dyssynergia. J Urol. 1976;116(4):493–5.
31. Schurch B, et al. Botulinum-A toxin as a treatment of detrusor-sphincter dyssynergia: a prospective study in 24 spinal cord injury patients. J Urol. 1996;155(3):1023–9.
32. de Seze M, et al. Botulinum a toxin and detrusor sphincter dyssynergia: a double-blind lidocaine-controlled study in 13 patients with spinal cord disease. Eur Urol. 2002;42(1):56–62.
33. Gallien P, et al. Placebo controlled, randomised, double blind study of the effects of botulinum A toxin on detrusor sphincter dyssynergia in multiple sclerosis patients. J Neurol Neurosurg Psychiatry. 2005;76(12):1670–6.
34. Maria G, et al. Relief by botulinum toxin of voiding dysfunction due to benign prostatic hyperplasia: results of a randomized, placebo-controlled study. Urology. 2003;62(2):259–64; discussion 264-5.
35. Chuang YC, et al. Botulinum toxin type A improves benign prostatic hyperplasia symptoms in patients with small prostates. Urology. 2005;66(4):775–9.
36. Chuang YC, et al. Sustained beneficial effects of intraprostatic botulinum toxin type A on lower urinary tract symptoms and quality of life in men with benign prostatic hyperplasia. BJU Int. 2006;98(5):1033–7. discussion 1337
37. McVary KT, et al. A multicenter, randomized, double-blind, placebo controlled study of onabotulinumtoxinA 200 U to treat lower urinary tract symptoms in men with benign prostatic hyperplasia. J Urol. 2014;192(1):150–6.
38. Marberger M, et al. A randomized double-blind placebo-controlled phase 2 dose-ranging study of onabotulinumtoxinA in men with benign prostatic hyperplasia. Eur Urol. 2013;63(3):496–503.
39. van de Merwe JP, et al. Diagnostic criteria, classification, and nomenclature for painful bladder syndrome/interstitial cystitis: an ESSIC proposal. Eur Urol. 2008;53(1):60–7.
40. Smith CP, et al. Botulinum toxin a has antinociceptive effects in treating interstitial cystitis. Urology. 2004;64(5):871–5. discussion 875
41. Kuo HC. Preliminary results of suburothelial injection of botulinum a toxin in the treatment of chronic interstitial cystitis. Urol Int. 2005;75(2):170–4.
42. Giannantoni A, et al. Botulinum a toxin intravesical injections in the treatment of painful bladder syndrome: a pilot study. Eur Urol. 2006;49(4):704–9.

43. Kuo HC, Chancellor MB. Comparison of intravesical botulinum toxin type A injections plus hydrodistention with hydrodistention alone for the treatment of refractory interstitial cystitis/painful bladder syndrome. BJU Int. 2009;104(5):657–61.
44. Pinto R, et al. Trigonal injection of botulinum toxin A in patients with refractory bladder pain syndrome/interstitial cystitis. Eur Urol. 2010;58(3):360–5.
45. Kuo HC, et al. Intravesical botulinum toxin-A injections reduce bladder pain of interstitial cystitis/bladder pain syndrome refractory to conventional treatment—a prospective, multicenter, randomized, double-blind, placebo-controlled clinical trial. Neurourol Urodyn. 2016;35(5):609–14.
46. Turner JA, et al. Primary care and urology patients with the male pelvic pain syndrome: symptoms and quality of life. J Urol. 2002;167(4):1768–73.
47. Zermann D, et al. Perisphincteric injection of botulinum toxin type A. A treatment option for patients with chronic prostatic pain? Eur Urol. 2000;38(4):393–9.
48. Gottsch HP, Yang CC, Berger RE. A pilot study of botulinum toxin A for male chronic pelvic pain syndrome. Scand J Urol Nephrol. 2011;45(1):72–6.
49. Fam M, Gilhooly P. The use of botulinum neurotoxin type a in a patient with refractory urge incontinence to facilitate the intravesical treatment of bladder carcinoma. Rev Urol. 2014;16(4):194–7.
50. Lockwood G, Durkee C, Groth T. Intravesical Botulinum toxin for persistent autonomic dysreflexia in a pediatric patient. Case Rep Urol. 2016;2016:4569684.
51. Gupta M, et al. Prospective randomized evaluation of periureteral botulinum toxin type A injection for ureteral stent pain reduction. J Urol. 2010;183(2):598–602.
52. Reitz A, et al. European experience of 200 cases treated with botulinum-A toxin injections into the detrusor muscle for urinary incontinence due to neurogenic detrusor overactivity. Eur Urol. 2004;45(4):510–5.
53. Patki PS, et al. Botulinum toxin-type A in the treatment of drug-resistant neurogenic detrusor overactivity secondary to traumatic spinal cord injury. BJU Int. 2006;98(1):77–82.
54. Moore C, Rackley R, Goldman H. Urologic applications of botox. Curr Urol Rep. 2005;6(6):419–23.
55. Grosse J, Kramer G, Stohrer M. Success of repeat detrusor injections of botulinum a toxin in patients with severe neurogenic detrusor overactivity and incontinence. Eur Urol. 2005;47(5):653–9.
56. Kuo HC. Bladder base/trigone injection is safe and as effective as bladder body injection of onabotulinumtoxinA for idiopathic detrusor overactivity refractory to antimuscarinics. Neurourol Urodyn. 2011;30(7):1242–8.
57. Samal V, Mecl J, Sram J. Submucosal administration of onabotulinumtoxinA in the treatment of neurogenic detrusor overactivity: pilot single-centre experience and comparison with standard injection into the detrusor. Urol Int. 2013;91(4):423–8.
58. Nitti VW. Botulinum toxin for the treatment of idiopathic and neurogenic overactive bladder: state of the art. Rev Urol. 2006;8(4):198–208.
59. Popat R, et al. A comparison between the response of patients with idiopathic detrusor overactivity and neurogenic detrusor overactivity to the first intradetrusor injection of botulinum-A toxin. J Urol. 2005;174(3):984–9.
60. Sahai A, et al. Repeated injections of botulinum toxin-A for idiopathic detrusor overactivity. Urology. 2010;75(3):552–8.
61. Dowson C, et al. Repeated botulinum toxin type A injections for refractory overactive bladder: medium-term outcomes, safety profile, and discontinuation rates. Eur Urol. 2012;61(4):834–9.
62. Herschorn S, et al. Efficacy of botulinum toxin A injection for neurogenic detrusor overactivity and urinary incontinence: a randomized, double-blind trial. J Urol. 2011;185(6):2229–35.
63. Rovner E, et al. OnabotulinumtoxinA improves urodynamic outcomes in patients with neurogenic detrusor overactivity. Neurourol Urodyn. 2013;32(8):1109–15.
64. Kalsi V, et al. Quality of life changes in patients with neurogenic versus idiopathic detrusor overactivity after intradetrusor injections of botulinum neurotoxin type A and correlations with lower urinary tract symptoms and urodynamic changes. Eur Urol. 2006;49(3):528–35.

65. Kessler TM, et al. Botulinum A toxin injections into the detrusor: an effective treatment in idiopathic and neurogenic detrusor overactivity? Neurourol Urodyn. 2005;24(3):231–6.
66. Kuo HC, Liao CH, Chung SD. Adverse events of intravesical botulinum toxin a injections for idiopathic detrusor overactivity: risk factors and influence on treatment outcome. Eur Urol. 2010;58(6):919–26.
67. Oeconomou A, et al. Is botulinum neurotoxin type A (BoNT-A) a novel therapy for lower urinary tract symptoms due to benign prostatic enlargement? A review of the literature. Eur Urol. 2008;54(4):765–75.
68. BOTOX (onabotulinumtoxinA) for injection, for intramuscular, intradetrusor, or intradermal use. 2016. 1/2016. http://www.allergan.com/assets/pdf/botox_pi.pdf.
69. Smith CP, Chancellor MB. Emerging role of botulinum toxin in the management of voiding dysfunction. J Urol. 2004;171(6 Pt 1):2128–37.
70. Sahai A, et al. Botulinum toxin for the treatment of lower urinary tract symptoms: a review. Neurourol Urodyn. 2005;24(1):2–12.
71. Leippold T, Reitz A, Schurch B. Botulinum toxin as a new therapy option for voiding disorders: current state of the art. Eur Urol. 2003;44(2):165–74.
72. Visco AG, et al. Cost-effectiveness analysis of anticholinergics versus Botox for urgency urinary incontinence: results from the anticholinergic versus Botox comparison randomized trial. Female Pelvic Med Reconstr Surg. 2016;22(5):311–6.
73. Wu JM, et al. Cost-effectiveness of botulinum toxin a versus anticholinergic medications for idiopathic urge incontinence. J Urol. 2009;181(5):2181–6.

The Role of Botulinum Toxin in the Gastrointestinal Tract

Kaveh Sharzehi and Ron Schey

Introduction

Botulinum toxin, produced by Clostridium botulinum, is a potent toxin that inhibits the release of acetylcholine from nerve terminals and causes paralysis of skeletal muscle. Although it has eight major serotypes, only two types (A and B) have long-lasting period of action and are used in clinical practice. Botulinum toxin (Botox) injections have been utilized in a multitude of clinical indications, including strabismus, hemifacial spasm, and cervical dystonia [1–3].

In 1993, it was hypothesized that onabotulinumtoxinA (Botox) may have a similar effect on gastrointestinal smooth muscle. This was tested by injecting Botox into the lower esophageal sphincter of five piglets and comparing the effect with the injection of normal saline [4]. A tone reduction of about 60% was observed without evidence of toxicity [4]. In the same year, Botox was injected for the first time in a therapy-resistant achalasia patient, and eventually 2 years later. In 1995, it was demonstrated that intrasphincteric injection of botulinum toxin in humans had the potential to be useful in the treatment of achalasia [5, 6]. Since then, Botox has been used increasingly in the GI tract in various applications described in this review.

Upper Esophageal Sphincter Dysfunction

Botox has been in use in the field of otorhinolaryngology and Neurology, as a relatively safe and efficacious treatment of facial nerve disorders such as hemifacial-spasm, laryngealdystonia, oromandibular dystonia, and spasmodic torticollis [7, 8].

K. Sharzehi, M.D., M.S. (✉) • R. Schey, M.D., F.A.C.G.
Section of Gastroenterology, Lewis Katz School of Medicine at Temple University and the Temple University Health System, Philadelphia, PA, USA
e-mail: kvshrz@yahoo.com; Ron.schey@tuhs.temple.edu

B. Jabbari (ed.), *Botulinum Toxin Treatment in Clinical Medicine*,
DOI 10.1007/978-3-319-56038-0_5

Dysphagia and deglutition problems combined with aspiration are caused by spasticity, hypertonus, or delayed relaxation of the upper esophageal sphincter (UES). UES dysfunction during swallowing has been reported in numerous acute and progressive neurological conditions including, but not limited to, brainstem stroke, motor neuron disease, Parkinson's disease, myasthenia gravis, and inclusion body myositis [9–13].

Management of impaired UES relaxation varies across individuals and intervention can be pharmacological, compensatory, rehabilitative, or surgical in nature [14]. Compensation includes the use of postural strategies and voluntary maneuvers. Rehabilitation programs are designed to target impaired UES and include jaw exercises, the Shaker exercises, and the Mendelsohn maneuver [14]. In cases where patients have demonstrated minimal benefit from a trial of compensatory therapy and rehabilitation, they may be considered for surgical or pharmacological interventions. Surgical intervention includes cricopharyngral myotomy and upper esophageal dilatation. The pharmacological intervention consists of injection of Botox into the cricopharyngeus.

The first use of Botox in this setting was described in 1994 in a series of seven patients. Conventional therapy (i.e., lateral cricopharyngotomy and laser dissection of the UES) was replaced by Botox injection with complete resolution of symptoms in five of seven patients [15]. Since this initial 1994 study, cricopharyngeal Botox injection has been reported in over 200 patients with dysphagia of varying etiologies with success rates ranging between 43% and 100%. However, a Cochrane database Systemic review published in 2014 concluded that no randomized controlled studies are available and there is insufficient evidence to recommend its use in clinical practice, hence, it was not possible to reach a conclusion on the efficacy and safety of botulinum toxin as an intervention for people with UES dysfunction [14].

Achalasia

Achalasia is a disorder characterized by a failure of the lower esophageal sphincter to relax with swallowing and by a lack of esophageal peristalsis. The etiology, for the most part, is unknown. It is characterized manometrically by insufficient relaxation of the lower esophageal sphincter (LES) and loss of esophageal peristalsis; radiographically by aperistalsis, esophageal dilation, with minimal LES opening, "bird-beak" appearance and poor emptying of barium; and endoscopically, by dilated esophagus with retained saliva, liquid, and undigested food particles in the absence of mucosal stricturing or tumor [16].

Achalasia was first described and termed by Sir Thomas Willis in 1672, when he suggested that the disease is due to the loss of normal inhibition in the distal esophagus [17].

Since then, new ideas on the etiology and pathophysiology of the disease have been promoted leading to various theories in identifying the nature of motor disturbances in esophageal regions. This includes cardiospasm, esophageal muscle failure, and physical obstruction [18]. Subsequently, a body of evidence has emerged showing that idiopathic achalasia is indeed caused primarily by the loss of the inhibitory innervation of the esophageal myenteric plexus. However, the initiating cause remains elusive [16].

These abnormalities stem from impairment of the inhibitory innervation to the esophageal smooth muscle and the lower esophageal sphincter [19]. The smooth muscle of the distal esophagus is innervated by the preganglionic vagus nerve fibers with cell bodies located in the dorsal motor nucleus [20]. The postganglionic excitatory neurons release acetylcholine while the inhibitory neurons release nitric oxide and vasoactive intestinal polypeptide resulting in esophageal and LES contractions and relaxations, respectively [21, 22]. The inhibitory neurons also play a role in normal peristalsis. At baseline, the esophageal muscle is in a contractile state. With swallowing, the inhibitory neurons are excited, which results in esophageal relaxation. A coordinated series of relaxation followed by contraction in a cephalic-caudal direction results in peristalsis [23]. In patients with achalasia, there is loss of the inhibitory neurons, resulting in failure of LES relaxation and loss of esophageal peristalsis [24].

Idiopathic achalasia is rare, has an insidious onset, and disease progression is gradual. Patients typically experience symptoms for years prior to seeking medical attention. A recent population-based study reported mean incidences of 0.3–1.63 per 100,000 people per year in adults [25, 26]. The mean duration of symptoms was 4–6 years prior to diagnosis [27]. Most frequent symptoms are dysphagia toward solids (91%) and liquids (85%), regurgitation (76%), heartburn (52%), chest pain (41%), and weight loss (35%) [28]. In the early stages of the disease, dysphagia may be very subtle and can be misinterpreted as dyspepsia, poor gastric emptying, or stress. The presence of heartburn due to food stasis can add to this confusion. As the disease progresses, difficulty swallowing characteristically occurs with both solid foods and liquids. The dysphagia is more to solids than liquids.

When achalasia is suspected, a primary barium esophagogram with fluoroscopy is a useful diagnostic test (Fig. 1) [29].

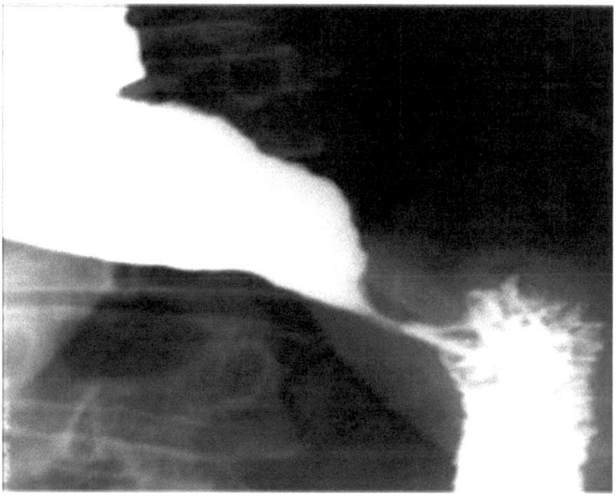

Fig. 1 Barium esophagogram showing "bird-beak" appearance of achalasia

Esophagogram findings include dilation of the esophagus, a narrow esophagogastric junction with "bird beak" appearance, aperistalsis, and poor emptying of barium. A variation of barium swallow, named "timed barium swallow," which includes measuring of a barium column height 1 and 5 min after upright ingestion of a large barium bolus, has been used to assess esophageal emptying after therapy [30]. The primary role of esophagogastroduodenoscopy (EGD) in the workup of achalasia is focused on ruling out a mechanical obstruction or pseudoachalasia as they can mimic achalasia. Endoscopic evaluation in these patients often demonstrates a dilated esophagus with retained food or saliva and a puckered gastroesophageal junction [16].

By definition, an assessment of esophageal motor function is essential for the diagnosis of achalasia. Achalasia is diagnosed on high-resolution manometry by an elevated median integrated relaxation pressure (IRP), which indicates impaired EGJ relaxation, and absence of normal peristalsis. According to the Chicago Classification (CC, version 3.0 [CC-3]) of patterns of esophageal pressurization on high-resolution manometry, achalasia is subtyped into Type I (classic achalasia), Type II, and Type III (spastic achalasia). These subtypes have important implications for management [31].

Achalasia is a chronic condition and current treatment options in achalasia are aimed at reducing the hypertonicity of the LES by pharmacologic, endoscopic, or surgical means.

For patients who are at low surgical risk, pneumatic dilation or surgical myotomy should be performed to treat achalasia. Per-oral endoscopic myotomy (POEM) is a promising new endoscopic technique for performing myotomy. The aim of all endoscopic and surgical treatments are to weaken the LES by cutting its circular muscle fibers [32]. Initial success rates are high with either modality (85% for pneumatic dilation and 90% for surgical myotomy); however, about one-third of patients have recurrence of symptoms within 4–6 years [33].

The two most frequently used pharmacological drugs are nitrates and calcium-channel blockers. Medical therapy is the least effective treatment option in patients with achalasia, and should be considered in patients who are unwilling or unable to tolerate invasive therapy and for patients who have failed Botox injections [34].

Botox therapy is strongly considered in patients who are not good candidates for more definitive therapy with pneumatic dilation or surgical myotomy. Botulinum toxin A, which blocks the release of acetylcholine from the nerve terminals, is directly injected into the LES. EGD for the injection of Botox is often performed under conscious sedation using a combination of intravenous fentanyl and versed or under monitored anesthesia care using predominantly propofol. The lower esophageal sphincter will be visualized endoscopically by identification of the sphincteric rosette, seen at the squamocolumnar junction. Botox is injected using a 5-mm or 7-mm sclerotherapy needle (other injection needles have been used based on the center) into the region of the lower esophageal sphincter. Aliquots of 1 ml each (20–25 units of botulinum toxin per milliliter of saline) are injected into quadrants, for a total of 80–100 units [35].

Table 1 Randomized trails comparing Botox injection to Balloon dilation and myotomy for treatment of achalasia

Author	Compared to	*N*	Response rate (30 day) Botox group vs. non-Botox group	Recurrence rate (12–24 month) Botox group vs. non-Botox group
Zaninotto et al. [42]	Surgical myotomy	80	66% vs. 82% ($p < 0.05$)	87.5% vs. 34% ($p < 0.05$)
Zhu et al. [41]	Balloon dilation and balloon dilation + Botox	90	75% vs. 85% vs. 93%	84% vs. 64% vs. 43%
Mikaeli et al. [40]	Balloon dilation	40	Not available	85% vs. 47% ($p < 0.05$)
Ghoshal et al. [39]	Balloon dilation	17	86% vs. 80% (p = NS)	71% vs. 25% ($p = 0.027$)
Vaezi et al. [38]	Balloon dilation	42	Not available	68% vs. 30% ($p < 0.01$)
Muehldorfer et al. [37]	Balloon dilation	24	75% vs. 83% (p = NS)	100% vs. 40% ($p < 0.05$)

More than 80% of cases have a clinical response by 1 month, but response fades rapidly, with less than 60% of patients in remission at 1 year [36]. Findings from six randomized trials comparing Botox with pneumatic dilatation and laparoscopic myotomy are shown in Table 1. These studies demonstrated comparable relief from dysphagia, but a rapid deterioration in patients treated with Botox after 6–12 months compared to the two other modalities [37–42].

The most common complications of esophageal Botox injections are mild and related to the injection procedure or the decreased LES pressure. The occurrence of transitory chest pain and gastroesophageal reflux has been reported after 0–30% of procedures. Thus far, no serious adverse events have been reported in secondary or pre-appraised publications. However, a number of case reports have been published on severe complications after esophageal Botox injections including one death due to pneumothorax [43].

Botox injection is less invasive compared with surgery and can be easily performed with endoscopy. As seen in Table 1, initial success rates with Botox are comparable to pneumatic dilation and surgical myotomy [44]. However, patients treated with Botox have more frequent relapses and a shorter time to relapse. Greater than 50% of patients with achalasia treated with Botox require retreatment within 6–12 months. Repeated Botox injections can negatively impact the outcome of subsequent myotomy [45].

Hypertensive Esophageal Disorders

This group of esophageal motility disorders is a somewhat rare but troublesome group of disorders that can lead to severe symptoms including nausea, regurgitation, dysphagia, and chest pain [46]. Using esophageal manometry, esophageal motility abnormalities are classified as achalasia (discussed previously) and other abnormal motility patterns, which are in turn subclassified into hypercontracting, hypocontracting, or discoordinated motility disorders. Since the introduction of Botox for the treatment of achalasia in 1995, its utility has been expanded to a spectrum of esophageal motility diseases, most importantly diffuse esophageal spasm (DES), nutcracker esophagus, and hypertensive lower esophageal sphincter. These conditions are also collectively called hypercontractile esophageal disorders.

There are limited data on the prevalence of hypercontractile esophageal disorders. The prevalence of these conditions among individuals with atypical chest pain appears to be between 4% and 13% [47]. The underlying pathophysiology for these conditions is relatively unknown. DES has been associated with an impairment of inhibitory innervation and malfunction in endogenous nitric oxide synthesis [48]. Nutcracker esophagus and hypertensive LES are due to overactivity of excitatory innervation or asynchrony of the smooth muscle response due to hypercholinergic state [49].

The typical symptoms of patients with DES are dysphagia associated with retrosternal chest pain. Many of the patients with nutcracker esophagus or hypertensive LES have no symptoms. The diagnosis of these patients is often made through esophageal manometry after a normal endoscopic examination. Each of these conditions has distinct manometric findings, and diagnosis is often made once manometric criteria are met.

Multiple therapies have been used to treat diffuse DES, nutcracker esophagus, and hypertensive LES, the most effective treatment has not been established yet. Calcium channel blockers and tricyclic antidepressants have been shown to be effective in the treatment of dysphagia and chest pain, respectively, and they have been considered as the first-line treatment for these conditions [50–52].

For patients who do not respond to the first-line treatment, injection of Botox or oral nitrates (isosorbide 10 mg or sildenafil 50 mg on an as-needed basis for pain) is considered as the next treatment option [53, 54].

Typically, 100 units of Botox is diluted in 4 ml saline. During the EGD, aliquots of 0.5 ml Botox are injected in the four quadrants at 2 cm above the gastroesophageal junction, and 5 cm more proximally using a standard sclerotherapy needle. In spastic esophageal motor disorders, Botox is injected at several levels close to the lower esophageal sphincter and in the distal esophageal body. It is important to avoid submucosal injection or injection outside the esophageal wall. Symptom relief occurs in 70–90% of patients within 30 days after the procedure. However, >50% of patients require repeat treatment within 6–24 months. The procedure is performed on a day-case basis and patients are allowed to eat as tolerated.

Botox injection in these patients has been shown to improve the symptoms of dysphagia significantly, but has no or minimal effect on chest pain, regurgitation, or heartburn [55]. Interestingly, injections into the esophageal body, application of more injection sites per procedure, history of previous injections, and increasing the dose did not increase the risk of complications [43].

Gastroparesis

Normal gastric motility results from a complex series of events that requires coordination of the sympathetic and parasympathetic nervous systems, neurons, and pacemaker cells of Cajal within the stomach and the smooth muscle cells. Abnormalities of this process can lead to a delay in gastric emptying [56]. Gastroparesis is defined by delayed gastric emptying in the absence of a mechanical obstruction [57]. The age-adjusted prevalence of gastroparesis is 9.6 per 100,000 persons for men and 38 per 100,000 persons for women [58].

The etiology for over half of the patients with gastroparesis in unknown and, therefore, these are classified as idiopathic gastroparesis. Both long-standing diabetes mellitus and hyperglycemia are associated with delayed gastric emptying. In the former, this occurs through diabetic neuropathy. Neuropathy causes abnormal postprandial proximal gastric accommodation and difficulties with antral motor function [59, 60]. Medications (including narcotics and dopamine agonists) have shown to delay gastric emptying [61]. Previous gastric and thoracic surgery can result in gastroparesis due to intentional or accidental injury to the vagus nerves [62]. Several common neurologic disorders are associated with gastroparesis, which include multiple sclerosis and Parkinson's disease [63].

Patients with gastroparesis can present with nausea, vomiting, abdominal pain, early satiety, postprandial fullness, bloating, and weight loss. The vomitus may contain food ingested several hours previously [57].

Initial evaluation of patients with gastroparesis includes endoscopy and cross-sectional imaging to exclude mechanical obstruction. The most commonly used and cost-effective modality to diagnose gastroparesis is a 4 h scintigraphic gastric emptying scan [64, 65].

Treatment options for gastroparesis include dietary changes, prokinetic drugs, antiemetics, correction of malnutrition and electrolyte disturbances, jejunal feeding, parenteral nutrition, gastric neurostimulation therapy, and surgery.

The first step in management is dietary counseling and nutritional support. For severe cases, enteral nutrition should be established, before consideration of medical, endoscopic, or surgical therapy [66, 67].

Dopamine type 2(D2) receptor antagonists have been the most studied and utilized family of medications for the treatment of gastroparesis. Notable in this family of drugs are metoclopramide and domperidone, of which, the former has been in use for close to 40 years [68–70]. Macrolides (erythromycin), 5-HT4 receptor agonists, ghrelin agonists, 5-HT3 receptor antagonists, and cannabinoid-1 agonists have been used as well with variable degrees of response in gastroparesis [66].

Invasive interventions include intra-pyloric botulinum toxin injection, venting gastrostomies, gastric electric stimulators, and pyloromyotomy (surgical or endoscopic). Since the late 1990s, there has been conflicting evidence regarding the efficacy of intra-pyloric botulinum toxin in the management of gastroparesis. The first data on the intrapyloric application of Botox in patients with gastroparesis was published in 2002 [71]. Injection of 100 units of Botox into the pylorus in patients with diabetic gastroparesis showed 50% improvement in their symptoms and gastric emptying tests. Further, open-labeled trials showed promising evidence of improvement in gastric emptying tests, symptoms, and SF-36 scores with an intra-pyloric injection of 200 units Botox [72, 73]. Miller et al. demonstrated the effectiveness of repeat injections but at the same time raised a question regarding long-term outcomes of the procedure [73]. Two additional randomized trials reported improvement on gastric emptying tests without significant symptomatic improvement [74, 75]. A small retrospective analysis of 21 patients with a mean follow-up of 2 years demonstrated a 62% response to treatment compared to 19% non-responders. The mean response duration was 4.2 months. Weight gain and increased insulin requirement were observed in the diabetic group with greater effectiveness in the diabetic population compared to idiopathic gastroparesis [76]. Thus far, one of the largest studies published was a retrospective trial of 179 patients including 81 with diabetic gastroparesis and 76 idiopathic gastroparesis cases, and suggested a better response in women, younger patients (<50 years old) and those with idiopathic gastroparesis [77]. Ukleja et al. concluded in a review article that it is important to emphasize that improvement in gastric emptying has not been shown to correlate with symptom improvement in this patient population. Hence, assessing response to Botox treatment based on gastric emptying studies has its own limitations [78]. Thus, despite the fact that it is currently not recommended, due to limited availability of medical treatment options, physicians should consider Botox as a trial therapy before directing patient with refractory gastroparesis for more aggressive treatment such as surgical interventions including placement of jejunostomy tube or gastric electrical stimulator and gastrectomy.

Sphincter of Oddi Dysfunction

Sphincter of Oddi dysfunction (SOD) refers to a clinical syndrome that occurs because of the abnormal sphincter of Oddi (SO) contractility. It has been defined by an excessively high baseline sphincter pressure of ≥40 mmHg [79]. Elevated pressure in the sphincter can lead to pancreatitis, chronic right upper quadrant pain, and elevated liver function tests. A subgroup of these patients has only elevated pressure above 40 mmHg with pain and is designated "sphincter of Oddi dysfunction type III." Controversy exists concerning the best management of this subgroup. Performing sphincterotomy during endoscopic retrograde cholangiopancreatography (ERCP) is considered one of the treatment options. The risks associated with sphincterotomy include bleeding perforation and pancreatitis, and the results following endoscopic sphincterotomy are often disappointing [80]. Therefore, the concept of trial of Botox prior to sphincterotomy has been entertained. Pilot studies have shown a substantial decrease in the SO pressure with the use of Botox injection [81], but there are no placebo-controlled studies available formally evaluating the effect of Botox injection on SOD type III. One study has shown that 50% of patients receiving Botox for SOD (type III) had some improvement of their pain. It has also served as a predictor to determine who may respond to endoscopic sphincterotomy [82].

However, long-term follow-up of patients with SOD type III has shown no benefit from ERCP and sphincterotomy to the extent that it has been recently proposed to discard the concept of SOD type III from GI functional gastrointestinal disorders (i.e., Rome IV criteria) [83]. This undermines the usefulness of any intervention of the SO (sphincterotomy or Botox) in patients with type III SOD.

New and novel indications for Botox injection in SO have been proposed. Recently, Botox has been successfully used to temporarily reduce the SO pressure after distal pancreatectomy to prevent pancreatic fistula formation. Injecting Botox pre-operatively has reduced the incidence of fistula formation significantly without any major or minor side effects [84].

Anal Fissure

An anal fissure is a common benign anorectal condition that may result from high anal pressure. Fissure is a tear in the anoderm distal to the dentate line. Anal fissures may be acute or chronic. Acute fissures may result from local trauma or may be secondary to an underlying medical/surgical condition. Chronic anal fissure fails conservative management and requires a more aggressive approach [85].

Fissure is the result of the stretching of the anal mucosa beyond its normal capacity. Once the tear occurs, it begins a cycle leading to repeated injury. The exposed internal sphincter muscle beneath the tear goes into spasm. This results in severe pain, pulling apart the edges of the fissure and subsequent impair healing of the wound. Repeated trauma results in a chronic anal fissure in 50% of patients [86].

Anal fissures most often affect infants and middle-age individuals, and the most common causes are the passage of hard stool, prolonged diarrhea, vaginal delivery, or anal sex [87].

Patients with an acute anal fissure present with sharp pain associated with the passage of bowel movements. Some describe a small amount of bright red blood on the stool or the toilet paper. Other less frequent complaints include perianal pruritus and/or skin irritation. Patients with a chronic fissure typically have less intense pain. The most common location of a fissure is posterior midline. Deep fissures can extend to the external anal sphincter. Chronic fissures are often characterized by sentinel pile and hypertrophic anal papillae resulting from chronic inflammation [88].

This first line of treatment for anal fissure is a combination of supportive measures and a topical vasodilator. Conservative measures include increase dietary fiber (or fiber supplements) and water intake to soften and bulk the stool, Sitz baths a few times a day, and topical analgesics such as 2% lidocaine jelly [89–91]. Commonly used topical vasodilators include nifedipine (0.2% or 0.3%) and nitroglycerin (0.2% or 0.4%) ointments. These therapies have a response rate ranging from 60% to 90%, and a recurrence rate of 30–40% [92, 93]. For patients who fail medical treatment, the next step is either Botox injection or a lateral sphincterotomy. One of the main concerns with surgical option for the management of anal fissures is incontinence. In patients with high risk of incontinence such as multiparous women and elderly, Botox injection is considered as the first line of treatment option for refractory fissures.

The first use of Botox in anal fissure was reported in 1993 when the first case was treated using 2.5 units of Botox injected into the external anal sphincter [94]. Injection of Botox into the anal sphincter can help relax the hypertonic anal sphincter muscle and, in turn, improve healing of anal fissures. Botox is typically injected into the internal anal sphincter on either side of the fissure using a 27-gauge needle [95]. The most common dose for injection is 10–20 units of Botox. A recent meta-analysis showed a range of 5–150 units of Botox being used in various settings [96]. The same study did not show any dose-dependent efficiency or complication rate.

Botox injection has been shown to be superior to topical vasodilators in the treatment of chronic anal fissure; however, in long-term follow-up may not differ significantly from vasodilators [97, 98]. Thus, botulinum toxin has proven to be a valid option in patients with chronic anal fissures who desire a non-surgical intervention or those with certain grades of incontinence.

Randomized trials have compared the efficacy and side-effect profile of Botox injection with lateral sphincterotomy. Sphincterotomy has a higher healing rate and a lower recurrence rate than the intra-sphincteric injection of Botox. Botox injection has a reported recurrence of up to 40–50% [99]. The risk of incontinence in Botox injection, however, is less than lateral sphincterotomy (7% vs. 35%) [100]; therefore, Botox injection appears to be a simple noninvasive technique that avoids the greater risk of incontinence and it could be used as the first therapeutic approach in patients without clinical risk factors of recurrence [101, 102].

References

1. Carruthers A, Carruthers J. Botulinum toxin products overview. Skin Therapy Lett. 2008;13(6):1–4.
2. Dressler D. Clinical applications of botulinum toxin. Curr Opin Microbiol. 2012;15(3):325–36.
3. Walker TJ, Dayan SH. Comparison and overview of currently available neurotoxins. J Clin Aesthet Dermatol. 2014;7(2):31–9.
4. Pasricha PJ, Ravich WJ, Kalloo AN. Effects of intrasphincteric botulinum toxin on the lower esophageal sphincter in piglets. Gastroenterology. 1993;105(4):1045–9.
5. Pasricha PJ, Ravich WJ, Hendrix TR, Sostre S, Jones B, Kalloo AN. Intrasphincteric botulinum toxin for the treatment of achalasia. N Engl J Med. 1995;332(12):774–8.
6. Pasricha PJ, Ravich WJ, Kalloo AN. Botulinum toxin for achalasia. Lancet (London, England). 1993;341(8839):244–5.
7. Mauriello JA Jr, Coniaris H, Haupt EJ. Use of botulinum toxin in the treatment of one hundred patients with facial dyskinesias. Ophthalmology. 1987;94(8):976–9.
8. Blitzer A, Brin MF, Fahn S, Lovelace RE. Localized injections of botulinum toxin for the treatment of focal laryngeal dystonia (spastic dysphonia). Laryngoscope. 1988;98(2):193–7.
9. Bian RX, Choi IS, Kim JH, Han JY, Lee SG. Impaired opening of the upper esophageal sphincter in patients with medullary infarctions. Dysphagia. 2009;24(2):238–45.
10. Colton-Hudson A, Koopman WJ, Moosa T, Smith D, Bach D, Nicolle M. A prospective assessment of the characteristics of dysphagia in myasthenia gravis. Dysphagia. 2002;17(2):147–51.
11. Higo R, Tayama N, Watanabe T, Nitou T. Videomanofluorometric study in amyotrophic lateral sclerosis. Laryngoscope. 2002;112(5):911–7.
12. TH O, Brumfield KA, Hoskin TL, Kasperbauer JL, Basford JR. Dysphagia in inclusion body myositis: clinical features, management, and clinical outcome. Am J Phys Med Rehabil. 2008;87(11):883–9.

13. Restivo DA, Palmeri A, Marchese-Ragona R. Botulinum toxin for cricopharyngeal dysfunction in Parkinson's disease. N Engl J Med. 2002;346(15):1174–5.
14. Regan J, Murphy A, Chiang M, McMahon BP, Coughlan T, Walshe M. Botulinum toxin for upper oesophageal sphincter dysfunction in neurological swallowing disorders. Cochrane Database Syst Rev. 2014;(5):Cd009968.
15. Schneider I, Thumfart WF, Pototschnig C, Eckel HE. Treatment of dysfunction of the cricopharyngeal muscle with botulinum A toxin: introduction of a new, noninvasive method. Ann Otol Rhinol Laryngol. 1994;103(1):31–5.
16. Ates F, Vaezi MF. The pathogenesis and management of achalasia: current status and future directions. Gut Liver. 2015;9(4):449–63.
17. Birgisson S, Richter JE. Achalasia: what's new in diagnosis and treatment? Dig Dis (Basel, Switzerland). 1997;15(Suppl 1):1–27.
18. Paterson WG. Etiology and pathogenesis of achalasia. Gastrointest Endosc Clin N Am. 2001;11(2):249–66. vi
19. Reynolds JC, Parkman HP. Achalasia. Gastroenterol Clin N Am. 1989;18(2):223–55.
20. Collman PI, Tremblay L, Diamant NE. The central vagal efferent supply to the esophagus and lower esophageal sphincter of the cat. Gastroenterology. 1993;104(5):1430–8.
21. Goyal RK, Rattan S, Said SI. VIP as a possible neurotransmitter of non-cholinergic non-adrenergic inhibitory neurones. Nature. 1980;288(5789):378–80.
22. Yamato S, Spechler SJ, Goyal RK. Role of nitric oxide in esophageal peristalsis in the opossum. Gastroenterology. 1992;103(1):197–204.
23. Crist J, Gidda JS, Goyal RK. Intramural mechanism of esophageal peristalsis: roles of cholinergic and noncholinergic nerves. Proc Natl Acad Sci U S A. 1984;81(11):3595–9.
24. Mearin F, Mourelle M, Guarner F, et al. Patients with achalasia lack nitric oxide synthase in the gastro-oesophageal junction. Eur J Clin Investig. 1993;23(11):724–8.
25. Farrukh A, DeCaestecker J, Mayberry JF. An epidemiological study of achalasia among the South Asian population of Leicester, 1986-2005. Dysphagia. 2008;23(2):161–4.
26. Sadowski DC, Ackah F, Jiang B, Svenson LW. Achalasia: incidence, prevalence and survival. A population-based study. Neurogastroenterol Motil. 2010;22(9):e256–61.
27. Eckardt VF, Kohne U, Junginger T, Westermeier T. Risk factors for diagnostic delay in achalasia. Dig Dis Sci. 1997;42(3):580–5.
28. Fisichella PM, Raz D, Palazzo F, Niponmick I, Patti MG. Clinical, radiological, and manometric profile in 145 patients with untreated achalasia. World J Surg. 2008;32(9):1974–9.
29. Richter JE. Achalasia—an update. J of Neurogastroenterol Motil. 2010;16(3):232–42.
30. de Oliveira JM, Birgisson S, Doinoff C, et al. Timed barium swallow: a simple technique for evaluating esophageal emptying in patients with achalasia. AJR Am J Roentgenol. 1997;169(2):473–9.
31. Pandolfino JE, Kwiatek MA, Nealis T, Bulsiewicz W, Post J, Kahrilas PJ. Achalasia: a new clinically relevant classification by high-resolution manometry. Gastroenterology. 2008;135(5):1526–33.
32. Kostic S, Johnsson E, Kjellin A, et al. Health economic evaluation of therapeutic strategies in patients with idiopathic achalasia: results of a randomized trial comparing pneumatic dilatation with laparoscopic cardiomyotomy. Surg Endosc. 2007;21(7):1184–9.
33. Boeckxstaens GE, Annese V, des Varannes SB, et al. Pneumatic dilation versus laparoscopic Heller's myotomy for idiopathic achalasia. N Engl J Med. 2011;364(19):1807–16.
34. Boeckxstaens GE, Zaninotto G, Richter JE. Achalasia. Lancet (London, England). 2014;383(9911):83–93.
35. Annese V, Bassotti G, Coccia G, et al. A multicentre randomised study of intrasphincteric botulinum toxin in patients with oesophageal achalasia. GISMAD Achalasia Study Group. Gut. 2000;46(5):597–600.
36. Leyden JE, Moss AC, MacMathuna P. Endoscopic pneumatic dilation versus botulinum toxin injection in the management of primary achalasia. Cochrane Database Syst Rev. 2006;(4):Cd005046.
37. Muehldorfer SM, Schneider TH, Hochberger J, Martus P, Hahn EG, Ell C. Esophageal achalasia: intrasphincteric injection of botulinum toxin A versus balloon dilation. Endoscopy. 1999;31(7):517–21.

38. Vaezi MF, Richter JE, Wilcox CM, et al. Botulinum toxin versus pneumatic dilatation in the treatment of achalasia: a randomised trial. Gut. 1999;44(2):231–9.
39. Ghoshal UC, Chaudhuri S, Pal BB, Dhar K, Ray G, Banerjee PK. Randomized controlled trial of intrasphincteric botulinum toxin A injection versus balloon dilatation in treatment of achalasia cardia. Dis Esophagus. 2001;14(3–4):227–31.
40. Mikaeli J, Fazel A, Montazeri G, Yaghoobi M, Malekzadeh R. Randomized controlled trial comparing botulinum toxin injection to pneumatic dilatation for the treatment of achalasia. Aliment Pharmacol Ther. 2001;15(9):1389–96.
41. Zhu Q, Liu J, Yang C. Clinical study on combined therapy of botulinum toxin injection and small balloon dilation in patients with esophageal achalasia. Dig Surg. 2009;26(6):493–8.
42. Zaninotto G, Annese V, Costantini M, et al. Randomized controlled trial of botulinum toxin versus laparoscopic heller myotomy for esophageal achalasia. Ann Surg. 2004;239(3):364–70.
43. van Hoeij FB, Tack JF, Pandolfino JE, et al. Complications of botulinum toxin injections for treatment of esophageal motility disorders. Dis Esophagus. 2016;30(3):1–5.
44. Campos GM, Vittinghoff E, Rabl C, et al. Endoscopic and surgical treatments for achalasia: a systematic review and meta-analysis. Ann Surg. 2009;249(1):45–57.
45. Bonavina L, Incarbone R, Reitano M, Antoniazzi L, Peracchia A. Does previous endoscopic treatment affect the outcome of laparoscopic Heller myotomy? Ann Chir. 2000;125(1):45–9.
46. Amarasinghe G, Sifrim D. Functional esophageal disorders: pharmacological options. Drugs. 2014;74(12):1335–44.
47. Dalton CB, Castell DO, Hewson EG, WC W, Richter JE. Diffuse esophageal spasm. A rare motility disorder not characterized by high-amplitude contractions. Dig Dis Sci. 1991;36(8):1025–8.
48. Konturek JW, Gillessen A, Domschke W. Diffuse esophageal spasm: a malfunction that involves nitric oxide? Scand J Gastroenterol. 1995;30(11):1041–5.
49. Korsapati H, Bhargava V, Mittal RK. Reversal of asynchrony between circular and longitudinal muscle contraction in nutcracker esophagus by atropine. Gastroenterology. 2008;135(3):796–802.
50. Cattau EL Jr, Castell DO, Johnson DA, et al. Diltiazem therapy for symptoms associated with nutcracker esophagus. Am J Gastroenterol. 1991;86(3):272–6.
51. Clouse RE, Lustman PJ, Eckert TC, Ferney DM, Griffith LS. Low-dose trazodone for symptomatic patients with esophageal contraction abnormalities. A double-blind, placebo-controlled trial. Gastroenterology. 1987;92(4):1027–36.
52. Cannon RO III, Quyyumi AA, Mincemoyer R, et al. Imipramine in patients with chest pain despite normal coronary angiograms. N Engl J Med. 1994;330(20):1411–7.
53. Eherer AJ, Schwetz I, Hammer HF, et al. Effect of sildenafil on oesophageal motor function in healthy subjects and patients with oesophageal motor disorders. Gut. 2002;50(6):758–64.
54. Miller LS, Parkman HP, Schiano TD, et al. Treatment of symptomatic nonachalasia esophageal motor disorders with botulinum toxin injection at the lower esophageal sphincter. Dig Dis Sci. 1996;41(10):2025–31.
55. Vanuytsel T, Bisschops R, Farre R, et al. Botulinum toxin reduces Dysphagia in patients with nonachalasia primary esophageal motility disorders. Clin Gastroenterol Hepatol. 2013;11(9):1115–1121.e2.
56. Camilleri M. Clinical practice. Diabetic gastroparesis. N Engl J Med. 2007;356(8):820–9.
57. Camilleri M, Parkman HP, Shafi MA, Abell TL, Gerson L. Clinical guideline: management of gastroparesis. Am J Gastroenterol. 2013;108(1):18–37. quiz 38
58. Jung HK, Choung RS, Locke GR III, et al. The incidence, prevalence, and outcomes of patients with gastroparesis in Olmsted County, Minnesota, from 1996 to 2006. Gastroenterology. 2009;136(4):1225–33.
59. Forster J, Damjanov I, Lin Z, Sarosiek I, Wetzel P, McCallum RW. Absence of the interstitial cells of Cajal in patients with gastroparesis and correlation with clinical findings. J Gastrointest Surg. 2005;9(1):102–8.
60. Vittal H, Farrugia G, Gomez G, Pasricha PJ. Mechanisms of disease: the pathological basis of gastroparesis—a review of experimental and clinical studies. Nat Clin Pract Gastroenterol Hepatol. 2007;4(6):336–46.

61. Jeong ID, Camilleri M, Shin A, et al. A randomised, placebo-controlled trial comparing the effects of tapentadol and oxycodone on gastrointestinal and colonic transit in healthy humans. Aliment Pharmacol Ther. 2012;35(9):1088–96.
62. Fich A, Neri M, Camilleri M, Kelly KA, Phillips SF. Stasis syndromes following gastric surgery: clinical and motility features of 60 symptomatic patients. J Clin Gastroenterol. 1990;12(5):505–12.
63. Jost WH. Gastrointestinal dysfunction in Parkinson's disease. J Neurol Sci. 2010;289(1–2): 69–73.
64. Camilleri M, Shin A. Novel and validated approaches for gastric emptying scintigraphy in patients with suspected gastroparesis. Dig Dis Sci. 2013;58(7):1813–5.
65. Sachdeva P, Malhotra N, Pathikonda M, et al. Gastric emptying of solids and liquids for evaluation for gastroparesis. Dig Dis Sci. 2011;56(4):1138–46.
66. Langworthy J, Parkman HP, Schey R. Emerging strategies for the treatment of gastroparesis. Expert Rev Gastroenterol Hepatol. 2016;10(7):817–25.
67. Malamood M, Parkman H, Schey R. Current advances in treatment of gastroparesis. Expert Opin Pharmacother. 2015;16(13):1997–2008.
68. McCallum RW, Ricci DA, Rakatansky H, et al. A multicenter placebo-controlled clinical trial of oral metoclopramide in diabetic gastroparesis. Diabetes Care. 1983;6(5):463–7.
69. Snape WJ Jr, Battle WM, Schwartz SS, Braunstein SN, Goldstein HA, Alavi A. Metoclopramide to treat gastroparesis due to diabetes mellitus: a double-blind, controlled trial. Ann Intern Med. 1982;96(4):444–6.
70. Tonini M, Cipollina L, Poluzzi E, Crema F, Corazza GR, De Ponti F. Review article: clinical implications of enteric and central D2 receptor blockade by antidopaminergic gastrointestinal prokinetics. Aliment Pharmacol Ther. 2004;19(4):379–90.
71. Ezzeddine D, Jit R, Katz N, Gopalswamy N, Bhutani MS. Pyloric injection of botulinum toxin for treatment of diabetic gastroparesis. Gastrointest Endosc. 2002;55(7):920–3.
72. Lacy BE, Crowell MD, Schettler-Duncan A, Mathis C, Pasricha PJ. The treatment of diabetic gastroparesis with botulinum toxin injection of the pylorus. Diabetes Care. 2004;27(10):2341–7.
73. Miller LS, Szych GA, Kantor SB, et al. Treatment of idiopathic gastroparesis with injection of botulinum toxin into the pyloric sphincter muscle. Am J Gastroenterol. 2002;97(7):1653–60.
74. Friedenberg FK, Palit A, Parkman HP, Hanlon A, Nelson DB. Botulinum toxin A for the treatment of delayed gastric emptying. Am J Gastroenterol. 2008;103(2):416–23.
75. Arts J, Holvoet L, Caenepeel P, et al. Clinical trial: a randomized-controlled crossover study of intrapyloric injection of botulinum toxin in gastroparesis. Aliment Pharmacol Ther. 2007;26(9):1251–8.
76. Rameshshanker RSL, Southern P, Whitelaw D, Beckett C. Gastroparesis and botulinum toxin. Gut. 2011;60:2.
77. Coleski R, Anderson MA, Hasler WL. Factors associated with symptom response to pyloric injection of botulinum toxin in a large series of gastroparesis patients. Dig Dis Sci. 2009;54(12):2634–42.
78. Ukleja A, Tandon K, Shah K, Alvarez A. Endoscopic botox injections in therapy of refractory gastroparesis. World Jof Gastrointest Endosc. 2015;7(8):790–8.
79. Friedenberg F, Gollamudi S, Parkman HP. The use of botulinum toxin for the treatment of gastrointestinal motility disorders. Dig Dis Sci. 2004;49(2):165–75.
80. Neoptolemos JP, Bailey IS, Carr-Locke DL. Sphincter of Oddi dysfunction: results of treatment by endoscopic sphincterotomy. Br J Surg. 1988;75(5):454–9.
81. Pasricha PJ, Miskovsky EP, Kalloo AN. Intrasphincteric injection of botulinum toxin for suspected sphincter of Oddi dysfunction. Gut. 1994;35(9):1319–21.
82. Wehrmann T, Seifert H, Seipp M, Lembcke B, Caspary WF. Endoscopic injection of botulinum toxin for biliary sphincter of Oddi dysfunction. Endoscopy. 1998;30(8):702–7.
83. Cotton PB, Elta GH, Carter CR, Pasricha PJ, Corazziari ES. Rome IV. Gallbladder and sphincter of Oddi disorders. Gastroenterology. 2016; pii:S0016-5085(16)00224-9. doi:10.1053/j.gastro.2016.02.033.

84. Hackert T, Klaiber U, Hinz U, et al. Sphincter of Oddi botulinum toxin injection to prevent pancreatic fistula after distal pancreatectomy. Surgery. 2016;161(5):1444–50.
85. Zaghiyan KN, Fleshner P. Anal fissure. Clin Colon Rectal Surg. 2011;24(1):22–30.
86. Madalinski MH. Identifying the best therapy for chronic anal fissure. World J Gastrointest Pharmacol Ther. 2011;2(2):9–16.
87. Oh C, Divino CM, Steinhagen RM. Anal fissure. 20-year experience. Dis Colon Rectum. 1995;38(4):378–82.
88. Madoff RD, Dykes SL. What's new in colon and rectal surgery. J Am Coll Surg. 2004;198(1):91–104.
89. American Gastroenterological Association. American Gastroenterological Association medical position statement: Diagnosis and care of patients with anal fissure. Gastroenterology. 2003;124(1):233–4.
90. Dodi G, Bogoni F, Infantino A, Pianon P, Mortellaro LM, Lise M. Hot or cold in anal pain? A study of the changes in internal anal sphincter pressure profiles. Dis Colon Rectum. 1986;29(4):248–51.
91. Jensen SL. Treatment of first episodes of acute anal fissure: prospective randomised study of lignocaine ointment versus hydrocortisone ointment or warm sitz baths plus bran. Br Med J (Clin Res Ed). 1986;292(6529):1167–9.
92. Ezri T, Susmallian S. Topical nifedipine vs. topical glyceryl trinitrate for treatment of chronic anal fissure. Dis Colon Rectum. 2003;46(6):805–8.
93. Lund JN, Scholefield JH. A randomised, prospective, double-blind, placebo-controlled trial of glyceryl trinitrate ointment in treatment of anal fissure. Lancet (London, England). 1997;349(9044):11–4.
94. Jost WH, Schimrigk K. Use of botulinum toxin in anal fissure. Dis Colon Rectum. 1993;36(10):974.
95. Maria G, Cassetta E, Gui D, Brisinda G, Bentivoglio AR, Albanese A. A comparison of botulinum toxin and saline for the treatment of chronic anal fissure. N Engl J Med. 1998;338(4):217–20.
96. Bobkiewicz A, Francuzik W, Krokowicz L, et al. Botulinum toxin injection for treatment of chronic anal fissure: is there any dose-dependent efficiency? A meta-analysis. World J Surg. 2016;40(12):3064–72.
97. Samim M, Twigt B, Stoker L, Pronk A. Topical diltiazem cream versus botulinum toxin a for the treatment of chronic anal fissure: a double-blind randomized clinical trial. Ann Surg. 2012;255(1):18–22.
98. Brisinda G, Cadeddu F, Brandara F, Marniga G, Maria G. Randomized clinical trial comparing botulinum toxin injections with 0.2 per cent nitroglycerin ointment for chronic anal fissure. Br J Surg. 2007;94(2):162–7.
99. Arroyo A, Perez F, Serrano P, Candela F, Lacueva J, Calpena R. Surgical versus chemical (botulinum toxin) sphincterotomy for chronic anal fissure: long-term results of a prospective randomized clinical and manometric study. Am J Surg. 2005;189(4):429–34.
100. Jost WH. One hundred cases of anal fissure treated with botulin toxin: early and long-term results. Dis Colon Rectum. 1997;40(9):1029–32.
101. Nasr M, Ezzat H, Elsebae M. Botulinum toxin injection versus lateral internal sphincterotomy in the treatment of chronic anal fissure: a randomized controlled trial. World J Surg. 2010;34(11):2730–4.
102. Chen HL, Woo XB, Wang HS, et al. Botulinum toxin injection versus lateral internal sphincterotomy for chronic anal fissure: a meta-analysis of randomized control trials. Tech Coloproctol. 2014;18(8):693–8.

Botulinum Toxin for Treatment of Spasticity in Cerebral Palsy

Kat Kolaski and L. Andrew Koman

Cerebral palsy (CP) is the most common cause of chronic childhood motor disability [1]. Cases of children with stiffness and orthopedic deformities attributed to difficulties during birth were first described in the mid-nineteenth century [2]. The term CP was coined in the late nineteenth century and persists as a diagnosis today, but it is applied to a heterogeneous group of disorders. Definitions of CP over the last century consistently describe it as a disorder of movement and posture resulting from a non-progressive abnormality in the brain acquired early in life [3, 4]. More recent descriptions of CP highlight that its symptoms may change over time; in addition, there has been increased recognition of the complexity of the clinical presentation. The currently accepted definition of CP from the American Academy of Cerebral Palsy and Developmental Medicine states that the motor disorder of CP is often accompanied by problems with sensation, perception, cognition, communication and behavior, seizures, and secondary musculoskeletal problems [5].

Epidemiology

The prevalence of CP among children is reported to be 2–3 per 1000 live births based on registry data from several European countries [1]. Based on information gathered in 2010 from four communities by the Centers for Disease Control and Prevention, the prevalence of CP in the US is similar, approximately 2.9 per 1000 live births [6]. Worldwide prevalence is 1–5 in every 1000 live births [7]. Almost all children with CP have a normal life expectancy, thus it also affects a large adult population [8, 9].

K. Kolaski, M.D. (✉) • L. Andrew Koman, M.D.
Department of Orthopaedic Surgery, Wake Forest School of Medicine, Medical Center Boulevard, Winston-Salem, NC 27157-1070, USA
e-mail: kkolaski@wakehealth.edu

B. Jabbari (ed.), *Botulinum Toxin Treatment in Clinical Medicine*,
DOI 10.1007/978-3-319-56038-0_6

The prevalence of CP is significantly higher in pre-term births (40–100 per 1000 live births) and increases with decreasing gestational age [1]. An estimated 8–10% of infants born at a gestational age of less than 28 weeks are diagnosed with CP [10, 11]. However, while prematurity is a significant risk factor, it does not account for the majority of children with CP who are born at or near term. Numerous studies provide evidence for the importance of prenatal factors in term infants who develop CP, with implications for multifactorial processes [12, 13]. Major birth defects, most commonly of the brain, were the most frequently occurring risk factor in children with CP born at a gestational age of at least 35 weeks, and birth defects combined with fetal growth restriction were associated with the highest relative risk [14]. The prevalence of CP in term infants has been stable, but has decreased in preterm infants [6, 15]. The overall prevalence of CP has remained stable to slightly increased over time because of the increased survival of preterm infants and the more severely affected children [16].

Etiology and Diagnosis

While there is no consensus on an upper age limit, it is generally accepted that the brain injury in CP occurs before the age of 2 years as opposed to later onset lesions acquired from trauma, injury, or specific disease processes affecting the central nervous system (CNS). The brain pathology of CP is dependent on the timing of events occurring after conception and before age 2 years that damage the brain and/or interfere with its development [17]. Cortical neurogenesis takes place during the first and second trimesters, and disturbances of this process result in brain maldevelopment. Causes include hypoxia, stroke, infection, and/or genetic factors. During the third trimester, growth and differentiation events predominate. Disturbances during this period are typically caused by hypoxic-ischemic, inflammatory, and/or infectious mechanisms [18]. Early in the third trimester, white matter is more susceptible, potentially causing damage to the motor tracts as is often seen with the classic lesions of prematurity, periventricular leukomalacia, and intraventricular hemorrhage. In the later third trimester, damage typically affects the cortical gray matter, basal ganglia, and thalamus [19]. Strokes also occur around the time of birth; middle cerebral artery territory infarction is most common [20].

Neuroimaging is not included in the definition of CP despite the fact that abnormalities on neuroimaging are found in more than 80% of children with CP [21, 22]. The pathogenic patterns found on neuroimaging are not always reliable for predicting severity; however, they are helpful for understanding the etiology of CP and its symptoms, and national guidelines support the use of neuroimaging in the diagnosis of CP [23]. In CP, damage to the brain occurs most commonly prenatally. The most frequent neuroimaging findings are periventricular white matter injury (56%), deep gray matter injury (18%), and brain maldevelopment (9%). Intrapartum events causing perinatal asphyxia are still commonly regarded as a leading cause of CP, but account for less than 10% of cases [12].

The best practice recommendation for diagnosis of CP entails the use of a combination of tools, including documentation of historical risk factors, neurological examination, standardized motor assessments, and neuroimaging [23, 24]. Of these tools, the General Movements assessment of movement quality has the best sensitivity for early detection of CP; in preterm infants, the combined sensitivity of abnormal General Movements and an abnormal MRI showing white matter injury is 100% [25]. In most cases, diagnosis is established when neuroimaging reveals abnormalities consistent with the history (e.g., premature birth) and clinical exam (e.g., abnormal movements on neurological exam). However, it is important to recognize those specific aspects of the history, physical examination, and neuroimaging findings (or lack thereof), referred to as "red flags," which strongly question a CP diagnosis [26, 27]. In such cases, serial neuroimaging, metabolic studies, and/or genetic test are needed in order to rule out diseases that can "masquerade" as CP. It is essential to differentiate a static from a progressive clinical course: loss of previously acquired motor milestones (regression) is characteristic of neurodegenerative and metabolic disorders.

CP is typically diagnosed around 12–24 months of age, which usually corresponds to the time when obvious failure to achieve motor milestones is observed. Given the lack of biomarkers, many clinicians are reluctant to diagnosis CP despite the fact that early diagnosis is possible in those children with identifiable risk factors as early as 12 weeks of age [28]. Early diagnosis allows access to diagnosis-specific interventions that promote neuroplasticity and is currently considered best practice. However, in cases with inconsistent findings or "red flags," diagnosis of CP may be one of exclusion, and observation until children are 4 years of age may be needed in order to establish a non-progressive course.

Clinical Features

Motor disorders associated with CP involve multiple neural components, including basal ganglia, cerebellum, cerebral cortex, brainstem, and descending spinal tracts [29]. Much of the terminology used to describe motor disorders seen in individuals with CP lacks precision and consistency due, in part, to their derivation from seemingly analogous signs in adult disorders. For example, motor signs in adults are often categorized as pyramidal or extra-pyramidal; while many of these same signs are present in individuals with CP, they often have a combination of pyramidal and extrapyramidal signs. An international task force has promoted improved understanding of childhood motor disorders as well as consensus on the terminology used to describe them [29–31]. They divide motor disorders of childhood (including CP) into three broad categories (hypertonia, hyperkinetic movements, and negative signs) and provide clinical definitions for specific disorders. Features of these motor disorders—as well as non-motor symptoms—of CP are reviewed below.

Hypertonia

Hypertonia is defined as abnormally increased resistance to externally imposed movement about a joint [30]. Two important aspects of this definition are: (1) Resistance is related to neuromuscular tone with explicit exclusion of resistance related to joint, ligament, or skeletal properties, and (2) Resistance is evaluated at rest by a passive movement. Spasticity causes hypertonia that increases with increasing velocity of movement or causes a spastic catch [29]. Spasticity is the most common motor disorder seen in CP. It can affect the entire body, including the trunk, face, and neck. It tends to be worse in the lower limbs of those with bilateral involvement, and in the upper limbs of those with unilateral involvement [32]. While spasticity is assessed at rest, active movements in spastic forms of CP can be impaired by a number of related neuro-pathologic influences, including co-contraction, postural reflexes, mirror movements, involuntary synergies, abnormal cutaneo-muscular reflexes, hyperreflexia, and reflex overflow [33].

Hyperkinetic Movements

Hyperkinetic movements cause excess or unwanted movements [31]. The hyperkinetic movements most commonly seen in CP include dystonia, chorea, and athetosis. In dystonia, there are involuntary sustained or intermittent muscle contractions causing twisting and repetitive movements and/or abnormal postures [33]. Dystonia can occur with spasticity; it also can cause resistance to passive joint movement, but, unlike spasticity, it does not change with varying speeds. Chorea refers to brief, random, discrete movements while athetosis is characterized by slow, continuous writhing movements. In CP, chorea and athetosis often occur together but may not be the prominent movement disorder [31].

Negative Signs

These are also known as deficit symptoms and include weakness, poor selective motor control, voluntary synergies, dependency on posture, impaired balance, loss of dexterity of movement, enhanced fatigability, ataxia, and apraxia/developmental dyspraxia [30, 34]. Any or all of these signs are present to some extent in all types of CP.

Non-motor Symptoms

In addition to motor symptoms, children with CP almost always have accompanying co-morbidities. These are sometimes—but not always—associated with the severity of the motor disorder. Occasionally, associated co-morbidities, such as difficulties with feeding, predominate over motor symptoms in infants and very young children [35]. Conditions that occur with the highest frequency and severity in children with CP are intellectual disability, vision impairment, speech and language disorders, incontinence, and seizures [2]. Behavior and sleep disorders and pain are also common, but are often under-recognized [36]. Other associated conditions include hearing loss, gastrointestinal and nutritional problems, drooling, dysphagia, and respiratory disorders [37]. While the treatment of the non-motor conditions associated with CP is not addressed in this chapter, they are important to consider in the planning and evaluation of treatments targeting the motor system. Moreover, these accompanying medical conditions may directly influence symptoms of the motor disorder, for example, constipation or seizures can effect global spasticity.

Motor System Developmental Issues

Although the brain injury causing CP is static, its associated motor signs and symptoms evolve over time. Of particular importance, individuals with CP experience progressive muscle weakness as well as reductions in passive joint range of motion and increasing joint stiffness (clinically referred to as contracture) with age [38–40]. Our current understanding of why this occurs is inadequate; nevertheless, animal and human research to date indicates that unique developmental adaptations—both neural and musculoskeletal—occur in individuals with CP related to early brain injury [41].

Based on animal models and studies of adult pathologies, it is known that spasticity is caused by complex, interdependent pathways that depend on the etiology, location, and timing of the upper motor neuron (UMN) lesion [42]. A common feature is deregulation of the descending motor tracts and reduced inhibition of the alpha motor neurons in the spinal cord, with later adaptations in the spinal networks. In CP, the primary brain lesion occurs before the motor system is developed. Maturation likely affects the subsequent reorganization of both supra-spinal and segmental spinal inputs which impacts symptoms over time; however, the exact mechanisms involved are unknown and pose significant challenges to investigation. Studies of the natural history of CP provide clues from which we can infer evolving neural mechanisms during development. For example, there is evidence that individuals with spastic CP are less able to activate their muscles maximally and activate greater amounts of antagonistic muscles (co-contraction) [39, 43]. Spasticity in CP decreases with age [44] suggesting possible alterations in maturing neural pathways and/or increased non-neural influences. In addition, movement disorders in CP often evolve from the neonatal period through childhood. In pre-term infants, hypotonia is commonly observed in the first year of life. Spasticity and hyperkinetic movements become more apparent over time, and hyperkinetic movement disorders tend to present later than spasticity, which suggests a relationship to progressive myelination [45, 46].

Table 1 Reported alterations in limb muscles of individuals with CP

Gross morphology
Muscle fascicle length
Muscle belly length
Muscle fascicle angle
Muscle cross-sectional area
Muscle volume
Muscle thickness
Microstructural properties
Increased sarcomere length
Extracellular matrix stiffness
Fiber type proportions
Biomechanical properties
Muscle fiber stiffness
Tendon slack length and compliance
Myogenetic properties
Reduced muscle growth rates
Altered transcriptional pathways
Lower number of satellite cells

With regard to the musculoskeletal system, there are multiple developmental considerations which we will simplify into three key areas:

1. Overall Growth: Primary motor impairments affecting muscle strength and balance may be exacerbated with growth because of additional biomechanical and postural demands imposed by increasing body dimensions.
2. Muscle Growth: In individuals with UMN lesions, affected muscles are unable to effectively contract and generate force while inherent tone abnormalities impede their ability to relax and maximally lengthen. Over time, decreased neuromechanical stimulation and muscle activation produce secondary changes that further compromise muscle function. In CP, these pathophysiologic processes occur before muscles are fully developed, thus contributing to weakness and stiffness, but also impaired muscle growth. In fact, it has been speculated that early brain lesions in CP may affect muscle fiber development prenatally given muscle fiber numbers approximately double from the third trimester to 4 months after birth [41]. Not surprisingly, a variety of macro- and microstructural, histologic, and biomechanical changes have been reported in muscles from limbs of children with spastic CP (Table 1). This research is largely preliminary; however, there is strong evidence for reduced muscle size in children with CP compared to normally developing children [47]. A difference in muscle growth is evident as early as 15 months of age and is independent of bone growth [48]. Overall, reported alterations of intrinsic and dynamic muscle-tendon properties support the hypothesis that impaired muscle growth is a major factor in contracture development in CP; specifically, decreased muscle volume reduces muscle length, as opposed to fixed muscle shortening from spastic muscle overactivity [49].

3. Skeletal Growth: In UMN syndromes, abnormal muscle contraction interferes with voluntary control and impairs function. In CP, the resultant decreased weight bearing forces and inadequate and/or imbalanced muscle forces acting on joints can adversely influence skeletal as well as muscle growth. Thus growing children with CP often experience failure of normal remodeling or abnormal modeling of bone. As a result, common osseous deformities seen in CP are hip subluxation and dislocation, torsional deformities of long bones, scoliosis, and foot deformities. In ambulatory individuals with CP, contractures and bony deformity cause abnormal joint movements during gait and produce what is known as lever-arm dysfunction [50].

A complex interplay of these pathophysiologic and biomechanical changes in the nervous and musculoskeletal system occurs over time in children growing with CP [47]. Currently, the exact mechanisms are not fully understood, but they are clearly implicated in the development and progression of muscle weakness and soft tissue contracture, joint contracture, and/or osseous deformity. These problems adversely affect motor function, potentially cause deformity and pain, and likely impact quality of life in individuals with CP.

Treatment Planning

Treatment planning for an individual with CP involves a comprehensive evaluation of motor and non-motor impairments along with the assessment of the other ICF domains, specifically activity and function, participation, and environmental factors. Ideally, this is accomplished by a multidisciplinary team of professionals with expertise in CP who provide patient and family focused care throughout the lifespan. Current management of CP can be categorized into three general areas of focus, child active rehabilitation, health and complication prevention, and compensatory and environmental adaptation [24]. Descriptions, features, and recommended timing of these approaches are detailed in Table 2.

Treatment should be based on the child and family's short- and long-term goals which should be re-evaluated frequently. Selection of appropriate interventions and tools for measuring progress involves understanding the child and family goals in terms of the World Health Organization's International Classification of Functioning, Disability and Health (ICF) [51]. The ICF is a multidimensional model of health and function with domains of body structure and function, activity and participation, and environmental and personal factors. Clinical tools that incorporate the ICF are available for goal setting [52]. These are valuable because it is known that evidence-based interventions for CP operating at one level (e.g., treatment of spasticity) do not necessarily have effects at other levels (e.g., improved ability to walk unassisted at school) [53]. The following sections will focus on the evaluation and treatment of abnormal muscle tone in CP. However, we emphasize muscle tone abnormalities are only one aspect of the motor dysfunction of CP; moreover, treat-

Table 2 Strategies for the management of cerebral palsy

Child active rehabilitation approaches
Description: Child is actively practicing real-life tasks during intervention for purpose of gaining or improving real-life skills
Features: Goal-based, task-specific practice, high-dose repetition, plasticity
Timing: Recommended during period of maximal motor potential, which, based on clinical and GMFCS data is up to 5–7 years of age
Health and secondary prevention approaches
Description: Interventions for management of the child's motor symptoms, general health and co-morbidities, and for prevention or limitation of secondary complications
Features: Treatment options may target whole body (generalized) or specific areas (focal)
Timing: Lifelong, with certain interventions recommended at specific ages for maximal benefit
Compensatory and environmental adaptation approaches
Description: Society provides environmental and task modification or specialized equipment to accommodate the child's disability, and to promote inclusion and independence
Features: Context-focused therapy, assistive technology
Timing: Lifelong, with shift to become primary focus after 5–7 years, especially for those who are in GMFCS III–V or similar levels using other functional classification systems

Adapted with permission from Novak I. Evidence-based diagnosis, health care, and rehabilitation for children with cerebral palsy. J of Child Neurol 2014;29 (8):1141–1156

ment of abnormal muscle tone does not address the non-motor impairments, and does not specifically target goals at the activity or participation levels of the ICF.

Motor Evaluation

Motor Disorder Classification

An essential part of the motor evaluation of children with CP is the classification of the CP because some treatments are indicated for specific types of CP or may only be feasible or appropriate for children at a certain level of function. CP has been traditionally classified by the type and location of the motor disorder. Currently, the most widely accepted system for movement disorder classification is the European Classification of CP [1]. This system has three categories: (1) Spastic CP occurs in the majority of individuals with CP; (2) Dyskinetic CP includes chorea, athetosis, and dystonia (referred to as "hyperkinetic" in the terminology used by the Task Force on Childhood Movement Disorders (31)); and (3) Ataxic/hypotonic CP. Although spasticity is often the dominant disorder, many children with CP demonstrate more than one of these movement disorders, most commonly mixed spasticity and dystonia. For epidemiologic purposes, cases of mixed movement disorder features are classified by the predominant disorder, with the listing of secondary disorders.

The traditional descriptions of limb distribution used in spastic CP are hemiplegia, diplegia, and quadriplegia/tetraplegia, and less commonly, monoplegia and triplegia. These imprecisely capture the extent of motor involvement and have poor inter-rater reliability [1]. Registries for CP surveillance have proposed alternative classification methods. Currently, the most widely used is the European system which describes spastic limb involvement as either unilateral or bilateral [1]. However, the topographical classification of CP remains controversial, and the use of the various topographical terms persists in most clinical settings despite a lack of consensus on their application [54, 55].

Functional Classification

Functional classification systems have evolved over the past two decades in response to the need for better epidemiological tools as well as the interest in describing all the ICF dimensions. These scales are independent of the CP motor type and distribution—i.e., impairment. The Gross Motor Functional Classification System (GMFCS) is age-dependent and describes five categories according to the patient's level of mobility [56]. The GMFCS-Expanded and Revised [57] includes children up to 18 years of age with descriptions of skills provided for five different age groups [57]. It classifies gross motor function on a 5-point scale (see Fig. 1). The GMFCS has been widely adopted in both research and clinical settings for classification, and analyses of GMFCS data has also been shown to provide prognostic information [58, 59]. Figure 2 depicts a summary of the proportions of CP by topography, and by severity using the GMFCS. The GMFCS has also served as a model for the development of other functional scales for CP. These also use a five-category system, and include the Manual Ability Classification System [60], the Communication Function Classification System [61], and the Eating and Drinking Abilities Classification System [62].

Evaluation of Hypertonia

Evaluation of hypertonia in CP requires differentiation of neural (dynamic) from non-neural influences [63, 64]. In spasticity-related hypertonia, resistance to passive stretch is encountered from premature and/or exaggerated muscle contraction that is caused by lack of modulation of the stretch reflex. Passive resistance can also be caused by peripheral biomechanical components [63]. As discussed above, alterations in the structural and mechanical properties of spastic muscles and tendons in children with CP contribute to increased stiffness. These changes are reported in very young children with CP and have been related to growth velocity rather than neural influences [64–66]. Thus, in CP, the non-neural contributions to resistance to

GMFCS E & R between 6th and 12th birthday: Descriptors and illustrations

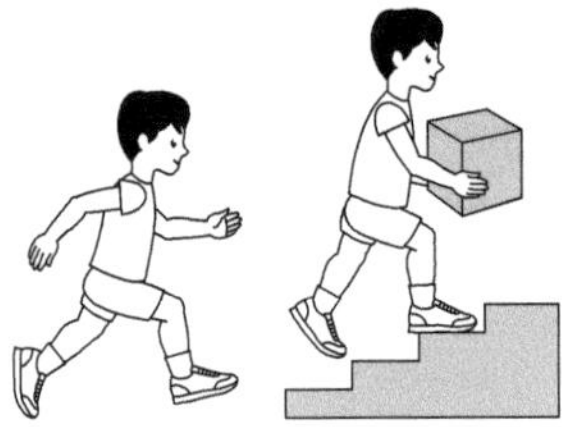

GMFCS Level I

Children walk at home, school, outdoors and in the community. They can climb stairs without the use of a railing. Children perform gross motor skills such as running and jumping, but speed, balance and coordination are limited.

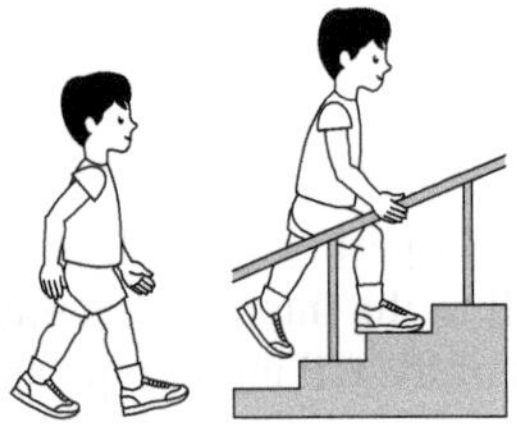

GMFCS Level II

Children walk in most settings and climb stairs holding onto a railing. They may experience difficulty walking long distances and balancing on uneven terrain, inclines, in crowded areas or confined spaces. Children may walk with physical assistance, a hand-held mobility device or used wheeled mobility over long distances. Children have only minimal ability to perform gross motor skills such as running and jumping.

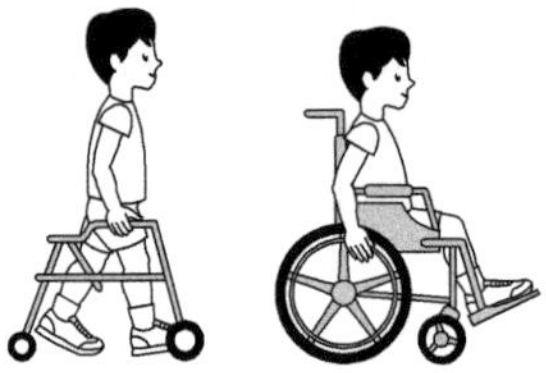

GMFCS Level III

Children walk using a hand-held mobility device in most indoor settings. They may climb stairs holding onto a railing with supervision or assistance. Children use wheeled mobility when traveling long distances and may self-propel for shorter distances.

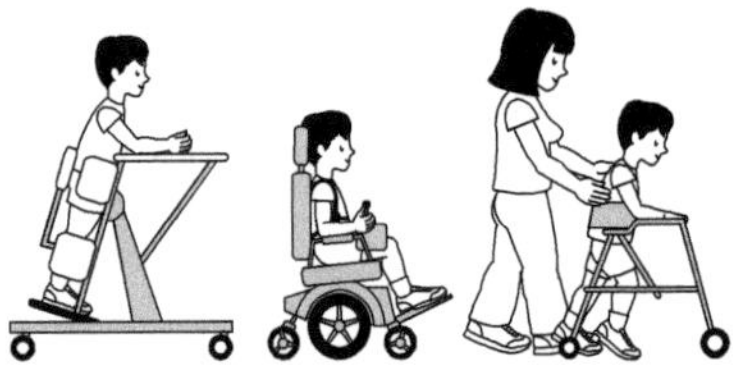

GMFCS Level IV

Children use methods of mobility that require physical assistance or powered mobility in most settings. They may walk for short distances at home with physical assistance or use powered mobility or a body support walker when positioned. At school, outdoors and in the community children are transported in a manual wheelchair or use powered mobility.

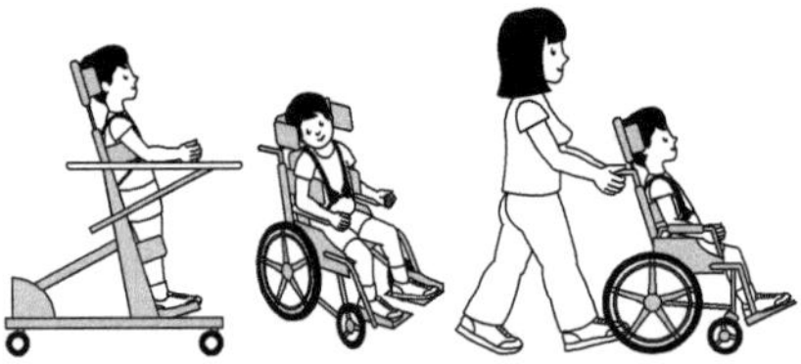

GMFCS Level V

Children are transported in a manual wheelchair in all settings. Children are limited in their ability to maintain antigravity head and trunk postures and control leg and arm movements.

GMFCS descriptors: Palisano et al. (1997) Dev Med Child Neurol 39:214-23
CanChild: www.canchild.ca

Illustrations Version 2 © Bill Reid, Kate Willoughby, Adrienne Harvey and Kerr Graham, The Royal Children's Hospital Melbourne ERC151050

Fig. 1 GMFCS illustrations

GMFCS E & R between 12th and 18th birthday: Descriptors and illustrations

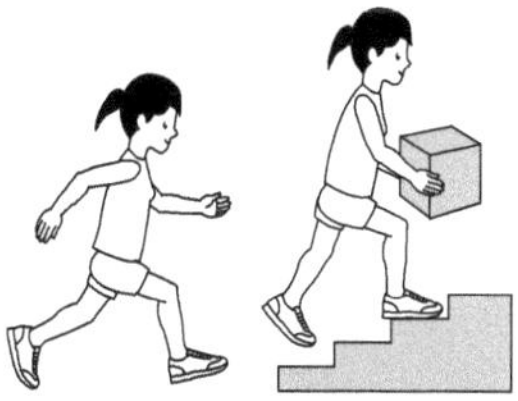

GMFCS Level I

Youth walk at home, school, outdoors and in the community. Youth are able to climb curbs and stairs without physical assistance or a railing. They perform gross motor skills such as running and jumping but speed, balance and coordination are limited.

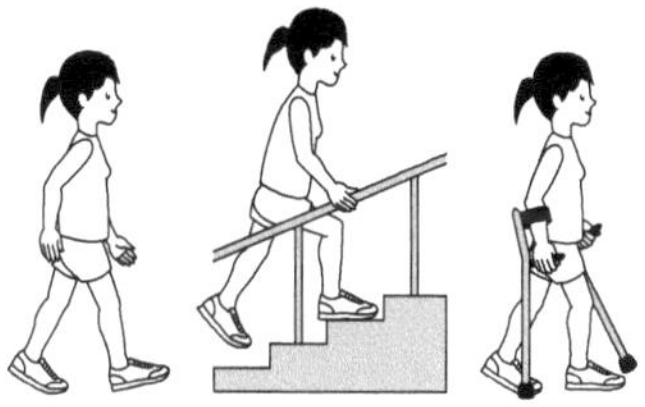

GMFCS Level II

Youth walk in most settings but environmental factors and personal choice influence mobility choices. At school or work they may require a hand held mobility device for safety and climb stairs holding onto a railing. Outdoors and in the community youth may use wheeled mobility when traveling long distances.

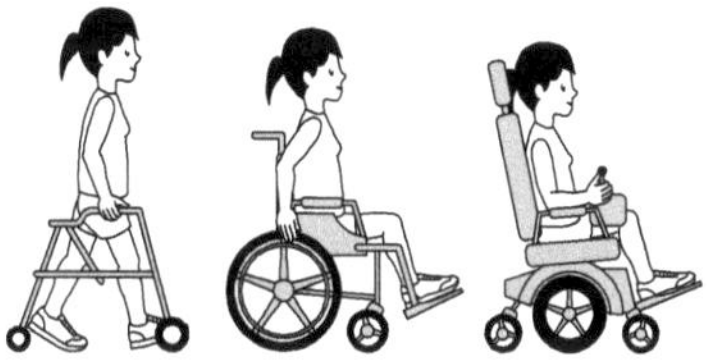

GMFCS Level III

Youth are capable of walking using a hand-held mobility device. Youth may climb stairs holding onto a railing with supervision or assistance. At school they may self-propel a manual wheelchair or use powered mobility. Outdoors and in the community youth are transported in a wheelchair or use powered mobility.

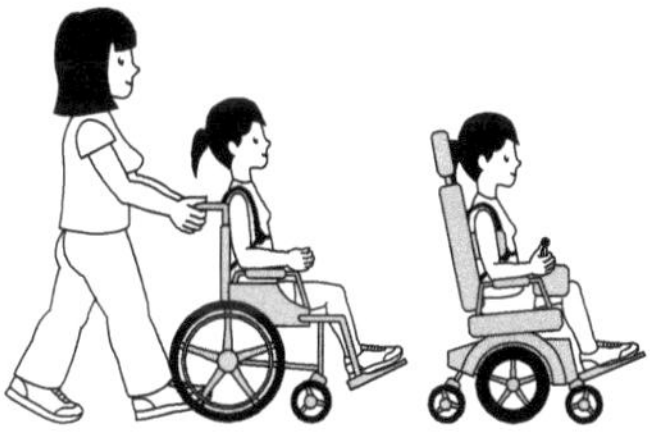

GMFCS Level IV

Youth use wheeled mobility in most settings. Physical assistance of 1–2 people is required for transfers. Indoors, youth may walk short distances with physical assistance, use wheeled mobility or a body support walker when positioned. They may operate a powered chair, otherwise are transported in a manual wheelchair.

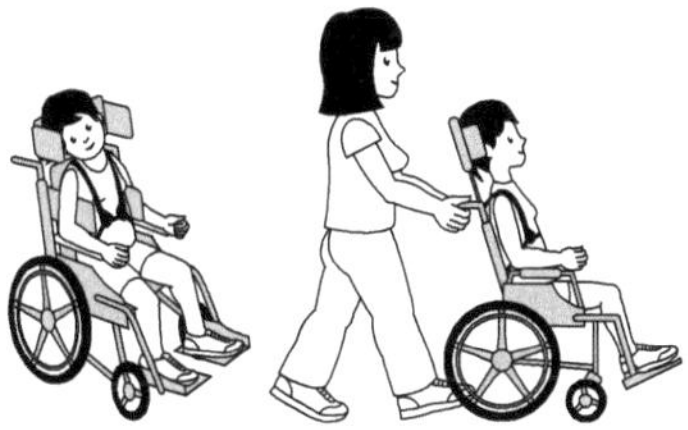

GMFCS Level V

Youth are transported in a manual wheelchair in all settings. Youth are limited in their ability to maintain antigravity head and trunk postures and control leg and arm movements. Self-mobility is severely limited, even with the use of assistive technology.

GMFCS descriptors: Palisano et al. (1997) Dev Med Child Neurol 39:214-23
CanChild: www.canchild.ca

Illustrations Version 2 © Bill Reid, Kate Willoughby, Adrienne Harvey and Kerr Graham, The Royal Children's Hospital Melbourne ERC151050

Fig. 1 (continued)

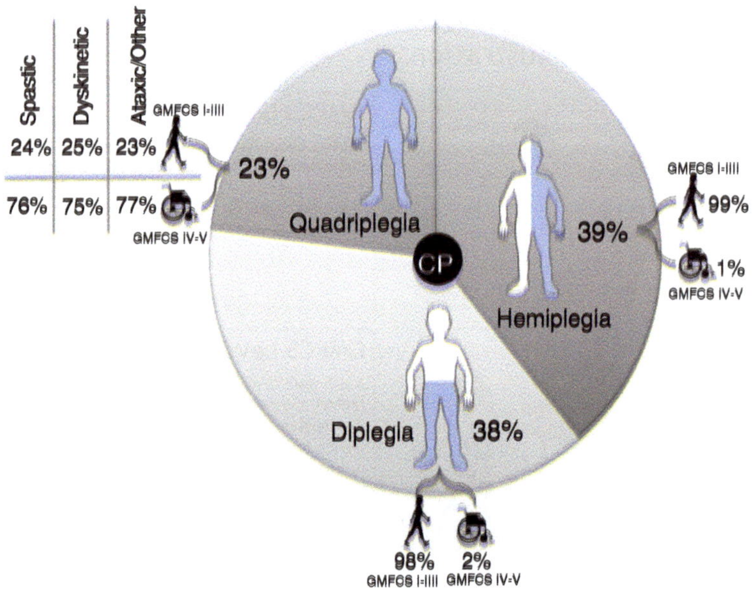

Fig. 2 Proportion of cerebral palsy by topography and severity. Reproduced with permission from Sage (Novak 2014)

passive movement are significant, and their relative contribution may become more significant over time.

Clinical evaluation of hypertonia in individuals with CP, like for other disorders, is largely subjective. Measurement of spasticity is most often done using the Modified Ashworth Scale (MAS) which grades tone from 0 to 4 [67]. The Modified Tardieu Scale (MTS) involves the movement of a joint at fast and slow speeds, with measurement of the angle at which resistance is felt initially (R1), as well as the end of passively available range of motion (R2) [63]. Main advantages of the MTS are its ability to detect velocity-dependent resistance and to distinguish spasticity from the end range of motion. Reliability and sensitivity of these clinical tests for assessment of spasticity is limited as they do not control the velocity of the stretch and level of muscle relaxation nor do they evaluate active movement [42]. Other measures of body structures and function used less commonly in studies of spasticity treatment in children with CP include dynamic electromyography, dynamic muscle length, selective motor control, and strength [68]. The Hypertonia Assessment Tool (HAT) was developed to differentiate types of hypertonia (spasticity, dystonia, and rigidity) in order to guide treatment [69]. The Barry-Albright Dystonia (BAD) Scale is a reliable clinical tool for quantifying the severity of posturing and abnormal movements seen in CP and other conditions causing secondary dystonia [70]. Instrumented assessments of spasticity [42, 71] and dystonia [72] are more objective, sensitive, and may be more responsive and predictive compared to clinical scales [64]; however, their use in children with CP to date has been limited to experimental and explorative studies.

Table 3 Commonly used functional outcome measures in studies of BoNT-A treatment effects in children with CP

Lower extremity	
Gait analysis	
	Kinetics. Kinematics, and/or time/distance parameters
Gait assessment	
	Physician rating, scale, observational gait analysis score, Edinburgh Visual Gait Score
Gross motor function measure	
Gross motor performance measure	
6 min walk test	
Upper extremity	
Melbourne assessment of unilateral upper limb function	
Quality of upper extremity skills test	
Global	
Pediatric evaluation of disability inventory	
Functional Independence measure for children (weeFIM)	
Individualized goal attainment	
Canadian Occupational Performance Measure	
Goal attainment scale	

In addition to these qualitative and quantitative measurements of motor disorders, a large number of reliable measures for CP are available to assess function (or activity) and participation, and to evaluate the quality of life, comfort, and caregiving burden. Table 3 lists the most commonly used functional outcome measures used in studies evaluating the effectiveness of treatment with botulinum toxin (BoNT) in children with CP. In this literature, there is a preponderance of measures which evaluate outcomes in the body structures and function and activity domains of the ICF, and the majority of activity measures report on gait analysis parameters [68]. This is not surprising because BoNT is a treatment for spasticity which is a body function. It is important to acknowledge that, while all of these measures are helpful to track changes over time and in response to treatment, they may not be practical to perform consistently in clinical settings. Outside of research and academic settings, the decision to treat spasticity or dystonia in children with CP is generally based on clinical indications, and assessment of outcomes after treatment may be based on patient and family feedback, without using any reliable measurement tool.

Treatment Options

There are many medical, surgical, and rehabilitative treatment options available for persons with CP. Treatments are often combined, and indications change over time based on changing needs and goals of the growing child and their family.

Table 4 Interventions for motor dysfunction and musculoskeletal co-morbidities in children with CP

	Strong evidence/effective	Moderate evidence/promising
Focal spasticity	Botulinum toxin	N/A
Generalized spasticity	Selective dorsal rhizotomy	Oral baclofen
	Diazepam	Intrathecal baclofen
Contracture management	Lower extremity casting	Upper extremity casting
		Hand surgery
		Orthotics
Skeletal Alignment	N/A	Orthopedic surgery
		Orthotics

Adapted with permission from Novak I. Evidence-based diagnosis, health care, and rehabilitation for children with cerebral palsy. J of Child Neurol 2014;29 (8):1141–1156

Fortunately, many commonly used treatments in CP have been the subject of systematic reviews (SR) which provide a basis for rational, informed treatment selection. In fact, the available evidence on treatments for CP was evaluated and summarized by Novak et al. [53] using the Grading of Recommendations Assessment, Development, and Evaluation (GRADE) system [73] providing additional confidence in the evidence-based literature. Table 4 displays treatments to improve motor function, decrease spasticity, and to address associated musculoskeletal co-morbidities; those found to have strong evidence are "recommended" and those with moderate evidence are considered "promising." Effective or promising treatments for generalized abnormal muscle tone in CP include oral medications, selective dorsal rhizotomy, and intrathecal baclofen. For focal spasticity, BoNT is the only treatment with strong evidence of efficacy in children with CP.

History of BoNT Use in CP

During the 1960s and 1970s, phenol and ethanol were used for the treatment of focal spasticity in children with CP. These agents are injected near a motor nerve where it enters a muscle or into a muscle near the nerve terminals [74]. Injections with these agents require technical skill as well as patient cooperation and may cause adverse effects. Currently, BoNT has largely replaced the use of these agents, but they continue to be used, mainly in combination with BoNT, in order to allow more muscles to be targeted in a single chemodenervation session [75, 76].

BoNT has been used clinically in the management of CP since 1987 when it was first applied to the treatment of limb spasticity [77]. Interestingly, the use of BoNT for the treatment of limb spasticity was inspired by its earlier use to treat muscle overactivity in other disorders such as torticollis and strabismus. The first study of BoNT in the US assessed 27 pediatric patients with CP who had dynamic deformities unresponsive to other non-operative treatments [77]. Following BoNT injections, all patients showed improvement in clinical assessments with minimal side effects. A randomized, controlled trial (RCT) by the same group then found five of six patients injected with BoNT-A showed improvement in dynamic equinus deformities as opposed to two of six patients in the placebo group [78]. Based on the positive results, a larger RCT was undertaken to study the safety and short-term efficacy of BoNT for dynamic equinus deformity; this study showed improvement in 61% of those treated versus 25% in the placebo group [79].

Since the release of the initial report in 1993 [77], there has been a rapid acceleration of research and interest in the use of BoNT for the treatment of spasticity in CP. The number of publications on the subject doubled during the 5-year period of 2003–2007 compared to 1998–2002 [80]. A wide range of positive outcomes and low incidence of adverse effects have been reported. Over the past decade, BoNT has been established as a standard of care for the treatment of focal limb spasticity in CP [53, 81, 82].

A major indication in CP continues to be the improvement of function by the weakening of focal spastic muscles. A population-based study showed children in GMFCS I-III were more likely to receive treatment with BoNT than those in Level IV and V [83]. However, the use of BoNT has expanded to address non-functional goals such as comfort, ease of caregiving, facilitation of seating and positioning, prevention of deformity, and cosmesis (Table 5). BoNT has been recommended as an effective treatment for children with CP who have generalized spasticity if there are problematic focal spastic muscle groups which may be causing specific problems [53]. For example, a patient with quadriplegic or bilateral spastic CP may have problematic hip adductor spasticity interfering with perineal hygiene and caregiving.

Table 5 Common indications for treatment with botulinum toxin in CP

Unilateral CP	Bilateral ambulant CP	Bilateral non-ambulant CP	Bilateral non-ambulant CP
Upper limb	Improved function Improved aesthetic appearance	N/A	Pain management Easier caring and positioning Functional and/or cosmetic improvement of hand position
Lower limb	Improved gait	Improved gait	Pain management Easier caring and positioning Improvement of weight bearing Prevention of hip dislocation
Spine	N/A	N/A	Postural management Care Pain management

Used with permission from Strobl W, Theologis T, Brunner R, Kocer S, Vichweger E, Pascual-Pascual et al. Best Clinical Practice in Botulinum Toxin treatment for children with cerebral palsy. Toxins 2015;7:1629–1848

Table 6 FDA-Approved BoNT products for movement disorders

	Trade name	Indications for adults	Indications for children ≥2 years	Product supplied
Onabotulinum-A	*Botox*™	Cervical dystonia UE[a] and LE[b] spasticity	Not available	100, 200 Unit vials[c]
Abobotulinumtoxin-A	*Dysport*™	UE[a] spasticity	LE[d] spasticity	300, 500 Unit vials[c]
Rimabotulinumtoxin-B	*Myobloc*™	Cervical dystonia	Not available	2500, 5000, 10,000 Unit vials[e]

UE upper extremity, *LE* lower extremity
[a]Elbow, wrist, finger and thumb flexors
[b]Ankle and toe flexors
[c]In powder form, requires reconstitution for injection
[d]Gastrocnemius and soleus
[e]In solution, does not require reconstitution

Safety and Dosing

Currently, BoNT is licensed for children at least 2 years of age in over 40 countries worldwide, but licensing and labeling varies. Table 6 summarizes the three BoNT products currently available in the US with safety and efficacy labeling. Their formulations and potencies are different, and the units are not interchangeable, even among the same serotype. Of the three commercially available products in the US, only abobotulinum-A (Dysport) is Federal Drug Administration (FDA)-approved for children older than 2 years for the treatment of lower limb spasticity, specifically the gastrocnemius and soleus muscles. None of the FDA-approved products are labeled for use in children for treatment of spasticity of upper extremity, trunk, or neck muscles or for dystonia in any location. Thus, the previous—and current—widespread use of BoNT in children with CP is mostly "off label." In addition, other "off-label" clinical problems in patients with CP are treated with BoNT; these include post-operative pain, drooling, and detrusor (bladder) muscle spasticity. This discussion will be confined to the use of BoNT for movement disorders associated with CP.

Given the heterogeneity of symptoms in CP and lack of manufacturer guidance on optimal dose ranges, doses of BoNT used over last two decades have varied significantly. Most early studies of BoNT treatment in children with CP determined the maximum units of toxin injected per kilogram of body weight. Recommended total doses since then have been based on expert opinion and the results of small clinical trials. Since the first published report in 1993, there has been an increase in the recommended total doses of BoNT-A, the most widely used serotype, with a significant rise from 2000 to 2008 as shown in Fig. 3 [84]. This reflects, in part, a trend during these years for increasing the use of BoNT-A in multi-level injection protocols, but

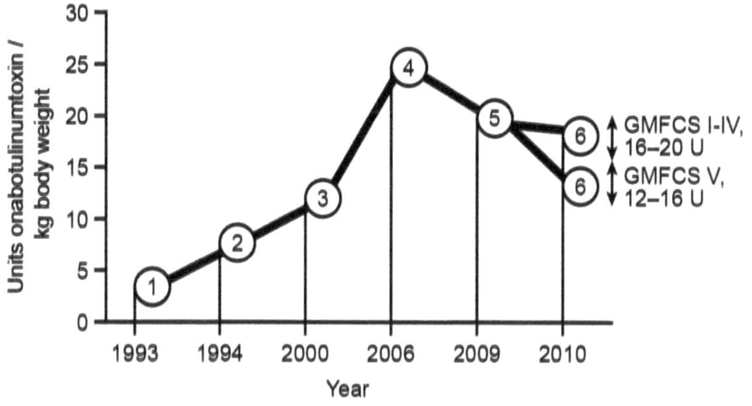

Fig. 3 Reported/recommended total dose of BoNT-A for the treatment of spasticity in children with cerebral palsy. (*GMFCS* - Gross Motor Function Classification System). Reproduced with permission from Strobl W, Theologis T, Brunner R, Kocer S, Vichweger E, Pascual-Pascual et al. Best Clinical Practice in Botulinum Toxin treatment for children with cerebral palsy. Toxins 2015;7:1629–1848

there was also an escalation in dosage for specific indications such as spastic equinus [85]. In the literature, the incidence of adverse events following injection of BoNT-A has remained relatively low during this period, and those adverse events reported were most commonly mild and include temporary injection site discomfort and local weakness. An SR published in 2009 reported a good overall short-term safety profile, but found that adverse events tend to be more common in CP patients compared to other populations treated with BoNT [86].

The situation regarding safety changed in 2008 when reports were released describing children with symptoms concerning for systemic spread of BoNT, including generalized weakness, diplopia, dysphagia, aspiration, pneumonia, and death. This resulted in a black box warning being applied to the label of all BoNT products by the FDA in 2009. Since then, the relationship between dosing and adverse events has continued to be debated, given confounding factors such as the use of anesthesia during BoNT administration and various medical co-morbidities [87]. Nevertheless, because children may be at higher risk for serious systemic adverse events, various panels and international consensus groups have lowered their total dose recommendations for BoNT [84]. In addition, many now recommend dosing based on GMFCS level and pre-existing medical co-morbidities. Risk factors include symptoms and signs of pseudobulbar palsy, swallowing difficulties, history of aspiration, and respiratory disease [82, 85].

Thus, it is important to consider the child's overall motor function when determining safe dose levels of BoNT. However, an appropriate dose or number of units must be injected in the target muscle(s) in order to neutralize neuromuscular junction (NMJ) activity. Other dosing considerations include motor disorder severity, goals of treatment, previous BoNT experience, the total number and size of the targeted muscle(s), and body region [88]. Smaller muscles in closer proximity (e.g., forearm) may require lower doses especially if the aim is for functional gains [88]. In addition, because only active muscle can take up BoNT, the dose should be modified if atrophy and/or fixed deformities are present. Various references are available with dosing recommendations for specific upper and lower limb muscles in children with CP [82, 88]. Labeling information for abobotulinum-A (Dysport) limits total dose per treatment session of 15 units/kg for unilateral and 30 units/kg for bilateral lower limb injections of the gastrocnemius and/or soleus muscles, or 1000 units, whichever is lower.

Procedure for Injections

In addition to determining the appropriate number of BoNT units for injection, several technique issues for administration of the injection must be considered in order to maximize clinical effectiveness of BoNT [89].

Injection Sites

Choice of injection sites is theoretically guided by the spatial distribution of the NMJs based on evidence from animal models and clinical studies showing injections of BoNT are more effective when located near the motor endplate [90]. Animal studies have shown the motor endplates are located at the midpoint of striated muscles fibers [91] with similar locations and distributions of NMJs in juvenile and adult muscles [92]. However, given the complex fiber structure of many limb muscles, the motor endplate region may not be well defined and their localization with electrophysiological techniques is tedious and time-consuming. For practical purposes, distributing the total BoNT dose within the center of the muscle by multiple injections of small or large volumes (depending on the size of the target muscle) may be equally or even more effective [93].

Dilution

Based on animal studies and clinical experience, approximately 4–5 cm of intramuscular diffusion of BoNT within the muscle and through the fascia can be expected, depending on the total dose and volume injected [93]. This was confirmed in a study of children with CP that found the spread of BoNT-A from foot flexors to antagonist extensors [94]. Thus an appropriate drug volume is required in order to optimize the delivery of the toxin to the NMJs and minimize unwanted spread. More diluted preparations of BoNT or larger volumes as well as increased number of injection sites may be needed for larger or more spastic muscles, or can be used when agonist or other target muscles are nearby and can benefit from diffusion. Conversely, less diluted or more concentrated preparations of BoNT are needed for smaller muscles or when spread to adjacent antagonist muscles needs to be limited.

Needle Placement and Muscle Localization

In order to maximize treatment effects, BoNT must be injected inside the fascial compartment which requires accurate placement of the needle in the target muscle. Manual intramuscular needle placements are usually based on a combination of visual inspection, identification of anatomical landmarks, and palpation. Many studies of BoNT in the treatment of children with CP refer to this method but do not provide further details of the process involved. Verification of the location of the needle after manual placement can be performed by active or passive movement [95, 96]. Enhanced localization techniques involve instrumentation using electrical stimulation (ES), ultrasonography (US), or electromyography (EMG). The use of EMG is limited in children with CP because of their difficulties with cooperation and selective control of movements. US offers non-invasive real-time imaging of muscles and surrounding structures to guide precise needle placement in the middle of the muscle belly and avoidance of nerves and vessels. ES provides actual confirmation that the needle is placed in a part of a muscle that can be activated.

In 2015, a SR provided evidence of improved efficacy of BoNT for spastic equinus in children with CP with the use of ES or US compared to non-instrumented techniques [97]. More recently, the use of a detailed protocol for manual needle placement using passive muscle stretching and relaxation, a non-instrumented technique, was evaluated in children undergoing BoNT injections [98]. Using ES for verification, the protocol was found to reliably localize the needle in the target lower extremity muscles; however, the use of general anesthesia may be needed in children, especially for multiple injections, so this technique may not offer much time or cost savings advantage over performance of injections under general anesthesia using ES for localization.

Evidence

There are unique challenges in interpreting the outcomes research on BoNT in CP. The treated population is diverse, includes multiple etiologies with varied severity and distribution of symptoms, and changes related to growth and maturation. There is a high variability in the treatment itself—different preparations, dosages, sites of injections, intervals between injections, and administration techniques. In addition, treatment with BoNT is usually repeated, but most studies report outcomes during or after a single cycle. A large range of outcomes are reported by studies of

Table 7 Systematic Reviews evaluating the efficacy of BoNT-A for improving spasticity or function in children with CP

First author, year (reference number)	SR methodology	First author, year (reference number)	SR methodology
UE spasticity		UE function	
Simpson 2008 [99]	AAN	Simpson 2008 [99]	AAN
Lukban 2009 [100]	AAN	Lukban 2009 [100]	AAN
Delgado 2010 [81]	AAN	Sakrewski 2009 [103]	PEDro
Fehlings 2010 [88]	AAN	Fehlings 2010 [88]	AAN
Hoare 2010 [101]	Cochrane, PEDro	Hoare 2010 [101]	Cochrane, PEDro
Novak 2013 [53]	GRADE	Novak 2013 [53]	GRADE
LE spasticity		LE function	
Simpson 2008 [99]	AAN	Simpson 2008 [99]	AAN
Lukban 2009 [100]	AAN	Lukban 2009 [100]	AAN
Delgado 2010 [81]	AAN	Love 2010 [84]	AAN
Koog 2010 [102]	AACPDM, meta-analysis	Koog 2010 [102]	AACPDM, meta-analysis
Novak 2013 [53]	GRADE	Ryll 2011 [104]	Cochrane, PEDro
		Novak 2013 [53]	Grade

SR systematic review, *UE* upper extremity, *LE* lower extremity, *AAN* American Academy of Neurology, *PEDro* physiotherapy evidence database, *GRADE* grading of recommendations assessment, development and evaluation, *AACPDM* American Academy of Cerebral Palsy and Developmental Medicine

treatment with BoNT in CP and often multiple measures are used. Because BoNT is typically not a stand-alone treatment, many studies report on comparative effects of BoNT in combination with other treatments vs BoNT or other treatments alone. Fortunately, the issue of BoNT-A efficacy in CP has been subject to critical appraisal in multiple SRs. Efficacy for spasticity reduction and functional improvement has been examined. This discussion is limited to SRs published in the last decade.

There are nine SRs addressing spasticity reduction after treatment with BoNT in childhood CP; of these, five report on UE and four on LE studies (Table 7). For the LE, they conclude BoNT is effective for spasticity reduction. For the UE, conclusions of the SRs are conflicting and inconclusive. Of note, these conclusions are based on a relatively low number of high-quality studies with small numbers of participants. Based on the evaluation of ten SRs, Novak et al. 2013 [53] concluded that BoNT is effective for LE spasticity, but available evidence is insufficient to confirm efficacy for UE spasticity.

There are ten SRs addressing functional improvement after treatment with BoNT in childhood CP, five report on UE studies, and five on LE studies (Table 7). For the LE, they conclude BoNT is effective for equinus gait. For the UE, they conclude BoNT alone and combined with occupational therapy (OT) are effective using individualized goal attainment measures as outcomes. Again, conclusions are based on low numbers of high-quality original studies with small numbers of participants. In addition, most outcomes were measured between 1 and 12 months, so no information can be inferred regarding long-term impact on function or other domains.

Based on the evaluation of seven SRs, Novak et al. [53] concluded that BoNT was effective for improving UE function in combination with OT, and probably effective for LE function in combination with physical therapy (PT).

Another SR evaluated the evidence to support repeated injections of BoNT-A in children with CP. They evaluated 19 original studies and concluded there was evidence for efficacy for spasticity reduction, especially after the first two injections/one repeat injection [105]. Other reviews have evaluated the effectiveness of BoNT in the treatment of specific subgroups of CP. In ambulatory children with CP, the efficacy of BoNT-A in combination with PT and BoNT in combination with serial casting was reviewed by examining the results of high-quality studies [106]. Limited evidence was found to support the belief that BoNT- related decreased spasticity potentiates these other interventions in reducing contracture. BoNT treatment of children with CP in GMFCS Level IV-V, a population likely to have goals other than improved function, was examined in an SR [107]. Only 1 of 19 original studies reviewed provided high-quality evidence. The conclusion was that there is insufficient evidence of BoNT efficacy for pain reduction, maintenance of hip integrity, functional changes, and goal attainment in this CP subgroup.

Three SRs have focused on very young children. Of these, two evaluated treatment effects; one limited their review to BoNT [108], the other included BoNT and other treatments [109]. Because of limited evidence, neither SR could make a conclusion about the therapeutic effects of BoNT in children less than 2 years of age. Another SR concluded the use of BoNT-A was safe in children less than 2 years of age, but included studies of children treated for conditions other than CP [110].

Potential Long-Term Benefits and Risks

The study of the long-term effects of BoNT in children with CP is additionally challenging for several reasons: (1) Repeat treatments are necessary to maintain decreased spasticity; (2) BoNT is typically part of a multi-modality intervention strategy; and (3) Influence of confounding factors such as co-morbidities, growth, aging, and personal and environmental factors. Not surprisingly, there is limited evidence-based information available on this crucial issue.

The potential goals of early treatment with BoNT (assuming effective spasticity reduction) are the prevention or reduction of contracture and deformity, decreased the need for orthopedic surgery, less pain and fatigue, and better function. Unfortunately, there is a dearth of evidence to conclude that treatment with BoNT produces these results. There is only one randomized controlled trial showing BoNT with bracing may slow progression but not prevent hip deformity [111]. There is inconclusive evidence from numerous low-quality studies that BoNT delays or prevents orthopedic surgery. However, the lack of evidence for BoNT affecting musculoskeletal morbidities in CP is not entirely unexpected considering the latest information about the development of contracture and bony deformity in CP as discussed above. Further support of this perhaps predictable lack of evidence is offered by a prospective clinical study of children with CP which found progressive loss of passive range of motion over time (up to 3 years) despite maintenance of decreased muscle tone with repeat BoNT treatments [112].

There are also questions about the long-term risks of BoNT treatment in children with CP, especially how BoNT affects muscle, the target organ of its mechanism of action. Histopathologic changes lasting months to years have been reported in recent studies of muscles treated with BoNT in children with CP [113–115]. These findings raise concerns, but are preliminary, and difficult to interpret as there is no information about adult outcomes based on childhood treatment with BoNT. This is now an active area of research which will provide more answers about the potential beneficial—and detrimental—effects of BoNT on muscle development in children with CP,

Evidence Summary

In summary, after over 20 years of experience, there is strong evidence that BoNT is effective for short-term reduction of upper and lower limb spasticity in children with CP. Nevertheless, there is less certain evidence that these effects translate into functional improvements. The available evidence does show beneficial functional effects—specifically decreased equinus gait and hand function—occur only when treatment with BoNT is combined with OT and PT. Thus it is important to communicate the need for stretching and strengthening to patients and their families when undergoing treatment with BoNT. Currently, there is insufficient evidence confirming the effectiveness of BoNT for spasticity reduction beyond 1 year, and inconclusive evidence for any long-term improvements or prevention of secondary musculoskeletal deformities. However, given the challenges of such studies, it is important to recognize there is a similar lack of evidence of long-term effectiveness of many other treatments used in children with CP.

References

1. Surveillance of Cerebral Palsy in Europe (SCPE). Surveillance of cerebral palsy in Europe: a collaboration of cerebral palsy surveys and registers. Dev Med Child Neurol. 2000;42:816–24.
2. Pakula AT, Van Naarden-Braun K, Yeargin-Alsopp M. Cerebral palsy: classification and epidemiology. Phys Med Rehabil Clin N Am. 2009;20(3):425–52.
3. Minear WL. A classification of cerebral palsy. Pediatrics. 1956;18(5):841–52.
4. Bax MC. Terminology and classification of cerebral palsy. Dev Med Child Neurol. 1964;6:295–7.
5. Rosenbaum P, Paneth N, Leviton A, Goldstein M, Bax M, Damiano D, et al. A report: the definition and classification of cerebral palsy April 2006. Dev Med Child Neurol Suppl. 2007 Feb;109:8–14.
6. Durkin MS, Benedict RE, Christensen D, Dubois LA, Fitzgerald RT, Kirby RS, et al. Prevalence of cerebral palsy among 8-year-old children in 2010 and preliminary evidence of trends in its relationship to low Birthweight. Paediatr Perinat Epidemiol. 2016;30(5):496–510.

7. Vincer MJ, Allen AC, Joseph KS, Stinson DA, Scott H, Wood E. Increasing prevalence of cerebral palsy among very preterm infants: a population-based study. Pediatrics. 2006;118(6):e1621–6.
8. Hutton JL, Pharoah PO. Life expectancy in severe cerebral palsy. Arch Dis Child. 2006;91:254–8.
9. Westbom L, Bergstrand L, Wagner P, Nordmark E. Survival at 19 years of age in a total population of children and young people with cerebral palsy. Dev Med Child Neurol. 2011;53(9):808–14.
10. McIntyre S, Taitz D, Keogh J, Goldsmith S, Badawi N, Blair E. A systematic review of risk factors for cerebral palsy in children born at term in developed countries. Dev Med Child Neurol. 2013;55(6):499–508.
11. Hirvonen M, Ojala R, Korhonen P, Haataja P, Erikkson K, Gissler M, et al. Cerebral palsy among children born moderately and late preterm. Pediatrics. 2014;134(6):e1584–93.
12. Jacobsson B, Hagberg G. Antenatal risk factors for cerebral palsy. Best Pract Res Clin Obstet Gynaecol. 2004;18(3):425–36.
13. Himmelmann K, Ahlin K, Jacobsson B, Cans C, Thorsen P. Risk factors for cerebral palsy in children born at term. Acta Obstet Gynecol Scand. 2011;90(10):1070–81.
14. Nelson KB, Blair E. Prenatal factors in singletons with cerebral palsy born at or near term. N Engl J Med. 2015;373(10):946–53.
15. Sellier E, Surman G, Himmelmann K, Andersen G, Colver A, Krageloh-Mann I, et al. Trends in prevalence of cerebral palsy in children born with a birthweight of 2500g or over in Europe from 1980 to 1998. Eur J Epidemiol. 2010;25(9):635–42.
16. Graham HK, Rosenbaum P, Paneth N, Dan B, Lin JP, Damiano DL, et al. Cerebral palsy. Nat Rev Dis Primers. 2016;2:15082.
17. Himmelmann K, Horber V, DeLaCruz J, Horridge K, Mejaski-Bosnjak V, Hollody K, et al. MRI classification system (MRIS) for children with cerebral palsy: development, reliability, and recommendations. Dev Med Child Neurol. 2016;89(1):57–4. [Epub ahead of print]
18. Edwards AD, Tan S. Perinatal infections, prematurity and brain injury. Curr Opin Pediatr. 2006;18(2):119–24.
19. Rutherford MA, Pennock JM, Schwieso JE, Cowan FM, Dubowitz LM. Hypoxic ischaemic encephalopathy: early magnetic resonance imaging findings and their evolution. Neuropediatrics. 1995;26(4):183–91.
20. Kirton A, de Veber G. Paediatric stroke: pressing issues and promising directions. Lancet Neurol. 2015;14(1):92–102.
21. Korzeniewski SJ, Birbeck G, DeLano MC, Potchen MJ, Paneth N. A systematic review of neuroimaging for cerebral palsy. J Child Neurol. 2008;23(2):216–27.
22. Reid SM, Dagia CD, Ditchfield MR, Carlin JB, Reddihough DS. Population-based studies of brain imaging patterns in cerebral palsy. Dev Med Child Neurol. 2014;56(3):222–32.
23. Ashwal S, Russman BS, Blasco PA, Miller G, Sandler A, Shevell M, et al. Practice parameter: diagnostic assessment of the child with cerebral palsy: report of the Quality Standards Subcommittee of the American Academy of Neurology and the Practice Committee of the Child Neurology Society. Neurology. 2004;62(6):851–63.
24. Novak I. Evidence-based diagnosis, health care, and rehabilitation for children with cerebral palsy. J Child Neurol. 2014;29(8):1141–56.
25. Spittle A, Brown N, Doyle LW, Boyd RN, Hunt RW, Bear M, et al. Quality of general movements is related to white matter pathology in very preterm infants. Pediatrics. 2008;121(5):e1184–9.
26. Lee RW, Poretti A, Cohen JS, Levey E, Gwynn H, Johnston MV, et al. A diagnostic approach for cerebral palsy in the genomic era. NeuroMolecular Med. 2014;16:821.
27. Wimalasundera N, Stevenson VL. Cerebral palsy. Pract Neurol. 2016;16(3):184–94.
28. McIntyre S, Morgan C, Walker K, Novak I. Cerebral palsy—don't delay. Dev Disabil Res Rev. 2011;17(2):114–29.
29. Sanger TD, Delgado MR, Gaebler-Spira D, Hallett M, Mink JW. Task force on childhood motor disorders. Classification and definition of disorders causing hypertonia in childhood. Pediatrics. 2003;111(1):e89–97.

30. Sanger TD, Chen D, Delgado MR, Gaebler-Spira D, Hallett M, Mink JW, et al. Definition and classification of negative motor signs in childhood. Pediatrics. 2006;118(5):2159–67.
31. Sanger TD, Chen D, Fehlings DL, Hallett M, Lang AE, Mink JW, et al. Definition and classification of hyperkinetic movements in childhood. Mov Disord. 2010;25(11):1538–49.
32. Sakrewski L, Ziyiani J, Boyd R. Systematic review and meta-analysis of therapeutic management of upper limb dysfunction in children with congenital hemiplegia. Pediatrics. 2009;123(6):e1111–22.
33. Becher JG. Pediatric rehabilitation in children with cerebral palsy: general management, classification of motor disorders. J Prosthet Orthot. 2002;14:143–9.
34. Russman BS, Gormley ME, Tilton A. Cerebral palsy: a rational approach to a treatment protocol, and the role of botulinum toxin treatment. In: Mayer NH BA, editor. Spasticity and other forms of muscle overactivity in the upper motor neuron syndrome: etiology, evaluation, management and the role of botulinum toxin. New York: WE MOVE; 2008.
35. Sewell MD, Eastwood DM, Wimalasundera N. Managing common symptoms of cerebral palsy in children. BMJ. 2014;349:g5474.
36. Hanna SE, Rosenbaum PL, Bartlett DJ, Palisano RJ, Walter SD, Avery L, et al. Stability and decline in gross motor function among children and youth with cerebral palsy aged 2 to 21 years. Dev Med Child Neurol. 2009;51(4):295–302.
37. Pruitt DW, Tsai T. Common medical comorbidities associated with cerebral palsy. Phys Med Rehabil Clin N Am. 2009;20:453–7.
38. Damiano DL, Martellotta TL, Sullivan DJ, Granata KP, Abel MF. Muscle force production and functional performance in spastic cerebral palsy: relationship of cocontraction. Arch Phys Med Rehabil. 2000;81(7):895–900.
39. Elder GC, Kirk J, Stewart G, Cook K, Weir D, Marshall A, et al. Contributing factors to muscle weakness in children with cerebral palsy. Dev Med Child Neurol. 2003;45(8):542–50.
40. Graham HK, Selber P. Musculoskeletal aspects of cerebral palsy. J Bone Joint Surg Br. 2003;85(2):157–66.
41. Barber LA, Boyd R. Growing muscles in children with cerebral palsy. Dev Med Child Neurol. 2016;58(5):431–2.
42. Bar-On L, Molenaers G, Aertbeliën E, Van Campenhout A, Feys H, Nuttin B, et al. Spasticity and its contribution to hypertonia in cerebral palsy. Biomed Res Int. 2015;2015:317047.
43. Stackhouse SK, Binder-Macleod SA, Lee SC. Voluntary muscle activation, contractile properties, and fatigability inchildren with and without cerebral palsy. Muscle Nerve. 2005;31(5):594–601.
44. Hägglund G, Wagner P. Development of spasticity with age in a total population of children with cerebral palsy. BMC Musculoskelet Disord. 2008;9:150.
45. Kuban KC, Leviton A. Cerebral palsy. N Engl J Med. 1994;330(3):188–95.
46. Smithers-Sheedy H, Badawi N, Blair E, Cans C, Himmelmann K, Krageloh-Mann I, et al. What constitutes cerebral palsy in the twenty-first century? Dev Med Child Neurol. 2014;56(4):323–8.
47. Barrett RS, Lichtwark GA. Gross muscle morphology and structure in spastic cerebral palsy: a systematic review. Dev Med Child Neurol. 2010;52(9):794–804.
48. Herskind A, Ritterband-Rosenbaum A, Willerslev-Olsen M, Lorentzen J, Hanson L, Lichtwark G, et al. Muscle growth is reduced in 15-month-old children with cerebral palsy. Dev Med Child Neurol. 2016;58(5):485–91.
49. Gough M, Shortland AP. Could muscle deformity in children with spastic cerebral palsy be related to an impairment of muscle growth and altered adaptation? Dev Med Child Neurol. 2012;54(6):495–9.
50. Gage JR, DeLuca PA, Renshaw TS. Gait analysis: principle and applications with emphasis on its use in cerebral palsy. Instr Course Lect. 1996;45:491–507.
51. World Health Organization. International classification of functioning, disability and health. Geneva: World Health Org.

52. Preston N, Clarke M, Bhakta B. Development of a framework to define the functional goals and outcomes of botulinum toxin A spasticity treatment relevant to the child and family living with cerebral palsy using the international classification of functioning, disability and health for children and youth. J Rehabil Med. 2011;43(11):1010–5. anization; 2001
53. Novak I, McIntyre S, Morgan C, Campbell L, Dark L, Morton N, et al. A systematic review of interventions for children with cerebral palsy: state of the evidence. Dev Med Child Neurol. 2013;55(10):885–910.
54. Gorter JW, Rosenbaum PL, Hanna SE, Palisano RJ, Bartlett DJ, Russell DJ, et al. Limb distribution, motor impairment, and functional classification of cerebral palsy. Dev Med Child Neurol. 2004;46(7):461–7.
55. Shevell MI. The terms diplegia and quadriplegia should not be abandoned. Dev Med Child Neurol. 2010;52(6):508–9.
56. Palisano R, Rosenbaum P, Walter S, Russell D, Wood E, Galuppi B. Development and reliability of a system to classify gross motor function in children with cerebral palsy. Dev Med Child Neurol. 1997;39(4):214–23.
57. Palisano R, Rosembaum P, Bartlett D, et al. GMFCS-E&R gross motor function classification system expanded and revised. Ontario, Canada: CanChild Centre for Childhood Disability Research; 2007.
58. Rosenbaum PL, Walter SD, Hanna SE, Palisano RJ, Russell DJ, Raina P, et al. Prognosis for gross motor function in cerebral palsy: creation of motor development curves. JAMA. 2002;288(11):1357–63.
59. McCormick A, Brien M, Plourde J, Wood E, Rosenbaum P, Mclean J. Stability of the gross motor function classification system in adults with cerebral palsy. Dev Med Child Neurol. 2007;49(4):265–9.
60. Eliasson AC, Krumlinde-Sundholm L, Rösblad B, Beckung E, Arner M, Ohrvall AM, et al. The Manual Ability Classification System (MACS) for children with cerebral palsy: scale development and evidence of validity and reliability. Dev Med Child Neurol. 2006;48(7):549–54.
61. Hidecker MJ, Paneth N, Rosenbaum PL, Kent RD, Lillie J, Eulenberg JB, et al. Developing and validating the Communication Function Classification System (CFCS) for individuals with cerebral palsy. Dev Med Child Neurol. 2011;53(8):704–10.
62. Sellers D, Mandy A, Pennington L, Hankins M, Morris C. Development and reliability of a system to classify the eating and drinking ability of people with cerebral palsy. Dev Med Child Neurol. 2014;56(3):245–51.
63. Boyd RN, Graham HK. Objective measurement of clinical findings in the use of botulinum toxin type A for the management of children with cerebral palsy. Eur J Neurol. 1999;6(suppl. 4):S23–35.
64. Bar-On L, Van Campenhout A, Desloovere K, Aertbeliën E, Huenaerts C, Vandendoorent B, et al. Is an instrumented spasticity assessment an improvement over clinical spasticity scales in assessing and predicting the response to integrated botulinum toxin type a treatment in children with cerebral palsy? Arch Phys Med Rehabil. 2014;95(3):515–23.
65. Barber L, Hastings-Ison T, Baker R, Barrett R, Lichtwark G. Medial gastrocnemius muscle volume and fascicle length in children aged 2 to 5 years with cerebral palsy. Dev Med Child Neurol. 2011;53(6):543–8.
66. Willerslev-Olsen M, Lorentzen J, Sinkjaer T, Nielsen JB. Passive muscle properties are altered in children with cerebral palsy before the age of 3 years and are difficult to distinguish clinically from spasticity. Dev Med Child Neurol. 2013;55(7):617–23.
67. Bohannon RW, Smith MB. Interrater reliability of a modified Ashworth scale of muscle spasticity. Phys Ther. 1987;67(2):206–7.
68. Baird MC, Vargus-Adams J. Outcome measures used in studies of Botulinum toxin in childhood cerebral palsy: a systematic review. J Child Neurol. 2010;25(6):721–7.
69. Jethwa A, Mink J, Macarthur C, Knights S, Fehlings T, Fehlings D. Development of the hypertonia assessment tool (HAT): a discriminative tool for hypertonia in children. Dev Med Child Neurol. 2010;52(5):e83–7.

70. Barry MJ, Van Swearingen JM, Albright AL. Reliability and responsiveness of the Barry-Albright Dystonia Scale. Dev Med Child Neurol. 1999;41:404–41.
71. Lin YC, Lin IL, Chou TFA, Lee HM. Quantitative evaluation for spasticity of calf muscle after botulinum toxin injection in patients with cerebral palsy: a pilot study. J Neuroeng Rehabil. 2016;13:25.
72. Bertucco M, Sanger TD. Current and emerging strategies for treatment of childhood dystonia. J Hand Ther. 2015;28(2):185–93.
73. Guyatt G, Oxman AD, Akl EA, Kunz R, Vist G, Brozek J, et al. GRADE guidelines: 1. Introduction-GRADE evidence profiles and summary of findings tables. J Clin Epidemiol. 2011;64(4):383–94.
74. Glenn MB. Nerve blocks. In: Glenn MB, Whyte J, editors. The practical management of spasticity in children and adults. Philadelphia: Lea & Febiger; 1990. p. 227–67.
75. Gooch JL, Patton CP. Combining botulinum toxin and phenol to manage spasticity in children. Arch Phys Med Rehabil. 2004;85(7):1121–4.
76. Kolaski K, Ajizian SJ, Passmore L, Pasutharnchat N, Koman LA, BPl S. Safety profile of multilevel chemical denervation procedures using phenol or botulinum toxin or both in a pediatric population. Am J Phys Med Rehabil. 2008;87(7):556–66.
77. Koman LA, Mooney JF III, Smith B, Goodman A, Mulvaney T. Management of cerebral palsy with botulinum-A toxin: preliminary investigation. J Pediatr Orthop. 1993;13(4):489–95.
78. Koman LA, Mooney JF III, Smith BP, Goodman A, Mulvaney T. Management of spasticity in cerebral palsy with botulinum-A toxin: report of a preliminary, randomized, double-blind trial. J Pediatr Orthop. 1994;14(3):299–303.
79. Koman LA, Mooney JF III, Smith BP, Walker F, Leon JM. Botulinum toxin type A neuromuscular blockade in the treatment of lower extremity spasticity in cerebral palsy: a randomized, double-blind, placebo-controlled trial. BOTOX Study Group. J Pediatr Orthop. 2000;20(1):108–15.
80. Seyler TM, Smith BP, Marker DR, Hanjun M, Shen I, Smih TL, et al. Botulinum neurotoxin as a therapeutic modality in orthopedic surgery: more than twenty years of experiences. J Bone Joint Surg Am. 2008;90(Suppl 4):133–45.
81. Delgado MR, Hirtz D, Aisen M, Ashwal S, Fehlings DL, Mclaughlin J, et al. Practice parameter: pharmacologic treatment of spasticity in children and adolescents with cerebral palsy (an evidence based review). Neurology. 2010;74(4):336–43.
82. Heinen F, Desloovere K, Schroeder AS, Berweck S, Borggraefe I, van Campenhout A, et al. The updated European consensus 2009 on the use of botulinum toxin for children with cerebral palsy. Eur J Paediatr Neurol. 2009;14(1):45–66.
83. Elkamil AI, Andersen GL, Skranes J, Lamvik T, Vik T. Botulinum neurotoxin treatment in children with cerebral palsy: a population-based study in Norway. Eur J Paediatr Neurol. 2012;16(5):522–7.
84. Strobl W, Theologis T, Brunner R, Kocer S, Viehweger E, Pascual-Pascual I, et al. Best clinical practice in botulinum toxin treatment for children with cerebral palsy. Toxins (Basel). 2015;7(5):1629–48.
85. Love SC, Novak I, Kentish M, Desloovere K, Heinen F, Molenaers G, et al. Botulinum toxin assessment, intervention and after-care for lower limb spasticity in children with cerebral palsy: international consensus statement. Eur J Neurol. 2010;17(Suppl 2):9–37.
86. Albavera-Hernández C, Rodríguez JM, Idrovo AJ. Safety of botulinum toxin type A among children with spasticity secondary to cerebral palsy: a systematic review of randomized clinical trials. Clin Rehabil. 2009;23(5):394–407.
87. Tilton AH. Evidence-based review of safety and efficacy in cerebral palsy. Toxicon. 2015;107:105–8.
88. Fehlings D, Novak I, Berweck S, Hoare B, Stott NS, Russo RN. Botulinum toxin assessment, intervention and follow-up for paediatric upper limb hypertonicity: international consensus statement. Eur J Neurol. 2010;17(Suppl 2):38–56.

89. Koman LA, Paterson Smith B, Balkrishnan R. Spasticity associated with cerebral palsy in children: guidelines for the use of botulinum toxin. Paediatr Drugs. 2003;5(1):11–23.
90. Gracies J-M, Weisz D-J, et al. Impact of botulinum toxin A (BTX-A) dilution and endplate targeting technique in upper limb spasticity. Ann Neurol. 2002;52(Suppl 1):S87.
91. Childers MK, Kornegay JN, Aoki R, Otaviani L, Bogan DJ, Petroski G. Evaluating motor end-plate-targeted injections of botulinum toxin type A in a canine model. Muscle Nerve. 1998;21:653–5.
92. Ma J, Smith BP, Smith TL, Walker FO, Rosencrance EV, Koman LA, et al. Juvenile and adult rat neuromuscular junctions: density, distribution and morphology. Muscle Nerve. 2002;26(6):804–9.
93. Schroeders AS, Berweck H, Lee SH, Heinen F. Botulinum toxin treatment of children with cerebral palsy— a short review of different injection techniques. Neurotox Res. 2006;9:189–96.
94. Frasson E, Dall'ora E, Bordignon M, Brigo F, Tocco P, Primon D, et al. Spread of botulinum neurotoxin type a at standard doses is inherent to the successful treatment of spastic equinus foot in cerebral palsy: short-term neurophysiological and clinical study. J Child Neurol. 2012;27(5):587–93.
95. Chin TY, Nattrass GR, Selber P, Graham HK. Accuracy of intramuscular injection of botulinum toxin A in juvenile cerebral palsy: a comparison between manual needle placement and placement guided by electrical stimulation. J Pediatr Orthop. 2005;25:286–91.
96. Warnink-Kavelaars J, Vermeulen R, Becher J. Study protocol: precision of a protocol for manual intramuscular needle placement checked by passive stretching and relaxing of the target muscle in the lower extremity during BTX-A treatment in children with spastic cerebral palsy, as verified by means of electrical stimulation. BMC Pediatr. 2013;13:129.
97. Grigoriu AI, Dinomais M, Rémy-Néris O, Brochard S. Impact of injection-guiding techniques on the effectiveness of botulinum toxin for the treatment of focal spasticity and dystonia: a systematic review. Arch Phys Med Rehabil. 2015;96(11):2067–78.
98. Warnink-Kavelaars J, Vermeulen RJ, Buizer AI, Becher JG. Botulinum neurotoxin treatment in children with cerebral palsy: validation of a needle placement protocol using passive muscle stretching and relaxing. Dev Med Child Neurol. 2016;58(12):1281–7. doi:10.1111/dmcn.13176. [Epub ahead of print]
99. Simpson DM, Gracies JM, Graham HK, Miyasaki JM, Naumann M, Russman B, et al. Assessment: Botulinum neurotoxin for the treatment of spasticity (an evidence-based review) report of the Therapeutics And Technology Assessment Subcommittee of the American Academy of Neurology. Neurology. 2008;70(19):1691–8.
100. Lukban MB, Rosales RL, Dressler D. Effectiveness of botulinum toxin A for upper and lower limb spasticity in children with cerebral palsy: a summary of evidence. J Neural Transm. 2009;116(3):319–31.
101. Hoare BJ, Wallen MA, Imms C, Villanueva E, Rawicki HB, Carey L. Botulinum toxin A as an adjunct to treatment in the management of the upper limb in children with spastic cerebral palsy (UPDATE). Cochrane Database Syst Rev. 2010;20(1):CD003469.
102. Koog YH, Min B-I. Effects of botulinum toxin A on calf muscles in children with cerebral palsy: a systematic review. Clin Rehabil. 2010;24(8):685–700.
103. Sakzewski L, Ziviani J, Boyd R. Review and meta-analysis of therapeutic management of upper-limb dysfunction in children with congenital hemiplegia. Pediatrics. 2009;123(6 Suppl):e1111–22.
104. Ryll U, Bastiaenen C, De Bie R, Staal B. Effects of leg muscle botulinum toxin A injections on walking in children with spasticity-related cerebral palsy: a systematic review. Dev Med Child Neurol. 2011;53(3):210–6.
105. Kahraman A, Seyhan K, Deger U, Kutluturk S, Mutlu A. Should botulinum toxin A injections be repeated in children with cerebral palsy? A systematic review. Dev Med Child Neurol. 2016;58(9):910–7.

106. Narayanan UG. Management of children with ambulatory CP: an evidence based review. J Pediatr Orthop. 2012;32(Suppl 2):S172–81.
107. Pin TW, Elmasry J, Lewis J. Efficacy of botulinum toxin A in children with cerebral palsy in gross motor function classification system levels IV and V: a systematic review. Dev Med Child Neurol. 2013;55(4):304–13.
108. Druschel C, Althuizes HC, Funk JF, Placzek R. Off label use of Botulinum toxin in children under two years of age: a systematic review. Toxins. 2013;5:60–72.
109. Ward R, Reynolds JE, Bear N, Elliott C, Valentine J. What is the evidence for managing tone in young children with, or at risk of developing, cerebral palsy: a systematic review. Disabil Rehabil. 2016;30:1–12.
110. Pascual-Pascual SI, Pascual-Castroviejo I. Safety of botulinum toxin type A in children younger than 2 years. Eur J Paediatr Neurol. 2009;13(6):511.
111. Graham HK, Boyd R, Carlin JB, Dobson F, Lowe K, Nattrass G, et al. Does botulinum toxin A combined with bracing prevent hip displacement in children with cerebral palsy and "hips at risk"? A randomized, controlled trial. J Bone Joint Surg Am. 2008;90(1):23–33.
112. Tedroff K, Granath F, Forssberg H, Haglund-Akerlind Y. Long-term effects of botulinum toxin A in children with cerebral palsy. Dev Med Child Neurol. 2009;51(2):120–7.
113. Williams SA, Reid S, Elliott C, Shipman P, Valentine J. Muscle volume alterations in spastic muscles immediately following botulinum toxin type-A treatment in children with cerebral palsy. Dev Med Child Neurol. 2013;55(9):813–20.
114. Barber L, Hastings-Ison T, Baker R, Kerr Grahm H, Barrett R, Lichtwark G. The effects of botulinum toxin injection frequency on calf muscle growth in young children with spastic cerebral palsy: a 12 month prospective study. J Child Orthop. 2013;7(5):425–33.
115. Valentine J, Stannage K, Fabian V, Ellis K, Reid S, Pitcher C, et al. Muscle histopathology in children with spastic cerebral palsy receiving botulinum toxin type A. Muscle Nerve. 2016;53(3):407–14.

Botulinum Toxin Treatment in Multiple Sclerosis

Yasaman Safarpour and Bahman Jabbari

Introduction

Multiple sclerosis (MS) is a chronic autoimmune-inflammatory and neurodegenerative disease of the central nervous system (CNS) in which the disease process typically destroys myelin sheets and axons. The prevalence of MS in the US as reported in recent large-scale studies varies from 130 (global survey) to 149 (insured population) in 100,000 [1]. It is believed that, currently, there are 400,000 people with MS living in the US and 2.1 million with MS live worldwide [2]. In the US, the cost per patient varies from $8000 to $52,000 per year [3]. Multiple sclerosis is the most common cause of non-traumatic disability in young adults [4]. The cause of multiple sclerosis is likely to involve a combination of genetic susceptibility and non-genetic factors (e.g., viral or bacterial infection, low vitamin D levels, etc.) resulting in a self-sustaining autoimmune disorder. Several clinical forms are described that include relapsing–remitting MS (RRMS), secondary progressive MS (SPMS), progressive relapsing MS (PRMS), and primary progressive MS (PPMS). The disease causes a multitude of symptoms leading to visual, motor, sensory, and autonomic dysfunctions. Treatment of multiple sclerosis (MS) focuses on two aims: (1) slowing down the progression of the disease and healing the existing myelin damage and (2) symptomatic treatment. Immunomodulatory therapy (IMT) for the underlying immune disorder and strategies to relieve or modify symptoms include administration of a variety of monoclonal antibodies with different functions: inhibition of

Y. Safarpour, M.D.
Research Scholar, Division of Nephrology and Hypertention, University of California, Irvine
e-mail: Yac.safarpour@gmail.com

B. Jabbari, M.D., FAAN (✉)
Department of Neurology, Yale University School of Medicine, New Haven, CT, USA

31 Silver Pine Drive, Newport Coast, CA 92657, USA
e-mail: Bahman.jabbari@yale.edu

B. Jabbari (ed.), *Botulinum Toxin Treatment in Clinical Medicine*,
DOI 10.1007/978-3-319-56038-0_7

migration of lymphocytes (natalizumab), depletion of lymphocytes (alemtuzumab), blocking the cytokine receptor interleukin (IL)-2 (daclizumab), inhibition of proliferation of activated lymphocytes (teriflunomide), and modulation of the sphingosine-receptor system (fingolimod). Dimethylfumarate combines features of immunomodulatory and immunosuppressive drugs [5]. Other commonly used pharmaceutical agents consist of interferons beta1a and b and glatiramer acetate.

Acute symptoms of multiple sclerosis can be arrested and reversed by 3–5 days of intravenous prednisone (Solumedrol). Chronic symptoms require symptomatic treatment with appropriate pharmacological agents. Botulinum neurotoxins are now used for treatment of a wide variety of symptoms and extensively for the management of upper and lower limb spasticity [6]. Among the symptoms of multiple sclerosis, spasticity, neuropathic pain, involuntary movements, bladder dysfunction, and autonomic disorders are responsive to botulinum toxin treatment.

Spasticity in Multiple Sclerosis

Spasticity is a clinical condition characterized by velocity-dependent increased stretch reflex associated with increased muscle tone in the absence of volitional activity [7]. It is caused by damage to the central nervous system. The pathophysiology of spasticity still needs clarification. In Gracies' extensive review of the subject [8, 9], two of the factors most relevant to the pathophysiology of spasticity are defined as decreased reciprocal Ia inhibition of α motor neurons via disynaptic interneuron and decreased nonreciprocal Ib inhibition (Golgi tendons limiting limb extension) [10, 11]. Furthermore, the hyperexcitable newly developed connections and sprouts play an important role in the emergence of the increased stretch reflexes. In spasticity, the response of motor neurons to stretch is more and longer than normal. The temperature, time of the day, fatigue, posture, and position of the limb influence the severity of spasticity [12].

Spasticity interferes with mobility, transfers, and personal care. It can manifest as muscle stiffness, pain, spasms, clonus, abnormal posture, dystonia (spastic dystonia), and co-contractions. If badly managed, it can cause shortening of muscles and tendons, movement limitations, and pressure sores [13].

In multiple sclerosis, demyelination and damage to descending spinal pathways (corticospinal, reticulospinal, vestibulospinal) can interrupt the control over alpha motor neurons via mono- and polysynaptic pathways. During the course of their disease, up to 80% of the patients with multiple sclerosis (MS) suffer from spasticity, which is often overlooked and undertreated in mild to moderate cases [14]. In one large registry, mild, moderate, and severe spasticity were found in 27.3%, 44.0%, and 28.7% of MS patients, respectively [15]. Lower limbs are more severely involved than either the arms or the trunk in lower MS spasticity [16] and are seen in one-half to two-thirds of patients with MS [17]. Multiple sclerosis-related spasticity has a fluctuating intensity and increases at night. Moderate and severe spasticity in MS impairs quality of life and is a major source of depression and considerable psychosocial stress.

Treatment usually combines physiotherapy with application of medications. The main oral anti-spasticity agents are those which act on the GABAergic system (baclofen, pregabalin, gabapentin, and benzodiazepines) and α-2 adrenergic system (tizanidine) and those that block calcium release into the muscles (dantrolene). Cannabinoids also have an anti-spasticity effect. Satisfaction with the currently available anti-spasticity agents is low [18]. In severe cases, phenol injection, baclofen pump, and selective dorsal rizotomy are employed.

Botulinum Toxin Treatment of Spasticity in Multiple Sclerosis

Snow et al. [19] were the first to study the efficacy of onabotulinumtoxinA in multiple sclerosis in a double-blind, placebo-controlled crossover study. Adductor brevis, longus, and magnus were injected with 100, 100, and 200 units, respectively. Among the patients, seven of nine were found to have significant reduction of spasticity and reported improvement of hygiene versus one out nine in the placebo group. In a similar study of five patients with multiple sclerosis, Grazko et al. [20] found that injection of a smaller dose into two adductors (total of 200 units of onaA, adductors brevis, and longus) resulted in improvement of spasticity (at least 2 grade improvement of Ashworth scale) and led to patient satisfaction. Later, a double-blind, parallel-designed study in 74 patients with MS [21] demonstrated improvement of spasticity and hygiene after administration of 1000 or 1500 units of abobotulinumtoxinA (Dysport) into adductor muscles with a significant increase of the distance between the knees during the passive movements (especially in the 1500 unit group).

Does spasticity of MS respond as well to botulinum toxin treatments compare to the spasticity of other conditions—for example, spasticity associated with stroke? This seems to be the subject of some controversy. In a study of 99 patients (33 MS, 33 stroke, and 33 cerebral palsy), the investigators found MS spasticity required substantially higher doses of BoNT to be effective [22]. Conversely, a large prospective registry of 508 patients with over 2000 injections reported no difference between different forms of spasticity (stroke, MS, CP, traumatic brain injury) in terms of the dose and magnitude of response to BoNTs [23].

Treatment of MS spasticity with BoNTs seems to be safe. The aforementioned studies report mild to moderate transient weakness in a small number of patients. A recent review found that treatment of spasticity even with high doses of onabotulinumtoxinA (800–1000 units) for MS spasticity caused transient weakness in 35% of the patients but no serious or life-threatening side effects [24]. Our own experience with over 100 patients with MS spasticity supports the effectiveness of this treatment in improving hygiene, quality of life, and, in some cases, even ambulation. Furthermore, many patients report a reduction of spasticity associated pain. We have observed no serious side effects with nearly a 1000 injections for MS spasticity. In the lower extremity, many patients respond well to injections of brevis and longus adductors only. With onabotulinumA (botox), we start with 75–100 units injected into each muscle (200–300 units for both sides). The adductor brevis is partly under the longus (Fig. 1), and both adductors can be injected close to the groin and at the medial part of the thigh after palpating the region. In severe spasticity, the combined muscle mass of the two feels like a tight rope, and injections in may not require EMG. If the first treatment is not satisfactory, subsequent injections can use higher doses and/or include the adductor magnus. For adductor injections in MS, we usually do not go beyond 500 units.

Case Report

A 34-year-old female with a history of remitting and relapsing multiple sclerosis developed progressive spastic paraparesis. On examination, both legs displayed significantly increased tone with prominent adductor spasticity forcing overadduction of the thighs. The patient complained of difficulty in dressing and undressing and in maintaining hygiene. She walked with a walker, slowly and with a scissoring gait. On palpation, both the adductor brevis and longus felt very tight. A total of 150 units of onabotulinumtoxinA, divided into two 75 units was injected on each side into the combined mass of adductor brevis and longus (Fig. 1b). Over a 5-year period of follow-up, the patient received injections every 3–4 months. Each treatment improved the adductor tone and relieved the patient's tightness and discomfort. She reported better ambulation and greater ease in performing cleaning tasks, with resulting improvement of her hygiene. To her surprise, her urinary urgency and frequency also improved, which she attributed to overall muscle relaxation in the region.

Pain

Pain is a common symptom in multiple sclerosis. Foley et al. [25] reported a prevalence of 63% for pain in MS, with 26% of the patients suffering from neuropathic pain. Truini et al. [26] described nine categories of pain in multiple sclerosis: trigeminal neuralgia, Lhermitte's phenomenon, ongoing extremity pain (dysaesthetic pain), painful tonic spasms, spasticity-associated pain, pain associated with optic neuritis, musculoskeletal pain, migraine, and treatment-induced pain. The first three are examples of central neuropathic pain.

The MS-associated neuropathic pain (usually central neuropathic pain, CNP) develops secondary to demyelination and plaque formation in the brain and spinal cord [27]. Dysaesthetic extremity pain has a prevalence of 12–28% in MS and often presents with tingling or burning, affects the legs predominantly, and worsens at night [26, 27]. Lhermitte's phenomenon, a paroxysmal electric shock-like pain usually evoked by neck flexion, begins in the back of the neck and spreads to the lower limbs. A prevalence of 41% for this phenomenon has been reported in MS in one recent study [28].

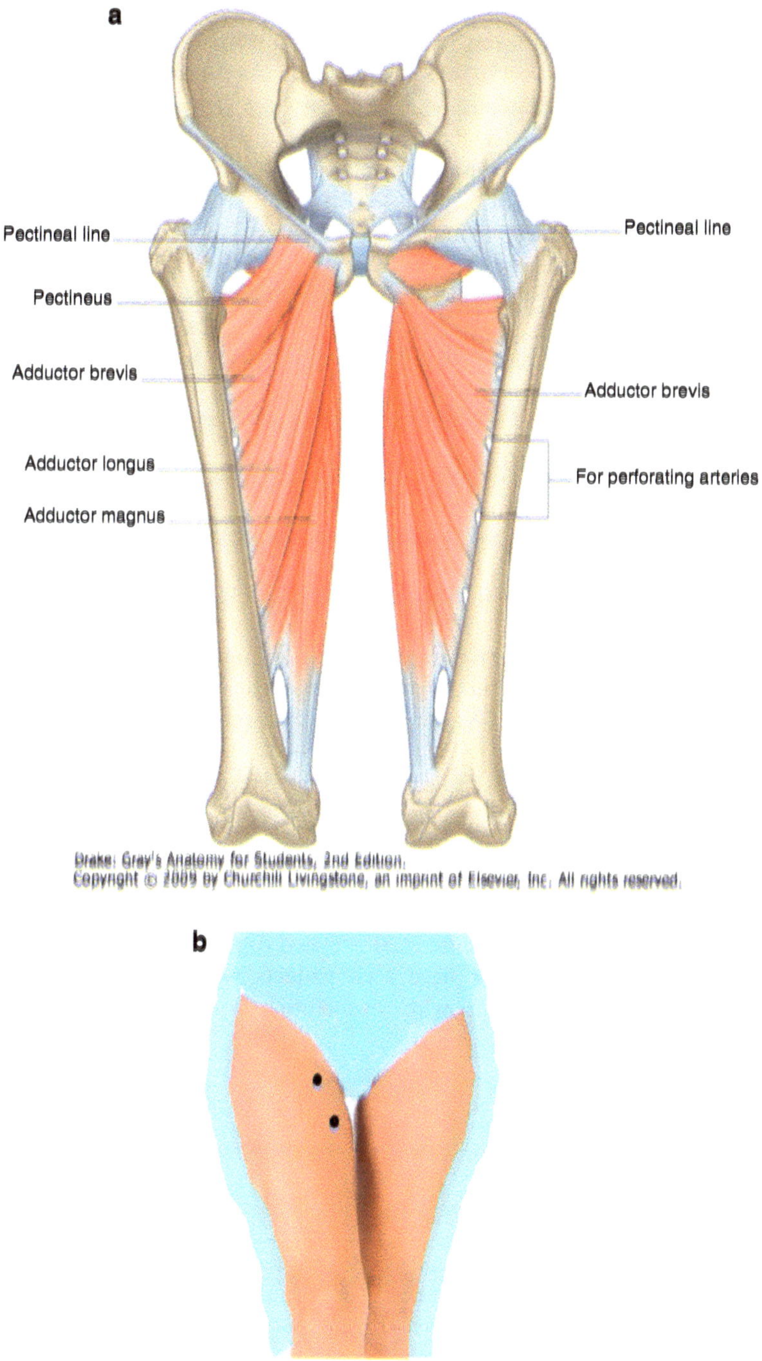

Fig. 1 (**a**) Anatomy of thigh adductors from Gray's anatomy for students reproduced with permission from Elsevier. (**b**) Site of injection into adductor brevis and longus (case report)

Trigeminal neuralgia (Tic Douloureux, TN) is characterized by a lancinating, sudden, usually unilateral, severe, stabbing pain in the distribution of one or more branches of the trigeminal nerve. TN frequently attacks the second or third division and rarely affects the ophthalmic branch of the nerve. The lifetime prevalence of trigeminal neuralgia is 0.3% [29] but in a patient with MS, this figure rises to 2–6% [30, 31]. Bilateral trigeminal neuralgia favors secondary form (e.g., MS) since classical (idiopathic) TN is rarely bilateral [32]. Based on Class I and II studies, the Therapeutic and Assessment Subcommittee of the American Academy of Neurology qualifies carbamazepine as an established and effective (Level A) and oxcarbamazepine as probably effective (Level B) treatment for TN. There is also limited evidence for the efficacy of baclofen, lamotrigine, and pimozide in TN (Level C) [33]. The recommendations of the International Association regarding the Study of Pain (IASP) for the treatment of neuropathic pain are shown in Table 1.

Botulinum Toxin Treatment of Neuropathic Pain and Trigeminal Neuralgia

Botulinum toxins have been shown to influence and alleviate pain through a variety of mechanisms. Some of our knowledge, gained from animal studies, includes peripheral and central inhibition of pain modulators and transmitters (substance P, calcitonin geese-related peptide, glutamate), decrease of local inflammation, and inhibition of sodium channels, among others [35–37].

In human pain, high-quality clinical trials (Class I and II) have shown efficacy in post-herpetic neuralgia, post-traumatic neuralgia, and diabetic neuropathy [38–40]. Four randomized, placebo-controlled, blinded studies have shown significant improvement of trigeminal neuralgia after botulinum toxin treatment (Table 2).

The clinical trials depicted in Table 2 represent investigations in classic trigeminal neuralgia. Clinical trials specific to MS-related trigeminal neuralgia with botulinum toxins do not exist. We have seen patients with MS-related trigeminal neuralgia in whom treatment with onabotulinumtoxinA improved the TN significantly.

Table 1 Recommended treatment of neuropathic pain—from Dworkin et al. [34]

First line	TCAs (e.g., nortriptyline), SNRIs (e.g., duloxetine and venlafaxine), voltage-gated calcium channel α2-8 subunit ligands (e.g., gabapentin and pregabalin), and topical lignocaine (Na + channel blocker).
Second line	Strong opioid analgesics (e.g., morphine, oxycodone, methadone, fentanyl) and tramadol (alone or in combination with a first-line agent).
Third line	Antiepileptic drugs (e.g., carbamazepine, lamotrigine, oxcarbazepine, topiramate, and valproic acid), mexiletine (orally active lignocaine analog), *N*-methyl-D-aspartate receptor antagonists (e.g., ketamine, memantine), and topical capsaicin, cannabinoids.

Table 2 Botulinum toxin treatment of trigeminal neuralgia Placebo-controlled, blinded clinical trials (RTCs)

Authors	Type/class	Number	Toxin	Units	Follow-up (weeks)	Outcome measure and results
Wu et al. 2012 [41]	DB/I	42	Chinese	75	13	VAS and PGIC ($p = 0.001$)
Zuniga et al. 2013 [43]	DB/I	36	onaA	60	8 and 12	VAS ($p = 0.01$ at 12 weeks)
Shehata et al. 2013 [42]	SB/III	20	onaA	40 and 60	12	VAS ($p = 0.0001$)
Zhang et al. 2014 [44]	DB/I	84	Chinese	25 and 75	1 and 8	VAS and PGIC ($p < 0.05$ at 8 weeks)—same efficacy for 25 and 75 units

DB double blind, *SB* single blind, *VAS* visual analog scale, *PGIC* patient global impression of change, *onaA* onabotulinumtoxinA (Botox)

Case Report

A 42-year-old female with a history of remitting and relapsing multiple sclerosis since age 18 was referred to Yale Botulinum Toxin Clinic with a complaint of bouts of disabling facial pain over the preceding 2 years. The pain occurred in brief episodes of few seconds, had a jabbing quality, and involved the left side of the face. It was severe and the patient described it as "intolerable, brings tears into my eyes." The frequency was several times per day. Touching the middle or lower part of the face (left side) often evoked the pain. Treatment with carbamazepine, oxcarbazepine, and gabapentin provided no satisfactory relief. She responded to the subcutaneous injection of onabotulinumtoxinA, 2.5 units into 12 sites (Fig. 2). The pain frequency dropped to 1–2 per month and the intensity from 9–10 to 1–3 on the VAS scale. Repeated injections every 3–4 months had the same effect.

Pain Associated with Spasticity

Spasticity is usually associated with significant discomfort and in one study 65% of the patients with spasticity complained of spasticity-related pain [45]. Three placebo-controlled, blinded studies of stroke cohorts have reported significant improvement of pain (measured by VAS) after treatment of spasticity with abobotulinumtoxinA [46–48]. In a recent prospective study of 131 patients with spasticity [45], of which 19% had multiple sclerosis, 60% of the patients reported significant improvement of spasticity-related pain after treatment with onabotlinumtoxinA.

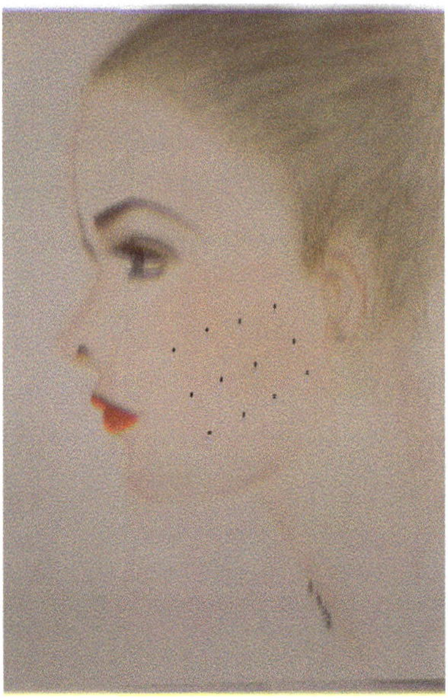

Fig. 2 Points of onabotulinumtoxinA injections for a patient with multiple sclerosis and trigeminal neuralgia (case described with trigeminal neuralgia). Each area was injected subcutaneously with 2.5 units. Drawing from Dr. Tahereh Mousavi

Migraine

Patients with multiple sclerosis suffer from migraine more often than the normal population. In a recent mail survey of 1300 patients with MS, 46% of the patients reported migraine, with 15% having headaches >15 days per month (chronic migraine) [49]. Gelfand et al. [50] critically reviewed the literature on this subject. Among ten cross-sectional studies, five clearly had a high incidence of migraine in patients with multiple sclerosis. The authors concluded, however, that the "effect size," is small and a causal relationship still remains to be determined. Although no RTCs have been reported regarding treatment of multiple sclerosis-associated migraine with botulinum toxins, because of the established efficacy of BoNTs in chronic migraine [51], it is likely that botulinum toxins will be effective in treating chronic migraine in MS patients.

Painful Tonic Spasms

Tonic spasms (previously called tonic seizures) occur in patients with multiple sclerosis and are attributed to ephatic transmission between demyelinated fibers in the spinal cord, brain stem, and cerebral white matter [52]. These spasms are painful and can occur frequently. Although in some cases they subside after a few weeks, those that persist can be the cause of significant discomfort. Restivo et al. [53] investigated the efficacy of onabotulinumtoxinA in five patients with multiple sclerosis and tonic spasms. The three men and two women, age 25–52 years, suffered from

Table 3 From Restivo et al. [53]

	Baseline	Day 8	Day 30	Day 90	Day 120
Intensity (0–3)	2.6	1.2	0.6	1.4	2.4
Pain frequency—episodes/month	12	2.8	2.8	4.2	12

multiple sclerosis for 3–16 years. Three patients had upper limb problems and 80 units of onabotulinumtoxinA was injected into their finger flexors and extensors. Two with lower limb spasms received 120 units in their gastrocnemius and 50 units into the toe flexors. A pain scale of 0–3 was used to assess the pain intensity. Patients were followed for 8, 30, 90, and 120 weeks. The effects of botulinumtoxinA injection on severity and frequency of the painful tonic spasms are shown in Table 3.

While the results of this observation are encouraging they need to be confirmed by larger future studies.

Bladder Disorders in Multiple Sclerosis

Anatomy—The human urinary system consists of the kidneys, ureters, urinary bladder, and the urethra. The transitional epithelial tissue lining the bladder, ureters, bladder, and part of the urethra is the urothelium which expands as needed during urine storage. Underneath the transitional epithelial lining of the bladder is the detrusor muscle, a smooth muscle that exerts the contractions necessary for bladder emptying during micturition. Proximally, at the junction between the bladder and the urethra is the internal sphincter, which consists of vertically oriented fibers of smooth muscle that provide the involuntary prevention of urine leakage. Distally, along the urethra, past the prostate gland in males, is the external sphincter, which consists of circular fibers of striated muscle encircling the urethra and which exerts secondary, and voluntary, prevention of urine leakage.

The functions of storing and emptying of urine are controlled by the sympathetic and parasympathetic nervous systems, respectively. Sympathetic input is mediated via the hypogastric nerve, which originates from T10 to L2 in the spinal cord. Parasympathetic input is mediated via the pelvic splanchnic nerve and originates from S2 to S4 in the spinal cord. The somatic input to the distal urethral sphincter originates from the anterior horn of S2 to S4 in the Onuf nucleus and is mediated via the pudendal nerve. General visceral afferent (GVA) fibers are part of the autonomic nervous system, which arise from the bladder and monitor minute pressure and stretch changes in the urothelium and carry sensory impulses to the sacral micturition center (SMC) and on to the periaqueductal gray, pontine micturition center (PMC) and cerebral cortex. Once the frequency of the afferent sensory impulses crosses a threshold, micturition becomes necessary.

During the filling phase, the internal sphincter remains tonic under sympathetic input. However, during micturition, the internal sphincter is allowed to relax via parasympathetic input. The detrusor muscle relaxes via sympathetic input during the filling phase and contracts through parasympathetic input during micturition. The detrusor muscle, in addition to several subtypes of muscarinic cholinergic receptors, also contains beta-adrenergic cathecholamine receptors. The internal sphincter also contains catecholamine receptors but of the alpha-adrenergic subtype. In the presence of cathecolamines, beta-adrenergic receptors trigger relaxation while the alpha-adrenergic receptors trigger contraction. The external urethral sphincter is under somatic control and contracts voluntarily to provide continence until micturition can be conveniently initiated [54].

The PMC, which is located in the dorsal pontine tegmentum, seems to be the main center for signaling the detrusor muscle to contract and the outer sphincter muscle to relax at the initiation of voiding PAG, which receives extensive input from the bladder, may turn voiding function on and off by signaling to PMC [55]. A complex cortical network communicates with these subcortical structures to maintain the storage and emptying bladder functions [56].

Dysfunction of the urinary system is common in multiple sclerosis. A recent review of 45 epidemiological articles reports a wide range of prevalence ranging from 6.9% to 95%, which reflects the inclusion of cohorts with different severity [57]. A survey conducted by the North American Research Committee on Multiple Sclerosis (NARCOMS) on 9702 patients with MS found that 65% complained of moderate to severe symptoms, which included increased frequency, urgency, nocturia, and leakage [58].

Wintner et al. [59] have reviewed the current knowledge about urinary system dysfunction in multiple sclerosis. In one study, 70% of the patients with multiple sclerosis stated that their voiding problem impacts moderately to severely on their quality of life [60]. Demyelinating lesions in multiple sclerosis that involve different levels of the central nervous system can lead to different types of voiding problems. Neurogenic detrusor overactivity (NDO) in a hyperreflexic bladder leads to problems with storage, small bladder, and common symptoms of urgency and incontinence. It is the most common urinary problem in multiple sclerosis [61].

Primary management of NDO should incorporate behavioral approaches such as increasing the frequency of micturition, limiting fluid intake in the evening, limiting intake of caffeine and alcohol, and using absorbent undergarments and bed pads. Anticholinergics are the first-line treatment to manage urinary symptoms of bladder overactivity, although conservative measures such as pelvic-floor muscle training and desmopressin spray may be beneficial, particularly in the early stages of the disease [61]. Anticholinergics are effective when detrusor overactivity is mild, but with increasing disability, these medications may lose efficacy. Decreased salivary production and dry mouth, decreased gastrointestinal motility and worsening of constipation, decreased sweating (which prevents cooling) and xerophthalmia are common side effects of anticholinergic drugs.

Detrusor-sphincter dyssynergia is another dysfunction of the voiding system observed in multiple sclerosis. Although less common than NDO, it can be the cause of significant discomfort. Here, the external sphincter cannot relax after detrusor contraction. The result, like NDO, is increased intravesicular pressure with potential damage to the upper urinary system. Muscle relaxants and alpha adrenergic blockers offer modest help. Drainage by catheterization is often required. A urethral stent may be helpful. Sphincterectomy can help but has the drawback of causing permanent incontinence. In women with MS, a weakened pelvic floor can cause laxity of the urethra and lead to stress incontinence. A variety of treatment approaches with limited efficacy exist to help this condition and alleviate the urinary incontinence [57].

Botulinum Toxin Treatment of Urinary Symptoms in Multiple Sclerosis

Following Carpenter's seminal observation in 1967 [62] that local injection of botulinumtoxinA can significantly decrease the acetylcholine content of the bladder tissue, investigators began to study the effect of this toxin on symptoms arising from bladder emptying and storage problems. Earlier studies focused on detrusor–sphincter dyssynergia. In 1990, two independent investigators reported small blinded studies denoting improvement of urinary symptoms in nine and five patients after injection of 100 units of botulinumtoxinA into the external urethral sphincter [63, 64]. Over the succeeding years, the attention of researchers was shifted to neurogenic detrusor overactivity (NDO), a problem which is more commonly encountered in neurogenic conditions such as multiple sclerosis and spinal cord injury. In January 2013, the FDA approved the use of onabotulinumtoxinA for the treatment of neurogenic detrusor overactivity based on two large multicenter studies (DIGNITY study) [65, 66]. Cruz and Nitti [67] have described the details of these studies in a recent article. In brief, a total of 691 patients with either multiple sclerosis or spinal cord injury were included in the study. The criteria for inclusion consisted of having >14 episodes of urinary incontinence per week and not being adequately managed by at least one anticholinergic medication. The three arms of the study included (1) injection of 200 units of onabotulinumtoxinA, (2) injection of 300 units of onabotulinumtoxinA, and (3) placebo injection. Injections were performed through endoscopy and into the bladder at 30 points, sparing the trigone. The primary outcome measure was the total number of urinary incontinence episodes at 6 weeks.

The pooled data from two studies showed significant improvement of incontinence episodes (IE) at 6 weeks (Table 4—Cruz et al. and Ginsberg et al. studies). Botulinum toxin groups also showed a significant increase in the quality of life and patient satisfaction scores (25 versus 11 and 78 versus 44, respectively). Side effects included urinary retention and urinary tract infection (defined by changes in the urine, not by patient symptoms). In regard to efficacy, there was no difference between spinal cord injury patients and those who had multiple sclerosis. Patient with multiple sclerosis, however, experienced more urinary retention (29.5% versus 4.6%) with a greater need for intermittent catheterization. Table 4 shows double-blind studies which have investigated the efficacy of botulinum toxins in alleviating detrusor overactivity of patients with multiple sclerosis.

Table 4 Double-blind studies of Botulinum toxin treatment of detrusor overactivity in multiple sclerosis

Authors	Number	Toxin	Units	Primary outcome	Results
Schurch et al. 2005 [69]	59	OnabotulinumtoxinA	200 and 300	Reduction of IEs/week	300: 10.5/week 200: 6.3/week Saline: 1.4/week $p = 0.04$
Hershorn et al. 2011 [70]	57[a]	OnabotulinumtoxinA	300	Reduction of IE at week 6	onaA: 4.7/week Saline: 1.3/week
Cruz et al. 2011 [65]	275 154 with MS	OnabotulinumtoxinA	300 and 200	Reduction of IEs at week 6	300: 19/week (0.047) 200: 21/week Saline 13/week
Ginsberg et al. 2012 [66]	416 222 with MS	OnabotulinumtoxinA	300 and 200	Reduction of IEs at week 6	300: 23/week 200: 21/week Saline: 9/week $p < 0.001$
Sussman et al. 2013 [71]	275[a]	OnabotulinumtoxinA	300 and 200	Mean improvement score in 16-item QoL6	300: 14.9 200: 12.4 $p > 0.001$) compared to placebo
Denys et al. 2016 [72]	47[a]	AbobotulinumtoxinA	750 Two groups: 15 and 30 injection sites	Reduction of IEs at week 12	Both groups reduced the IE/week > more than placebo (statistically not significant)

IE incontinence episode, *QOL* quality of life
[a]The studied cohort includes MS patients but the number of MS patients in the cohort has not been defined

Injection Technique

The FDA-approved dose of onabotulinumtoxinA for NDO treatment is 200 units, injected submucosally into 30 locations. Injections are performed through an endoscope via a flexible needle. Each vial of 100 units is diluted with 10 cc of saline without preservative. The bladder's trigone is spared. However, in different institutions, experts modify dose and technique. For example, Dr. C. Smith from Baylor Medical College routinely includes trigone in the plan of injection to influence the abundant nerve fibers in this area. He uses 100 units of onabotulinumtoxinA for the spontaneously voiding patients and 200 units for those who are already catheterizing [68].

Treatment of Detrusor-Sphincter Dyssynergia (DSD) with BoNTs in MS Patients

Small, blinded studies conducted with spinal cord injury patients suggested improvement of bladder function in DSD after injection of 100 units of onabotulinumtoxinA into the external sphincter [63, 64]. In multiple sclerosis, a multicenter, double-blind RTC of 86 patients showed no difference between the toxin (onabotulinumtoxinA) and placebo in regard to post-voiding residual urine (primary outcome at 4 weeks, single injection of 100 units). However, the BoNT group showed a significant increase in the voiding volume and a significant reduction in detrusor pressure [73].

Botulinum Toxin Treatment of Movement Disorders in Multiple Sclerosis

Tremor

Tremor is estimated to occur in 25–58% of the patients with multiple sclerosis [74]. In most patients the tremor is postural and intentional, although resting tremor and midbrain tremor (Holmes tremor) can be seen also, albeit in a smaller number of patients. In a large survey of 777 patients with multiple sclerosis and tremor, less than half of the patients (46%) were happy with their symptomatic treatment and considered their tremor a cause of significant functional impairment [75]. Tremor was considered severe by 15% of the patients who participated in this survey. Cerebellum and cerebellar circuits have been implicated as a major site of intentional tremor in multiple sclerosis. Limited postmortem and magnetic resonance imaging data in patients with MS and tremor have shown demyelinating lesions affecting cerebellar white matter, superior cerebellar peduncles, and cerebellar connections inside the brain stem. Pharmacological treatment of cerebellar tremor is difficult, and clinical trials for MS-related cerebellar tremor are rare. In one study propranolol, isoniazide, and alcohol failed to improve MS-related cerebellar tremor [76].

Botulinum Toxin Treatment of Tremor in Multiple Sclerosis

Injection of onabotulinumtoxinA into the forearm muscles with a fixed dose and fixed number of muscles has been shown to improve essential tremor and resting tremor of Parkinson disease but causes unacceptable weakness in 30–40% of the patients [77, 78]. More recently, however, it has been shown that using a customized approach (flexible dose and variable number of muscles), satisfactory tremor improvement can be achieved with a much lower incidence of finger weakness (<10%) [79, 80]. No RTCs have been conducted assessing the efficacy of botulinum toxins in multiple sclerosis-related tremor. Clark [81] reported the results of treating five patients with intention tremor in multiple sclerosis with onabotulinumtoxinA. Flexor and extensor muscles of the forearm were injected with 40 units. Two of the five patients received another 100 units 2 months later. No statistically significant improvement of tremor was noted at 2 and 8 weeks after injection. The physicians' impression of change, however, showed a trend toward improvement in the toxin group. Patients, in contrast, reported more weakness in the injected extremities.

We had a satisfactory response in a patient with multiple sclerosis and Holmes (midbrain) tremor using substantially higher doses of onabotulinumtoxinA (400 units) in the affected extremity.

Case Report

A 38-year-old man with a history of multiple sclerosis characterized by several episodes of motor, sensory, and visual deficits and typical MS-type signal abnormalities on MRI was referred to the Yale Botulinum Toxin Clinic for "uncontrollable shakes of the left arm." On examination, the patient was quadriparetic, walked with crutches, and had decreased sensations in both lower limbs. The left hand demonstrated a resting tremor of 3–4 Hz, which increased in amplitude during posture and intentional movements, and at times, assumed very high amplitude ballistic oscillations. Movements of the neck and torso and sometimes the right upper limb also enhanced the tremor and resulted in ballistic movements of the whole left arm. The sensitivity of the left arm to neck and torso movements interfered with the patient's sleep and alimentation and substantially impaired his quality of life. Treatment with baclofen and benzodiazepines provided limited relief. A total of 400 units of onabotulinumtoxinA was injected, including 75 units into the left biceps, left triceps, pectoralis major, and flexor carpi ulnaris, 40 units into the left trapezius, and 20 units into flexor carpi radialis, pronator teres, and finger flexors. In a clinic visit 2 weeks later, the patient's resting tremor was reduced and movements of the neck and torso no longer caused ballistic movements of the left hand. The left upper limb was diffusely weaker, but the patient reported satisfaction with the treatment on the patient's global-impression-of-change scale (6 out of 7). Repeat injections over the next 2 years produced similar results.

Facial Myokymia

The term "myokymia" was first coined by Schultze in 1895 (myokymie) and refers to a clinical phenomenon characterized by undulating, rippling movements like tiny snakes under the skin [82]. Andermann et al. [83] are credited for the first detailed description of facial myokymia including the description of the electrophysiological features. Single motor unit discharges of 50–150 Hz are electrical counterparts of myokymia and often occur in doublets and triplets with the regular frequency of up to several times per second. The characteristic clinical and electrical features of myokymia differentiate it from fasciculations, facial dyskinesias, and neuromyotonia. Myokymia can be focal or diffuse. Multiple sclerosis and pontine glioma are common causes of focal and facial myokymia, whereas Guilain–Barre syndrome, episodic ataxia type I, and exposure to radiation can cause focal or generalized myokymia. The myokymic movements are painless but can be the cause of significant stress, especially when they involve the face.

Jacobs et al. [84] have studied the site of the demyelinating lesions responsible for continuous facial myokymia in 12 patients with multiple sclerosis. In 11 of the 12 patients, lesions were identified on MRI. In all 11 patients, the demyelinating plaque involved the postero-lateral pontine tegmentum affecting the intra-axial part of the facial nerve after emerging from the nucleus and after the genu of the nerve. Pharmacological treatment of myokymia is usually unsuccessful. Transient improvement has been reported with intravenous prednisolone [85]. Increasing serum-ionized calcium decreases the intensity of the myokymia of peripheral origin but not in central myokymia [86].

Botulinum Toxin Treatment

Reported observations on significant improvement of facial myokymia in multiple sclerosis after injection of BoNT into the facial muscles are outlined in Table 5.

Our experience agrees with these observations in facial myokymia. We had two patients with facial myokymia, one due to multiple sclerosis and the other due to pontine glioma in whom injection of similar doses of onabotulinumtoxinA stopped the movements.

Table 5 Published cases of facial myokymia in multiple sclerosis treated with BoNT

Name	Age/ sex	Side	Toxin	Total dose	Result	Follow-up
Sedano et al. 2000 [85]						
Case 1	26/M	*Left*	onaA	10 units[a]	Ceased in 7 days	19 months
Case 2	42/M	*Left*	onaA	12.5 units[b]	Ceased in 7 days	Not stated
Habek et al. 2012 [87]	28/F	Right	onaA	10 units[c]	Ceased in 10 days	Not stated

[a]2.5 units in upper and lower lids and perioral region
[b]2.5 units into five locations around the left eye
[c]2.5 units into each location; upper lid, lower lid, zygomaticus, mentalis

Other Potential Indications of Botulinum Toxins in Multiple Sclerosis

Dysphagia: Restivo et al. [88] injected onabotulinumtoxinA percutaneously into the hyperactive cricopharyngeal muscle of 14 patients with multiple sclerosis and severe oropharyngeal dysphagia. The penetration/aspiration scale (PAS) was assessed, at weeks 1, 4, 12, 16, 18, and 24 after toxin injections. All patients showed significant improvement. The authors concluded that onabotulinumtoxinA injections into cricopharyngeal muscle might help MS patients with upper esophageal sphincter spasticity.

Internuclear ophthalmoplegia: Internuclear ophthalmoplegia (INO) resulting from lesion(s) of medial longitudinal fasciculus is common in multiple sclerosis patients with brain stem lesions. Injection of botulinumtoxinA into one or more extra-ocular muscles of 16 patients with MS has improved double vision in 87% of the patients. The effect on recovery of convergence and stereopsis was less satisfactory (18% and 12%). The study concluded that injection of BoNT-A into extra ocular muscles can help patients with multiple sclerosis with INO who suffer from disturbing double vision [89].

Sialorrhea: Sialorrhea is a common symptom in MS patients with dysphagia. Sialorrhea responds well to both type A and type B botulinum toxins [90]. Although it is likely that sialorrhea of dysphagic MS patients will respond to BoNT treatment, data relevant to this issue do not yet exist.

Conclusion

Several symptoms associated with multiple sclerosis have been shown responsive to botulinum toxin treatment. The bladder's detrusor overactivity, spasticity, and trigeminal neuralgia are indications in which efficacy has been established via randomized, double-blind clinical trials. Encouraging reports suggest efficacy in dysphagia, myokymia, tonic spasms, and internuclear ophthalmoplegia. Sialorrhea is also a potential indication, although information specific to multiple sclerosis has not been reported. With recommended doses, BoNT treatment seems to be safe in multiple sclerosis and side effects are reported to be transient.

References

1. Dilokthornsakul P, Valuck RJ, Nair KV, Corboy JR, Allen RR, Campbell JD. Multiple sclerosis prevalence in the United States commercially insured population. Neurology. 2016;86:1014–21.

2. Zwibel HL, Smrtka J. Improving quality of life in multiple sclerosis: an unmet need. Am J Manag Care. 2011;17(Suppl 5 Improving):S139–45.
3. Adelman G, Rane SG, Villa KF. The cost burden of multiple sclerosis in the United States: a systematic review of the literature. J Med Econ. 2013;16:639–47.
4. Compston A, Wekerle H, McDonald I. The origin of multiple sclerosis: a synthesis. In: Compston A, editor. McAlpine's multiple sclerosis. 4th ed. New York: Churchill Livingstone; 2006. p. 273–84.
5. Diebold M, Derfuss T. Immunological treatment of multiple sclerosis. Semin Hematol. 2016;53(Suppl 1):S54–7.
6. Moeini-Naghani I, Hashemi-Zonouz T, Jabbari B. Botulinum toxin treatment of spasticity in adults and children. Semin Neurol. 2016;36:64–72.
7. Lance JW. The control of muscle tone, reflexes, and movement: Robert Wartenberg lecture. Neurology. 1980;30:1303–13.
8. Gracies JM. Pathophysiology of spastic paresis. I: paresis and soft tissue changes. Muscle Nerve. 2005;31(5):535–51.
9. Gracies JM. Pathophysiology of spastic paresis. II: emergence of muscle over activity. Muscle Nerve. 2005;31(5):552–71.
10. Gioux M, Petit J. Effects of immobilizing the cat peroneus longus muscle on the activity of its own spindles. J Appl Physiol (1985). 1993;31(5):552–71.
11. Crone C, Johnsen LL, Biering-Srensen F, Nielsen JB. Appearance of reciprocal facilitation of ankle extensors from ankle flexors in patients with stroke or spinal cord injury. Brain. 2003;126(pt 2):495–507.
12. Kheder A, Nair KPS. Spasticity: pathophysiology, evaluation and management, practical. Neurology. 2012;12:289.
13. Yelnik AP, Simon O, paratte B, et al. How to clinically assess and treat muscle overactivity in spastic paresis. J Rehabil Med. 2010;42:801–7.
14. Pozzilli C. Advances in the management of multiple sclerosis spasticity: experiences from recent studies and everyday clinical practice. Expert Rev Neurother. 2013;13(12 Suppl):49–54.
15. Rizzo MA, Hadjimichael OC, preingerova J, Vollmer TL. Prevalence and treatment of spasticity reported by multiple sclerosis patients. Mult Scler. 2004;10:589–95.
16. Zwibel HL. Contribution of impaired mobility and general symptoms to the burden of multiple sclerosis. Adv Ther. 2009;26(12):1043–57.
17. Martin A, Abogunrin S, Kurth H, Dinet J. Epidemiological, humanistic, and economic burden of illness of lower limb spasticity in adults: a systematic review. Neuropsychiatr Dis Treat. 2014;10:111–22.
18. Flachenecker P, Henze T, Zettl UK. Spasticity in patients with multiple sclerosis—clinical characteristics, treatment and quality of life. Acta Neurol Scand. 2014;129(3):154–62.
19. Snow BJ, Tsui JK, Bhatt MH, Varelas M, Hashimoto SA, Calne DB. Treatment of spasticity with botulinum toxin: a double-blind study. Ann Neurol. 1990;28:512–5.
20. Grazko MA, Polo KB, Jabbari B. Botulinum toxin A for spasticity, muscle spasms, and rigidity. Neurology. 1995;45:712–7.
21. Hyman N, Barnes M, Bhakta B, Cozens A, Bakheit M, Kreczy-Kleedorfer B, Poewe W, Wissel J, Bain P, Glickman S, Sayer A, Richardson A, Dott C. Botulinum toxin (Dysport) treatment of hip adductor spasticity in multiple sclerosis: a prospective, randomised, double blind, placebo controlled, dose ranging study. J Neurol Neurosurg Psychiatry. 2000;68:707–12.
22. Phadke CP, Davidson C, Ismail F, Boulias C. The effect of neural lesion type on botulinum toxin dosage: a retrospective chart review. PM R. 2014;6:406–11.
23. Schramm A, Ndayisaba JP, Auf dem Brinke M, Hecht M, Herrmann C, Huber M, Lobsien E, Mehnert S, Reuter I, Stenner A, van der Ven C, Winterholler M, Kupsch A, Wissel J. Spasticity treatment with onabotulinumtoxin A: data from a prospective German real-life patient registry. J Neural Transm (Vienna). 2014;121:521–30.
24. Nuanthaisong U, Abraham N, Goldman HB. Incidence of adverse events after high doses of onabotulinumtoxinA for multiple indications. Urology. 2014;84:1044–8.

25. Foley PL, Vesterinen HM, Laird BJ, Sena ES, Colvin LA, Chandran S, Mac Leod MR, Fallon M. Prevalence and natural history of pain in adults with multiple sclerosis: systematic review and meta-analysis. Pain 2013;154:632–42.
26. Truini A, Barbanti P, Pozzilli C, Cruccu G. A mechanism-based classification of pain in multiple sclerosis. J Neurol. 2013;260:351–67.
27. Nurmikko TJ, Gupta S, Maclver K. Multiple sclerosis-related central pain disorders. Curr Pain Headache rep. 2010;14:189–95.
28. Al-Araji AH, Oger J. Reappraisal of Lhermitte's sign in multiple sclerosis. Mult Scler. 2005;11:398–402.
29. Mueller D, Obermann M, Yoon MS, et al. Prevalence of trigeminal neuralgia and persistent idiopathic facial pain: a population-based study. Cephalalgia. 2011;31:1542–8.
30. Broggi G, et al. Operative findings and outcomes of microvascular decompression for trigeminal neuralgia in 35 patients affected by multiple sclerosis. Neurosurgery. 2004;55:830–8. discussion 838–9
31. Katusic S, Williams DB, Beard CM, Bergstralh EJ, Kurland LT. Epidemiology and clinical features of idiopathic trigeminal neuralgia and glossopharyngeal neuralgia similarities and differences, Rochester, Minnesota, 1945-1984. Neuroepidemiology. 1991;10:276–81.
32. Cruccu G, Finnerup NB, Jensen TS, Scholz J, Sindou M, Svensson P, Treede RD, Zakrzewska JM, Nurmikko T. Trigeminal neuralgia: new classification and diagnostic grading for practice and research. Neurology. 2016;87:220–8.
33. Cruccu G, Gronseth G, Alksne J, et al. AANEFNS guidelines on trigeminal neuralgia management. Eur J Neurol. 2008;15:1013–28.
34. Dworkin RH, O'Connor AB, Audette J, Baron R, Gourlay GK, Haanpää ML, Kent JL, Krane EJ, Lebel AA, Levy RM, Mackey SC, Mayer J, Miaskowski C, Raja SN, Rice AS, Schmader KE, Stacey B, Stanos S, Treede RD, Turk DC, Walco GA, Wells CD. Recommendations for the pharmacological management of neuropathic pain: an overview and literature update. Mayo Clin Proc. 2010;85 (3 Suppl):S3–14.
35. Meng J, Wang J, Lawrence G, Dolly JO. Synaptobrevin I mediates exocytosis of CGRP from sensory neurons and inhibition by botulinum toxins reflects their anti-nociceptive potential. J Cell Sci. 2007;120(16):2864–74.
36. Cui M, Khanijou S, Rubino J, Aoki KR. Subcutaneous administration of botulinum toxin A reduces formalin-induced pain. Pain. 2004;107:125–33.
37. Shin MC, Wakita M, Xie DJ, et al. Inhibition of membrane Na+ channels by a type botulinum toxin at femtomolar concentrations in central and peripheral neurons. J Pharmacol Sci. 2012;118:33–42.
38. Xiao L, Mackey S, Hui H, Xong D, Zhang Q, Zhang D. Subcutaneous injection of Botulinum toxin A is beneficial in postherpetic neuralgia. Pain Med. 2010;11:1827–33.
39. Ranoux DA, Attal N, Morain F, Bouhassira D. Botulinum toxin type a induces direct analgesic effects in chronic neuropathic pain. Ann Neurol. 2008;64:274–83.
40. Yuan RY, Sheu JJ, YuJ M, Chen WT, Tseng IJ, Chang HH, Hu CJ. Botulinum toxin for diabetic neuropathic pain: a randomized double-blind crossover trial Neurology. 2009;72: 1473–8.
41. Wu CJ, Lian YJ, Zheng YK, et al. Botulinum toxin type A for the treatment of trigeminal neuralgia: results from a randomized, double-blind, placebo-controlled trial. Cephalalgia. 2012;32:443–50.
42. Shehata HS, El-Tamawy MS, Shalaby NM, Ramzy G. Botulinum toxin-type A: could it be n effective treatment option in intractable trigeminal neuralgia? J Headache Pain. 2013;14:92.
43. Zuniga C, Piedimonte F, Diaz S, Micheli F. Acute treatment of trigeminal neuralgia with onabotulinum toxin A. Clin Neuropharmacol. 2013;36:146–50.
44. Zhang H, Lian Y, Ma Y, et al. Two doses of botulinum toxin type A for the treatment of trigeminal neuralgia: observation of therapeutic effect from a randomized, double-blind, placebo-controlled trial. J Headache Pain. 2014;15:65.
45. Shaikh A, Phadke CP, Ismail F, Boulias C. Relationship between Botulinum toxin, spasticity, and pain: a survey of patient perception. Can J Neurol Sci. 2016;43:311–5.

46. Marco E, Duarte E, Vila J, Tejero M, Guillen A, Boza R, Escalada F, Espadaler JM. Is botulinum toxin type A effective in the treatment of spastic shoulder pain in patients after stroke? A double-blind randomized clinical trial. Rehabil Med. 2007;39: 440–7.
47. Shaw LC, Price CI, van Wijck FM, Shackley P, Steen N, Barnes MP, Ford GA, Graham LA, Rodgers H; BoTULS Investigators. Botulinum toxin for the upper limb after stroke (BoTULS) trial: effect on impairment, activity limitation, and pain. Stroke. 2011;42:1371–9.
48. Rosales RL, Kong KH, Goh KJ, Kumthornthip W, Mok VC, Delgado-De Los Santos MM, Chua KS, Abdullah SJ, Zakine B, Maisonobe P, Magis A, Wong KS. Botulinum toxin injection for hypertonicity of the upper extremity within 12 weeks after stroke: a randomized controlled trial. Neurorehabil Neural Repair. 2012;26: 812–21.
49. Moisset X, Ouchchane L, Guy N, Bayle DJ, Dallel R, Clavelou P. Migraine headaches and pain with neuropathic characteristics: comorbid conditions in patients with multiple sclerosis. Pain. 2013;154:2691–9.
50. Gelfand AA, Gelfand JM, Goadsby PJ. Migraine and multiple sclerosis: epidemiology and approach to treatment. Mult Scler Relat Disord. 2013;2:73–9.
51. Dodick DW, Turkel CC, DeGryse RE, Aurora SK, Silberstein SD, Lipton RB, Diener HC, Brin MF; PREEMPT Chronic Migraine Study Group. OnabotulinumtoxinA for treatment of chronic migraine: pooled results from the double-blind, randomized, placebo-controlled phases of the PREEMPT clinical program. Headache. 2010; 50:921–36.
52. Shibasaki H, Kuroiwa Y. Painful tonic seizures in multiple sclerosis. Arch Neurol. 1974;30:47–51.
53. Restivo DA, Tinazzi M, Patti F, Palmeri A, Maimone D. Botulinum toxin treatment of painful tonic spasms in multiple sclerosis. Neurology. 2003;61:719–20.
54. Yonnet GJ, Fjeldstad AS, Carlson NG, Rose JW. Advances in the management of neurogenic detrusor overactivity in multiple sclerosis. Int J MS Case. 2013;15:66–72.
55. Holstege G. Descending motor pathways and spinal motor system.: limbic and non-limbic components. Prog Brain Res. 1991;87:307–421.
56. Griffiths D. Neural control of micturition in humans: a working model. Nat Rev Urol. 2015;12:695–705.
57. Ruffion A, Castro-Diaz D, Patel H, Khalaf K, Onyenwenyi A, Globe D, et al. Systematic review of the epidemiology of urinary incontinence and detrusor overactivity among patients with neurogenic overactive bladder. Neuroepidemiology. 2013;41:146–55.
58. Mahajan ST, Patel PB, Marrie RA. Under treatment of overactive bladder symptoms in patients with multiple sclerosis: an ancillary analysis of the NARCOMS Patient Registry. J Urol. 2010;183:1432–7.
59. Wintner A, Kim MM, Bechis SK, Kreydin EI. Voiding dysfunction in multiple sclerosis. Semin Neurol. 2016;36:34–40.
60. de Sèze M, Ruffion A, Denys P, Joseph PA, Perrouin-Verbe B, GENULF. The neurogenic bladder in multiple sclerosis: review of the literature and proposal of management guidelines. Mult Scler. 2007;13:915–28.
61. Fowler CJ, Panicker JN, Drake M, et al. A UK consensus on the management of the bladder in multiple sclerosis. J Neurol Neurosurg Psychiatry. 2009;80:470–7.
62. Carpenter FG. Motor responses of the urinary bladder and skeletal muscle in botulinum intoxicated rats. J Physiol. 1967;188:1–11.
63. Schurch B, Hauri D, Largo M, Kreienbühl B, Meyer E, Rossier AB. Effects of Botulinum a toxin on the periurethral striated sphincter of the neurogenic bladder. Preliminary study. 63. J Urol (Paris). 1990;96:375–80.
64. Dykstra DD, Sidi AA. Treatment of detrusor-sphincter dyssynergia with botulinum A toxin: a double-blind study. Arch Phys Med Rehabil. 1990;71:24–6.
65. Cruz F, Herschorn S, Aliotta P, Brin M, Thompson C, Lam W, Daniell G, Heesakkers J, Haag-Molkenteller C. Efficacy and safety of onabotulinumtoxinA in patients with urinary incontinence due to neurogenic detrusor overactivity: a randomised, double-blind, placebo-controlled trial. Eur Urol. 2011;60: 742–50.

66. Ginsberg D, Gousse A, Keppenne V, Sievert KD, Thompson C, Lam W, Brin MF, Jenkins B, Haag-Molkenteller C. Phase 3 efficacy and tolerability study of onabotulinumtoxinA for urinary incontinence from neurogenic detrusor overactivity. J Urol. 2012;187:2131–9.
67. Cruz F, Nitti V. Chapter 5: clinical data in neurogenic detrusor overactivity (NDO) and overactive bladder (OAB). Neurourol Urodyn. 2014;33(Suppl 3):S26–31.
68. Smith CP, Chancellor MB. Botulinum toxin to treat neurogenic bladder. Semin Neurol. 2016;36:5–9.
69. Schurch B, de Sèze M, Denys P, Chartier-Kastler E, Haab F, Everaert K, Plante P, Perrouin-Verbe B, Kumar C, Fraczek S, Brin MF; Botox Detrusor Hyperreflexia Study Team. Botulinum toxin type a is a safe and effective treatment for neurogenic urinary incontinence: results of a single treatment, randomized, placebo controlled 6-month study. J Urol. 2005; 174:196–200.
70. Herschorn S, Gajewski J, Ethans K, Corcos J, Carlson K, Bailly G, Bard R, Valiquette L, Baverstock R, Carr L, Radomski S. Efficacy of botulinum toxin A injection for neurogenic detrusor overactivity and urinary incontinence: a randomized, double-blind trial. J Urol. 2011;185:2229–35.
71. Sussman D, Patel V, Del Popolo G, Lam W, Globe D, Pommerville P. Treatment satisfaction and improvement in health-related quality of life with onabotulinumtoxinA in patients with urinary incontinence due to neurogenic detrusor overactivity. Neurourol Urodyn. 2013;32:242–9.
72. Denys P, Del Popolo G, Amarenco G, Karsenty G, Le Berre P, Padrazzi B, Picaut P; Dysport Study Group. Efficacy and safety of two administration modes of an intra-detrusor injection of 750 units dysport® (abobotulinumtoxinA) in patients suffering from refractory neurogenic detrusor overactivity (NDO): a randomised placebo-controlled phase IIa study. Neurourol Urodyn. 2016; 36(2):457–62. [Epub ahead of print].
73. Gallien P, Reymann JM, Amarenco G, Nicolas B, de Sèze M, Bellissant E. Placebo controlled, randomised, double blind study of the effects of botulinum A toxin on detrusor sphincter dyssynergia in multiple sclerosis patients. J Neurol Neurosurg Psychiatry. 2005;76:1670–6.
74. Meador W, Salter AR, Rinker JR II. Symptomatic management of multiple sclerosis-associated tremor among participants in the NARCOMS registry. Int J MS Care. 2016;18:147–53.
75. Koch M, Mostert J, Heersema D, et al. Tremor in multiple sclerosis. J Neurol. 2007;254:133–45.
76. Koller WC. Pharmacologic trials in the treatment of cerebellar tremor. Arch Neurol. 1984;41:280–1.
77. Jankovic J, Schwartz K, Clemence W, Aswad A, Mordaunt J. A randomized, double-blind, placebo-controlled study to evaluate botulinum toxin type A in essential hand tremor. Mov Disord. 1996;11:250–6.
78. Rahimi F, Bee C, Debicki D, Roberts AC, Bapat P, Jog M. Effectiveness of BoNT A in Parkinson's disease upper limb tremor management. Can J Neurol Sci. 2013;40:663–9.
79. Rostami R, Chow C, Richardson D, Jabbari B, Machado D. Botulinum toxin treatment of essential tremor—a customized approach—AAN—poster S27-002, AAN meeting, April 18, 2016.
80. Mittal OS, Rostami R, Machado D, Richardson D, Jabbari B. A double blind investigation of efficacy and safety of incobotulinumtoxinA in Parkinson disease tremor—a customized injection approach. Abstract # 1896. Platform presentation S40-007, AAN meeting April 18, 2016.
81. Clarke CE. Botulinum toxin type A in cerebellar tremor caused by multiple sclerosis. Eur J Neurol. 1997;4:68–71.
82. Gutmann L, Gutmann L. Myokymia and neuromyotonia. J Neurol. 2004;251:138–42.
83. Andermann F, Cosgrove JBR, Lloyd-Smith DL, Gloor P, McNaughton FL. Facial myokymia in multiple sclerosis. Brain. 1961;84:31–44.
84. Jacobs L, Kaba S, Pullicino P. The lesion causing continuous facial myokymia in multiple sclerosis. Arch Neurol. 1994;51:1115–9.
85. Sedano MJ, Trejo JM, Macarrón JL, Polo JM, Berciano J, Calleja J. Continuous facial myokymia in multiple sclerosis: treatment with botulinum toxin. Eur Neurol. 2000;43:137–40.
86. Gutmann L, Brick JF, Riggs JE. Calcium and myokymia of brainstem origin. Neurology. 1986;36:26–30.

87. Habek M, Adamec I, Gabelić T, Brinar VV. Treatment of facial myokymia in multiple sclerosis with botulinum toxin. Acta Neurol Belg. 2012;112:423–4.
88. Restivo DA, Marchese-Ragona R, Patti F, Solaro C, Maimone D, Zappalá G, Pavone A. Botulinum toxin improves dysphagia associated with multiple sclerosis. Eur J Neurol. 2011;18:486–90.
89. Murthy R, Dawson E, Khan S, Adams GG, Lee J. Botulinum toxin in the management of internuclear ophthalmoplegia. J AAPOS. 2007;11:456–9.
90. Hosp C, Naumann MK, Hamm H. Botulinum toxin treatment of autonomic disorders: focal hyperhidrosis and Sialorrhea. Semin Neurol. 2016;36:20–8.

Clinical Uses of the Botulinum Toxin and Ophthalmology

Jennifer A. Galvin

Introduction

Since 1980, botulinum toxin has become an influential treatment in many medical sub-specialties, especially in ophthalmology [1–3]. Botulinum toxin is a potent neurotoxin which blocks the release of acetylcholine at the neuromuscular junction of cholinergic nerves [4]. When used appropriately, it will weaken the force of muscular contraction or inhibit glandular secretion. Recovery occurs over three to four months from nerve terminal sprouting and regeneration of inactivated proteins necessary for degranulation of acetylcholine vesicles [4, 5].

Clinically applicable ophthalmic conditions include but are not limited to: (1) dystonic movement disorders such as benign essential blepharospasm and hemifacial spasm, (2) strabismus, (3) nystagmus, (4) apraxia of the eyelid opening, (5) eyelid myokyomia, (6) facial nerve synkinesis, (7) lacrimal hypersecretion syndromes, (8) eyelid retraction, (9) spastic entropion, and (10) corneal protective ptosis. In this chapter, I briefly review the history of botulinum toxin development in clinical medicine and review the above ten indications for ophthalmology-related conditions, as well as periorbital/facial aesthetic use. In addition, I will address botulinum toxin-related complications.

J.A. Galvin, M.D. (✉)
Department of Ophthalmology and Visual Science, Yale University School of Medicine, New Haven, CT, USA

Pediatric Ophthalmology and Strabismus, Yale University School of Medicine, New Haven, CT, USA
e-mail: gennygalvin@gmail.com

B. Jabbari (ed.), *Botulinum Toxin Treatment in Clinical Medicine*,
DOI 10.1007/978-3-319-56038-0_8

Historical Background

Nearly 200 years ago, in Germany, Dr. Justinius Kerner categorized many cases of botulism, which he described as sausage poisoning, because the Latin word for sausage is *botulus* [6]. Since then, researchers have discovered that the botulinum toxin is an exotoxin produced by the bacterium *Clostridium botulinum*, an anaerobic Gram-positive sporulating organism and considered the most potent biological toxin in nature. Of note, Kerner identified a fatty acid as the poisonous agent and he hypothesized that the toxin may have a therapeutic role in an overactive nervous system [6]. In 1895, Dr. van Ermengen first isolated the bacterium *Clostridium botulinum* from the remnants of a preserved ham meal, which poisoned musicians in Belgium [6]. In 1928, Dr. Sommer purified the botulinum neurotoxin as a stable acid precipitate in the USA and Dr. Schantz at the US National Academy of Sciences laboratory in Maryland prepared large drug quantities for governmental use and institutional use during World War II. After the war, in 1949, Dr. Burgen discovered that botulinum toxin blocks neurotransmitter release at the neuromuscular junction and in 1950s, Dr. Brooks discovered that acetylcholine was the blocked neurotransmitter at the nerve terminal [6].

In 1980, the first report of clinical use in strabismus was published by Dr. Alan Scott and Dr. Schantz who tested botulinum toxin in monkeys to determine its effectiveness to treat strabismus [1]. In the 1980s, Dr. Scott formed a company to produce botulinum toxin type A, called Oculinum, and started FDA-clinical trials for the toxin's use in strabismus and blepharospasm. For approximately 20 years, Oculinum in a dose of 150 mg was the source worldwide [1, 6]. In 1989, the FDA approved Oculinum for use in patients 12 years and older to treat strabismus, blepharospasm, and hemifacial spasm. Later, in 1991, Allergen purchased the right to market the toxin and changed the name to Botox and in 1997, they produced a new bulk batch with a higher specific potency, reducing its antigenic potential [6]. Subsequent FDA approval was granted in 2000 for its use for cervical dystonia and spastic dysphonia and Elan Pharmaceuticals marketed botulinum toxin type B under the name of Myobloc for cervical dystonia that same year [6].

Regarding its aesthetic use, in 1987, Canadian dermatologist Dr. Alastair Carruthers reported the successful treatment for forehead frown lines with Botox and in 2002, the FDA approved this drug for the treatment of glabellar furrows [7]. Since 1989, botulinum toxin has been approved to be an effective treatment for more than 100 clinical disorders associated with involuntary muscle activity, excessive muscle tone, pain syndromes, and hypersecretory conditions.

Movement Disorders and Focal Dystonias

Patients with benign essential blepharospasm have a focal cranial dystonia which involves both the eyelid and forehead muscles. Patients with this disorder have involuntary orbicularis muscle contractions, which results in increased frequency of

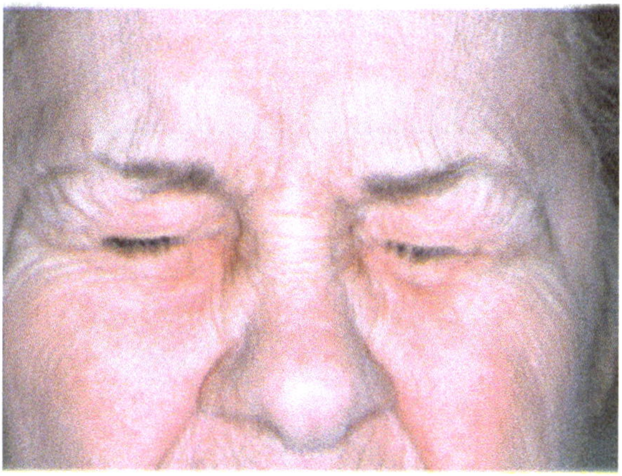

Fig. 1 External photograph of a patient with essential blepharospasm involving the orbicularis muscle and the protractors of the medial brow. Reprinted with permission from Dutton JJ, Buckley EG, American Medical Association, 1986.

blinking. In patients with a severe case, blinking is so forceful and repetitive that the patient cannot open his or her eyes, resulting in functional blindness (Fig. 1). Of note, the etiology is unknown, but researchers think it may involve dysfunction of the central coordination of visual sensory input and motor output to the eyelids [6]. In this way, severely affected patients have increased sensitivity to visual stimuli and an exaggerated motor response with excessive blinking and forced eyelid closure. Since the early 1980s, botulinum toxin has been used in the treatment of blepharospasm; it remains the treatment of choice for the successful control of eyelid spasms [3, 8–14]. In a review of 29 published reports, researchers reported that botulinum toxin type A as an effective treatment in 70–100% of patients, with a mean of 93.3% success [11]. The average dose of toxin type A is 12.5–25 units per eye, injected just beneath the skin into the orbicularis muscle. The most common injection pattern is noted in Fig. 2: into the medial and lateral portion of the upper and lower, lid pre-tarsal orbicularis. Of note, avoiding the central lid region minimizes the risk of ptosis [14, 15]. The treatment benefit in patients has been reported to last an average of 13 weeks [3, 12–14]. If patients develop resistance to type A, clinicians can use botulinum toxin type B, using 1000–2500 units per eye [6]. In comparison to type A, type B is used in much higher doses and has a shorter duration of effect of 8–10 weeks, with a greater tendency to diffuse to adjacent areas of the orbicularis muscle [3, 11]. Complications to its use for benign essential blepharospasm include ptosis, dry eyes, diplopia, eyelid edema, facial weakness, lagophthalmos, and ecchymoses [10–16]. Ptosis is the most common complication related to the injection technique and the spread of the chemodenervation to the levator muscle. Clinicians describe ptosis as a complication in 10–15% of treated patients [3, 13–16]. Typically, for most patients, complications are mild and transient and resolve with recovery of the levator function. For other complications involving dry eyes and a poor blink response from the treatment of the orbicularis muscle weakening and lagophthalmos, lubrication of the eyes with artificial tears can be used for beneficial therapy.

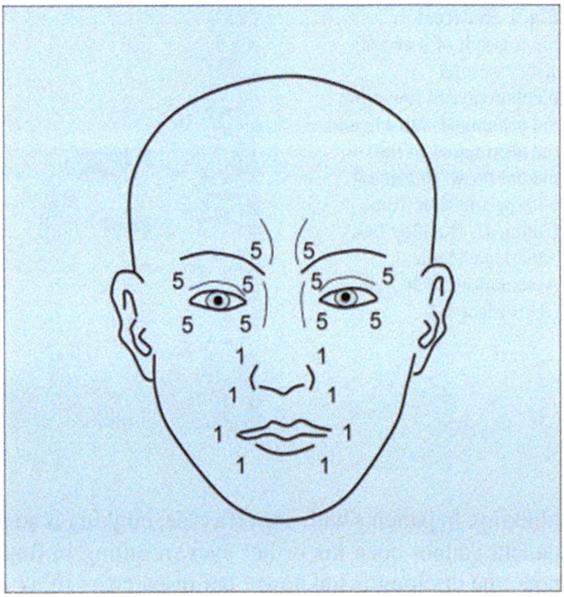

Fig. 2 Average injection pattern of botulinum toxin type A for benign essential blepharospasm. Reprinted with permission from Dutton JJ, Fowler AM, Elsevier, 2007.

When focal movement disorders affect the lower face, patients have spasms along the sides of the nose, the mouth, and chin, described as oromandibular dystonia [6, 11]. These patients are severely affected when they eat and/or speak. Treatment for oromandibular dystonia is a smaller dose of type A, 1–2 units injected into the affected facial muscles, with no more than 10 units on each side [3, 8, 11]. Of note, because the lower face muscles are small, complications such as overdosage and facial weakness can cause patients to develop drooling or cheek biting [3, 6, 16].

When a patient has a regional dystonia from two adjacent facial dystonias, benign essential blepharospasm and oromandibular dystonia, they are suffering from Meige Syndrome [3, 6, 8, 16, 17]. These patients typically present initially with orbicularis muscle spasm; months to years later, spasms spread to the lower face and neck. Facial spasms become less severe with 1–2 unit injections of botulinum toxin type A to the orbicularis muscle in combination with the middle and lower facial muscles [14–17]. As with the treatment of oromandibular dystonia, type A injection should be limited to no more than 10 units on each side [3, 8, 11].

Unilateral recurrent spasms are characterized as the neuromuscular disorder of hemifacial spasm, where there are unilateral recurrent twitches of the facial muscles innervated by the facial nerve as seen in Fig. 3a. Of note, unlike benign essential blepharospasm, these hemifacial spasms persist during sleep and are not related to hypersensory input [6, 18–20]. Researchers describe the etiology as a mechanical irritation of the facial nerve at its exit root by a sagging arterial branch and typically, treatment with botulinum type A toxin is successful, with an average of 25–35 units on the affected facial side lasting typically 16 weeks [6, 8–20]. Treatment is successful in 90% of the cases as seen in Fig. 3b [6].

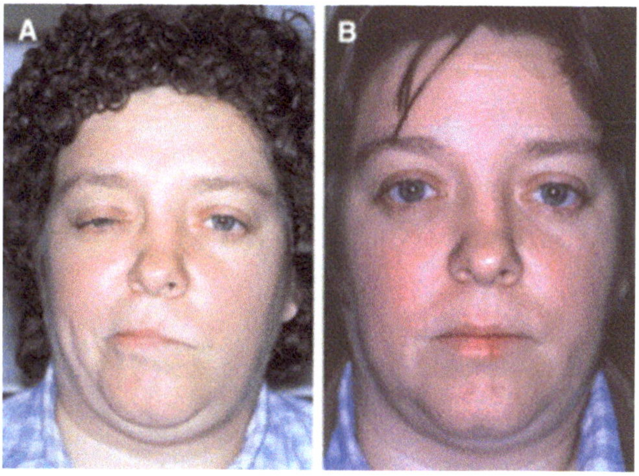

Fig. 3 External photograph of a patient with hemifacial spasm (**a**) before and (**b**) 2 weeks after injection with botulinum toxin. Reprinted with permission from Dutton JJ, Buckley EG, American Medical Association, 1986. All rights reserved

Strabismus

Botulinum toxin was first used in ophthalmology by Dr. Alan Scott to treat strabismus [1, 2]. The idea was to weaken the force of contraction of specific opposing muscles to straighten the eye. It was also hoped that permanent muscle weakness would result from the treatment [1, 2, 6]. Injection into the muscle usually requires the use of electromyography (EMG)-guided placement of the needle to ensure the toxin is accurately delivered (Fig. 4a, b), although an open sky technique without EMG-guidance is often used [1, 2, 6]. Researchers noted that for patients with infantile esotropia, early treatment to the bilateral medial rectus muscles was effective in restoration of motor and sensory fusion with good long-term results as compared to surgical intervention [21]. Another study noted improved alignment in all children younger than 7 months of age at the initial treatment for esotropia [22]. Researchers evaluating older children, with a mean age of 5.4 years, with an acute onset esotropia less than 30 prism diopters, noted improved alignment in 79% of the children with the initial treatment with botulinum toxin [23]. Similarly, another study with both children and adults with small angle esotropia, less than 15 prism diopters, had successful treatment of strabismus, with 60% achieving binocularity [24].

In the treatment of paretic strabismus, and in particular, sixth nerve palsy, botulinum toxin has been evaluated over the last two decades [25–27]. Successful treatment to weaken the medial rectus muscle in patients with traumatic sixth nerve palsy, in the acute phase, within 6 months from the traumatic onset, recovery of abduction, and recovery of binocular fusion has been found in up to 70% of patients in some studies [25, 26]. However, the researcher found that chronic sixth nerve palsy did not benefit from botulinum toxin treatment alone, but rather the use of

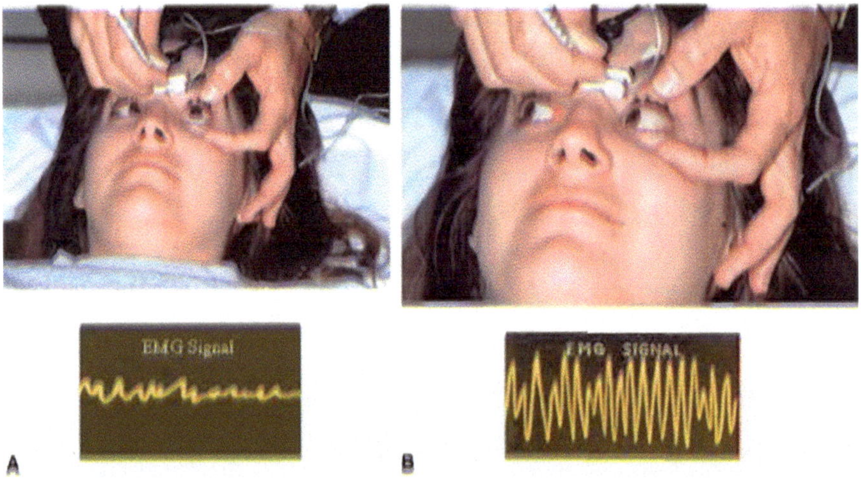

Fig. 4 External photograph of demonstration of a botulinum toxin injection with electromyography (EMG) guidance in the left medial rectus muscle for left cranial nerve sixth palsy. (**a**) The patient looks out of the field of action during the injection with minimal EMG signal prior injection. (**b**) The patient looks into the field of action with an increase in the EMG signal with the injection. Reprinted with permission of Buckley EG, Trigler L, Hess DB, Lippincott Williams & Wilkins, 1993. All rights reserved

botulinum toxin as an adjunct to strabismus surgery improved alignment and relief of diplopia for patients [27, 28].

In patients with sensory strabismus, we would expect to have limited success with long-term alignment due to the decreased visual acuity in the misaligned eye. One study in which botulinum toxin treatment was used to prevent muscle contracture [29] noted an improved alignment in 73% of the patients with sensory strabismus with follow-up of 6 months.

Treatment of secondary paralytic strabismus associated with sixth nerve palsies in children with brain tumors with botulinum toxin was not beneficial, however [30]. In another study of fourth nerve palsies due to trauma, authors also noted no benefit in using botulinum toxin injections to the inferior oblique muscle, requiring 83% of the patients to have strabismus surgery to improve ocular alignment and relieve diplopia [31].

In patients with larger strabismus angles, such as in one study with a mean angle of esotropia at 40 prism diopters, botulinum toxin type A was an effective long-term treatment for improved alignment and relief of diplopia in 72% of the patients after an 18-month follow-up [32]. However, for chronic and larger angle strabismus, botulinum toxin treatment to the rectus muscles is usually used as an adjunct to strabismus surgery for improved ocular alignment.

In addition to treating esotropia, the treatment of exotropia has been evaluated by researchers. In particular, one study of patients with intermittent exotropia with a mean angle at 45 prism diopters achieved fusional control and improved ocular alignment with botulinum toxin treatment to the lateral rectus muscles in 86% of the

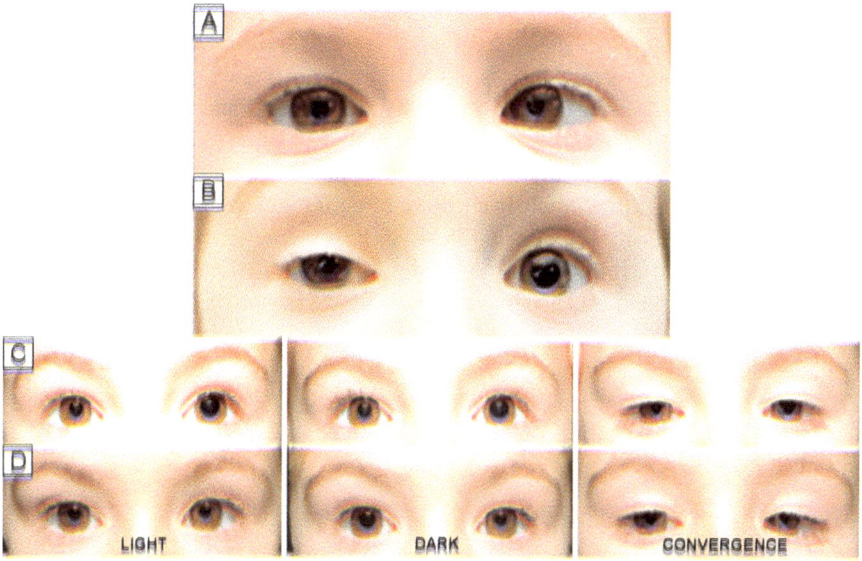

Fig. 5 External photographs in a patient who developed a tonic left pupil after botulinum toxin-A injection of both medial rectus muscles. (**a**) Pre-injection. (**b**) 2 weeks after injection. (**c**) 55 days after injection. (**d**) 55 days after injection, post-pilocarpine. In this patient, affected pupils showed minimal responsiveness to light but constriction with fixation on a near accommodative target. At 55 days post-injection, anisocoria was reversed after treatment of both eyes with pilocarpine 0.125%, diagnostic for tonic pupil. Reprinted with permission from Christiansen SP, Chandler DL, Lee KA et al, Elsevier, 2016. All rights reserved

patients at 6-month follow-up [33]. Other exodeviations have also been studied. One study of adult patients with convergence insufficiency showed improved reading symptoms with resolved diplopia after botulinum toxin treatment to the bilateral or unilateral lateral rectus muscle(s) [34].

Complications from botulinum toxin use in strabismus include ptosis, localized pain, subconjunctival hemorrhage at the conjunctival injection site, over-correction of the ocular alignment, blurry vision, diplopia, and tonic pupil. Such complications have been reported in one recent NIH-sponsored study of botulinum toxin treatment for pediatric esotropia [35] (Fig. 5).

Congenital and Acquired Nystagmus and Oscillopsia

Patients with nystagmus suffer from inability to maintain foveal fixation, and hence, experience blurry vision. If this occurs during the first decade of life, amblyopia, decreased vision during visual development, can occur. Patients with congenital nystagmus can have significant long-term consequences on binocularity, vision, and often have a compensatory head tilt or face turn to achieve better vision. Identification of the pattern and type of nystagmus is important to determine the etiology. Often, patients with congenital motor nystagmus and acquired nystagmus have shown decreased or dampening of their eye movements with injection of botulinum toxin directly into multiple rectus muscles, both the antagonist and agonist of the pulley system [36, 37]. More specifically, researchers have found that the decreased nystagmus amplitude improves vision in 43% of patients treated [37].

Although used today with great reservation, previous studies of patients with oscillopsia treated with retrobulbar injection of botulinum toxin reported improved vision in up to 66% of the patients [38–40]. However, other researchers reported concern regarding the injection of the botulinum toxin into the retrobulbar space; it was not successful and patients experienced complications of ptosis and diplopia [41].

Apraxia of Eyelid Opening

Patients with apraxia of eyelid opening suffer from a non-paralytic inability to raise the upper eyelid. Of note, these patients do not have traumatic injury to the orbicularis muscle or levator muscle. Initially, this disease was described among patients with a supranuclear injury who could not achieve activation of the levator muscle. Apraxic eyelids have been described in patients with several different disorders such as dystonic Parkinson syndrome, progressive supranuclear palsy, and isolated loss of levator muscle control. A fourth type is found in some patients with blepharospasm, referred to as blepharospastic apraxia. These patients have subclinical contractions of the pre-tarsal orbicularis muscle which persist into the post-blink phase and cause suppression of levator muscle contraction [42]. For patients with blepharospastic apraxia, injecting 5 units of botulinum toxin type A into the pretarsal orbicularis and Riolan's muscles along the upper eyelid margin has had beneficial results [43]. Researchers have noted that it is unclear if the problem is an abnormal co-contraction of the levator and orbicularis muscles or a failure of the relaxation of the orbicularis during the levator contraction [42, 43].

Eyelid Myokymia

Patients with eyelid myokymia have an uncontrollable twitching of the orbicularis muscle, typically involving the lower eyelid. The twitching is triggered by stress, fatigue, caffeine, or alcohol. While researchers do not completely understand the mechanism, in most patients, it is benign and self-limiting condition in which the affected muscle shows a slow, undulating fine movement in the most superficial muscle layers [44]. EMG studies have reported rhythmic bursts of normal-appearing potentials in group discharges [44]. For patients with eyelid myokymia, injection of 5 units of botulinum toxin type A into the superficial orbicularis muscle temporarily relaxes the muscle until the condition resolves spontaneously [45].

Facial Nerve Synkinesis After Facial Nerve Palsy

Patients with resolved facial nerve palsy, a benign condition, often have long-term motor dysfunction, including increased blinking and blepharospasm-like activity on the non-facial nerve palsy side. Researchers think that this post-peripheral facial nerve synkinesis results from increased excitability of the facial motorneurons of the trigeminal reflexes [6, 46]. Abnormal axonal branching leads to synkinesis, with patients having involuntary contraction of muscles innervated by one branch of the facial nerve when attempting to voluntarily activate muscles previously innervated by other branches [46, 47]. In this way, patients can have facial deformity, inappropriate eyelid closure, drooling, muscle twitching, or muscle spasms [6, 46–48]. Treatment with injection of 1–2 units of botulinum type A toxin has been shown to be highly effective in reducing synkinetic movements for 3–9 months in these patients [46–48].

Lacrimal Hypersecretion Syndromes

In the early stages of treatment with botulinum toxin for patients with hemifacial spasm, researchers observed decreased facial sweating on the treated side as a side effect [49]. This finding led to the use of botulinum toxin in the management of hyperhidrosis of the face, axilla, and the palms [49, 50]. Patients who suffer from Frey syndrome experience a gustatory facial sweating from the aberrant regeneration of facial nerve secretomotor fibers to sweat glands after a parotidectomy [50–52]. Researchers have found success in the management of hypersecretion with the injection of botulinum type A toxin into the postganglionic sympathetic cholinergic nerves to eccrine sweat glands in the affected areas [49, 50]. Typically, 0.5–0.8 units/cm^2 of type A toxin is injected intradermally at 10–25 sites. Large clinical studies noted greater than 50% reduction in sweating compared to baseline [50, 51]. Benefits from this treatment can last 3–5 months; higher doses can extend the benefits for up to 12 months [50, 51].

Gustatory epiphora, often called crocodile tears, may occur due to excessive lacrimation associated with salivatory stimulation [49–52]. For example, patients may have had a prior proximal facial nerve injury leading to aberrant regeneration of secretomotor fibers and mid-directed new fibers attach to lacrimal rather than salivary glands. [50–52]. Another more common secondary form of lacrimal hypersecretion is seen in patients who have ocular surface irritation from trichiasis or eyelid malposition, corneal exposure, or blepharitis.

Primary idiopathic lacrimal hypersecretion, often intermittent, may also be experienced in the absence of any obvious ocular surface abnormality. For patients suffering from lacrimal hypersecretion from any cause, injection of 2.5–5 units of botulinum type A toxin into the palpebral lobe of the lacrimal gland results in a clinically significant reduction in tear production and symptom improvement in 75% of patients [52]. Among these patients, relief of epiphora has been reported to last 3–4 months [52].

Eyelid Retraction

Patients with upper eyelid retraction associated with thyroid eye disease experience exposure keratopathy and in significant cases, corneal ulceration. Previous studies have shown that injection with 5–10 units of botulinum toxin type A into the levator muscle, with either transcutaneous or transconjunctival approach, can provide significant improvement in eyelid retraction with a drop in the eyelid position by 2.0–3.0 mm and results lasting for 12–14 weeks [53–57]. Complications involve over-correction with ptosis as well as diplopia noted in 10% of patients, due to involvement of the superior rectus muscle [55]. Other researchers also noted with increased retraction of the contralateral eyelid associated with the lowering of the treated eyelid with botulinum toxin (Herring's law) [56].

Spastic Entropion

Patients with spastic entropion experience a turning in of the lower eyelid with the riding up of the pre-tarsal orbicularis muscle. Usually, patients with pre-existing eyelid laxity experience corneal irritation which can cause orbicularis muscle spasm resulting in lower eyelid entropion. For these patients, relief can be achieved by weakening the pre-tarsal orbicularis muscle with injection of 5–8 units of botulinum toxin type A which reportedly eliminates the entropion for up to 3–4 months [58].

Corneal Protective Ptosis

For patients with a poor blink response or lagophthalmos, corneal exposure keratopathy can cause vision loss and compromise the health of the cornea. Protection of the cornea can be achieved by inducing ptosis with botulinum toxin treatment. Injection of 2.5–5 botulinum toxin units directly into the levator muscle through a transcutaneous approach in the superior sulcus or through a transconjunctival approach can achieve this goal without the need to surgically modify the eyelid margin via tarsorrhaphy [59, 60]. Reportedly, in 75–80% of patients, a protective ptosis results in sufficient corneal healing [60]. Of note, the botulinum toxin therapy is considered an adjunct to the treatment of the primary cause of exposure keratopathy and/or lagophthalmos.

Aesthetic Uses

Over the past decade, the use of botulinum toxin in facial rejuvenation has increased significantly [61–63]. Initially, treatment for facial wrinkles with botulinum toxin was for dynamic glabellar folds. Subsequently, treatment for the furrows created by repetitive corrugator supercillii contraction, or glabellar frown lines, were the first to show improvement with localized botulinum toxin type A treatment [61]. In particular, injection with 15–30 units of botulinum toxin type A into the corrugator muscle in a V-shaped pattern, to include both the transverse and oblique heads, between the eyebrows is effective [61–63]. The aesthetic use of this drug has now expanded to applications of many other areas of the face, including the lateral periocular rhytids (crows feet), transverse brow and forehead furrows, perioral rhytids (smokers lines), mesolabial folds (marionette lines), and platysmal bands. Moreover, the creation of a chemical brow lift with botulinum toxin can be accomplished by targeting the brow depressors, the depressor supercilii medially with the tail of the orbicularis laterally [63]. Treatment strategies for aesthetic uses vary widely and managing the expectations of the patients is very important. Complications include localized pain, facial numbness and brow droop, and ptosis.

Conclusions

The use of botulinum toxin in ophthalmologic clinical practice over the past three decades has significantly changed the ophthalmologist's management of many ocular conditions. We have benefited most from the successful treatment of our patients with benign essential blepharospasm, hemifacial spasm, acute sixth nerve palsy, small and moderate angle strabismus, and aesthetic wrinkle reduction. Care should be taken in counseling patients about this treatment modality as well as discussion of complications from the injection technique and chemodenervation of adjacent muscle groups.

References

1. Scott AB. Botulinum toxin injection of eye muscles to correct strabismus. Trans Am Ophthalmol Soc. 1981;79:734–70.
2. Scott AB, Magoon EH, McNeer KW, Stager DR. Botulinum treatment of strabismus in children. Trans Am Ophthalmol Soc. 1989;87:174–84.
3. Dutton JJ, Buckley EG. Long-term results and complications of botulinum A toxin in the treatment of blepharospasm. Ophthalmology. 1988;95:1529–34.
4. Humeau Y, Doussau F, Grant NJ, et al. How botulinum and tetanus neurotoxins block neurotransmitter release. Biochemistry. 2000;82:427–46.
5. Vissenberg I, Dieleman-Smet H, Tassignon MJ. Botulinum A toxin therapy in ophthalmology: a report of patients with facial dystonias. Bull Soc Belge Ophthalmol. 1993;248:77–82.
6. Dutton JJ, Fowler AM. Botulinum Toxin in Ophthalmology. Surv Ophthalmol. 2007;52:13–31.
7. Carruthers A, Carruthers J. Botulinum toxin type A for the treatment of glabellar rhytides. Dermatol Clin. 2004;22:137–44.
8. Scott AB, Kennedy RA, Stubbs HA. Botulinum A toxin injection as a treatment for blepharospasm. Arch Ophthalmol. 1985;103:347–50.
9. Shorr N, Seiff SR, Kopelman J. The use of botulinum toxin in blepharospasm. Am J Ophthalmol. 1985;99:542–6.

10. Cohen DA, Savino PJ, Stern MB, et al. Botulinum injection therapy for blepharospasm: a review and report of 75 patients. Clin Neuropharmacol. 1986;9:415–29.
11. Dutton JJ, Buckley EG. Botulinum toxin in the management of blepharospasm. Arch Neurol. 1986;43:380–2.
12. Engstrom PF, Arnoult JB, Mazow ML, et al. Effectiveness of botulinum toxin therapy for essential blepharospasm. Ophthalmology. 1987;17:971–5.
13. Elston JS. Long-term results of treatment of idiopathic blepharospasm with botulinum toxin injection. Br J Ophthalmol. 1987;71:664–8.
14. Carruthers J, Stubbs HA. Botulinum toxin for benign essential blepharospasm, hemifacial spasm and age-related lower eyelid ectropion. Can J Neurol Sci. 1987;14:42–5.
15. Cakmur R, Ozturk V, Uzunel F, et al. Comparison of pre-septal and pre-tarsal injections of botulinum toxin in the treatment of blepharospasm and hemifacial spasm. J Neurol. 2002;249:64–8.
16. Calace P, Cortese G, Piscopo R, et al. Treatment of blepharospasm with botulinum neurotoxin type A: long-term results. Eur J Ophthalmol. 2003;13:331–6.
17. Osako M, Keltner JL. Botulinum A toxin (Oculinum) in ophthalmology. Surv Ophthalmol. 1991;36:28–46.
18. Gonnering RS. Treatment of hemifacial spasm with botulinum A toxin: results and rationale. Ophthal Plast Reconstr Surg. 1986;2:143–6.
19. Taylor JD, Kraft SP, Kazdan MS, et al. Treatment of blepharospasm and hemifacial spasm with botulinum A toxin: a Canadian multicentre study. Can J Ophthalmol. 1991;26:133–8.
20. Sorgun MH, Yilmaz R, Akin YA, Mercan FN, et al. Botulinum toxin injections for the treatment of hemifacial spasm over 16 years. J Clin Neurosci. 2015;22(8):1319–25.
21. McNeer KW, Tucker MG, Guerry CH, et al. Incidence of stereopsis after treatment of infantile esotropia with botulinum toxin. J Pediatr Ophthalmol Strabismus. 2003;40:288–92.
22. Campos EC, Schiavi C, Bellusci C. Critical age of botulinum toxin treatment in essential infantile esotropia. J Pediatr Ophthalmol Strabismus. 2000;37:328–32.
23. Dawson EL, Marshman WE, Adams GG. The role of botulinum toxin A in acute-onset esotropia. Ophthalmology. 1999;106:1727–30.
24. Dawson EL, Lee JP. Does botulinum toxin have a role in the treatment of small angle esotropia? Strabismus. 2004;12:257–60.
25. Holmes JM, Droste PJ, Beck RW, et al. The natural history of acute traumatic sixth nerve palsy or paresis. J AAPOS. 1998;2:265–8.
26. Holmes JM, Beck RW, Kip KE, et al. Botulinum toxin treatment versus conservative management in acute traumatic sixth nerve palsy or paresis. J AAPOS. 2000;4:145–9.
27. Holmes JM, Leske DA, Christiansen SP. Initial treatment outcomes in chronic sixth nerve palsy. J AAPOS. 2001;5:370–6.
28. Rowe FL, Noonan CP. Botulinum toxin for the treatment of strabismus (review). Cochrane Database Syst Rev 2012(2):1–33. Wiley, Art. No:CD006499.
29. Han SH, Lew H, Jeong CW, et al. Effect of botulinum toxin A chemodenervation in sensory strabismus. J Pediatr Ophthalmol Strabismus. 2001;38:68–71.
30. Kerr NC, Hoehn MB. Botulinum toxin for sixth nerve palsies in children with brain tumors. J AAPOS. 2001;5:21–5.
31. Garnham LM, Lawqson JM, O'Neill D, et al. Botulinum toxin in fourth nerve palsies. Aust NZ J Ophthalmology. 1986;93:917–23.
32. Flores-Reyes EM, Castillo-Lopez MG, Toledo-Silva R, et al. Botulinum toxin type A as a treatment of partially accommodative esotropia. Arch Soc Esp Oftalmol. 2016;91(3):120–4.
33. Etezad Razavi M, Sharifi M, Armanfar F. Efficacy of botulinum toxin in the treatment of intermittent exotropia. Strabismus. 2014;22(4):176–81.
34. Saunte JP, Holmes JM. Sustained improvement of reading symptoms following botulinum toxin A injection for convergence insufficiency. Strabismus. 2014;22(3):95–9.
35. Christiansen SP, Chandler DL, Lee KA, et al. Tonic pupil after botulinum toxin-A injection for treatment of esotropia in children. J AAPOS. 2016;20(1):78–81.
36. Caruthers J, Carruthers A, et al. The treatment of congenital nystagmus with Botox. J Pediatr Ophthalmol Strabismus. 1995;32:306–87.

37. Repka MX, Savino PJ, Reinecke RD. Treatment of acquired nystagmus with botulinum neurotoxin A. Arch Ophthalmol. 1994;112:1320–4.
38. Helveston EM, Pogrebniak AE. Treatment of acquired nystagmus with botulinum A toxin. Am J Ophthalmol. 1988;106:584–6.
39. Ruben S, Dunlop IS, Elston J. Retrobulbar botulinum for treatment of oscillopsia. Aust NZ J Ophthalmol. 1994;22:65–7.
40. Ruben ST, Lee JP, O'Neil D, et al. The use of botulinum toxin for the treatment of oscillopsia. Ophthalmology. 1994;101:783–7.
41. Tomsak RL, Remler BF, Averbuch-Heller L, et al. Unsatisfactory treatment of acquired nystagmus with retrobulbar injection of botulinum toxin. Am J Ophthalmol. 1995;119:489–96.
42. Forget R, Tozlovanu V, Iancu A, et al. Botulinum toxin improves lid opening delays in blepharospasm-associated apraxia of lid opening. Neurology. 2002;58:1843–6.
43. Boghen D, Tozlovanu V, Iancu A, et al. Botulinum toxin therapy for apraxia of lid opening. Ann N Y Acad Sci. 2002;956:482–3.
44. Banik R, Miller NR. Chronic myokymia limited to the eyelid is a benign condition. J Neuroophthalmol. 2004;24:290–2.
45. Jordan DR, Anderson RL, Thiese SM, et al. Intractable orbicularis myokymia: treatment alternatives. Ophthalmic Surg. 1989;20:280–3.
46. Mountain RE, Murray JA, Quaba A. Management of facial synkinesis with botulinum toxin injection. Clin Otolaryngol Allied Sci. 1992;17:223–4.
47. Roggenkamper P, Laskawi R, Damanz W, et al. Orbicular synkinesis after facial paralysis: treatment with botulinum toxin. Doc Ophthalmol. 1994;86:395–402.
48. Chua CN, Quhill F, Jones E, et al. Treatment of aberrant facial nerve regeneration with botulinum toxin A. Orbit. 2004;23:213–8.
49. Kinkelin I, Hund M, Naumann M, et al. Effective treatment of frontal hyperhidrosis with botulinum toxin A. Br J Dermatol. 2000;143:824–7.
50. Kyrmizakis DE, Pangalos A, Papadakis CE, et al. The use of botulinum toxin type A in the treatment of Frey and crocodile tears syndromes. J Oral Maxillofac Surg. 2004;62:840–4.
51. Hofmann RJ. Treatment of Frey's syndrome (gustatory sweating) and crocodile tears (gustatory epiphora) with purified botulinum toxin. Ophthal Plast Reconstr Surg. 2000;16:289–91.
52. Keegan DJ, Geerlin G, Lee JP, et al. Botulinum toxin treatment for hyperlacrimation secondary to aberrant regenerated seventh nerve palsy or salivary gland transplantation. Br J Ophthalmol. 2002;86:43–6.
53. Scott AB. Injection treatment of endocrine orbital myopathy. Doc Ophthalmol. 1989;58:141–5.
54. Biglan AW. Control of eyelid retraction associated with Graves' disease with botulinum A toxin. Ophthalmic Surg. 1994;25:186–8.
55. Traisk F, Tallstedt L. Thyroid associated ophthalmology: botulinum toxin A in the treatment of upper eyelid retraction—a pilot study. Acta Ophthalmol Scand. 2001;79:585–8.
56. Morgenstern KE, Evanchan J, Foster JA, et al. Botulinum toxin type A for dysthyroid upper eyelid retraction. Ophthal Plast Reconstr Surg. 2004;20:181–5.
57. Shih MJ, Liao SL, Lu HY. A single transcutaneous injection with Botox for dysthyroid lid retraction. Eye. 2004;18:466–9.
58. Neetens A, Rubbens MC, Smet H. Botulinum A-toxin treatment of spasmodic entropion of the lower eyelid. Bull Soc Belge Ophthalmol. 1987;224:105–9.
59. Adams GG, Kirkness CM, Lee JP. Botulinum toxin A induced protective ptosis. Eye. 1987;1:603–8.
60. Ellis MF, Daniell M. An evaluation of the safety and efficacy of botulinum toxin type A when used to produce protective ptosis. Clin Experiment Ophthalmol. 2001;29:394–9.
61. Carruthers J, Fagien S, Matarasso SL, et al. Consensus recommendations on the use of botulinum toxin type A in facial aesthetics. Plast Reconstr Surg. 2004;114:1S–22S.
62. Fagien S. Botulinum toxin type A for facial aesthetic enhancement: role in facial shaping. Plast Reconstr Surg. 2003;112:6S–18S.
63. Chen AH, Frankel AS. Altering brow contour with botulinum toxin. Facial Plast Surg Clin North Am. 2003;11:457–64.

Botulinum Toxin Treatment of Migraine and Other Headaches

Sara M. Schaefer and Bahman Jabbari

Introduction

Headache is a common human ailment. Approximately 47% of the adult population in America is believed to have a headache at least once per year [1].

Over the past 15 years, there have been substantial developments in the pharmacological treatment of primary headaches (migraine and others), but still a large number of patients remain unsatisfied. The International Headache Society has classified headaches into primary and secondary headaches [2].

In this review, we describe common human headaches, their pathophysiology, and current accepted treatment strategies. We then provide data on botulinum toxin treatment of headaches with the focus on primary headache disorders (Table 1) and emphasize the data derived from prospective, double-blind, placebo-controlled studies.

Migraine

Migraine is the most common neurological disorder, and the third most prevalent condition overall in the world, after anemia and hearing loss [3]. In the largest and most recently published epidemiological study of migraine (12,000 participants), the overall prevalence of migraine was 12% (17% among women, 6% among men) [4]. This study noted that chronic migraine causes moderate to severe disability in 78% of women and 66% of men. Migraine headache often has a characteristic throbbing quality, is of moderate to severe intensity, and often affects one side of the head more than the other. Most patients complain of photophobia, phonophobia,

S.M. Schaefer, M.D. • B. Jabbari, M.D., FAAN (✉)
Department of Neurology, Yale University School of Medicine, New Haven, CT, USA
e-mail: Sara.schaefer@yale.edu; Bahman.jabbari@yale.edu

B. Jabbari (ed.), *Botulinum Toxin Treatment in Clinical Medicine*,
DOI 10.1007/978-3-319-56038-0_9

Table 1 Primary Headache Disorders, From International Headache Society Classification of Headache Disorders, 2nd Edition

Type	Subtype	Frequency	Duration	Characteristics	Associated symptoms
Migraine	Chronic	≥15 days per month for >3 months	4–72 h	Unilateral, pulsating, moderate to severe intensity	Photophobia, phonophobia, nausea, vomiting, avoidance of activity, ±aura
Migraine	Episodic	<15 days per month	4–72 h	As above	As above
Tension	Episodic (infrequent or frequent)	<1–15 days per month	30 min to 7 days	Bilateral, non-pulsating, mild to moderate intensity	No photophobia, phonophobia, nausea or vomiting. Not aggravated by routine activity
Tension	Chronic	≥15 days per month	Hours to continuous	As above	As above
Trigeminal autonomic cephalalgia (TAC)	Cluster headache	Every other day to 8 per day, occur in clusters	15–180 min	Unilateral, severe intensity, orbital, supraorbital, and/or temporal	Ipsilateral autonomic symptoms (lacrimation, conjunctival injection, edema, sweating, miosis, ptosis), restlessness
TAC	Paroxysmal hemicrania	3–200 per day	5–240 s	As above	Ipsilateral autonomic symptoms as above
TAC	Short-lasting, unilateral neuralgiform headache attacks with conjunctival injection and tearing (SUNCT)	5 per day for more than half the time	2–30 min	Unilateral, severe intensity, orbital, supraorbital and/or temporal, stabbing or pulsating	Ipsilateral conjunctival injection and lacrimation

and/or gastrointestinal distress during the attacks. Those with a severe migraine attack often seek a quiet, dark room because routine activities exacerbate the headache. Migraine may occur with or without aura, the most common of which are visual, sensory, or dysphasic. Episodic migraine is characterized by a headache frequency of less than 15 days per month and chronic migraine with a frequency of 15 or more days per month. The direct and indirect annual costs of migraine have been reported to be as high as $17 billion dollars in the United States in 2005 [5] and 27 billion Euros/year in Europe in 2004 [6].

The pathophysiology of migraine includes a cascade of events that begins with the phenomenon of cortical spreading depression (CSD), travelling across the cortex at a speed of 3–6 mm/s. This electrical phenomenon often involves the occipital cortex, leading to visual aura [7]. During CSD, the release of potassium, nitric oxide, adenosine, and other agents causes inflammation and vasodilation in the cortex and meningeal vessels with consequent sensitization of the trigemino-vascular system (TVS) [8]. Sensitized TVS sends enhanced afferent impulses to the trigeminal ganglion, trigeminal nucleus caudalis, superior salivatory nucleus, and parasympathetic efferent fibers [9]. The release of calcitonin gene-related peptide (CGRP), which corresponds to dural vasodilation, seems to be another major player in the process [10]. Recent studies have demonstrated a potential role of transient receptor potential vanilloid type-1 receptor (TRPV1) and transient receptor potential ankyrin 1 (TRPA1) channels in the pathophysiology of migraine pain. It has been shown that TRPV1 increases in the peri-arterial nerve fibers from scalp artery specimens in migraine patients as compared to controls, irrespective of whether or not the patient had a migraine at the time of sampling, implying a more chronic uptake in TRPV1 receptors among these patients [11]. Cutaneous allodynia during a migraine attack may mark a transition of pain from peripheral to central, since the peripherally activating agents such as triptans are ineffective once patients develop allodynia [12]. Cernuda-Morollon et al. found that, compared to asymptomatic controls, serum levels of calcitonin gene-related peptide (CGRP) are 2.5 times higher in patients with chronic migraine (CM) compared to asymptomatic controls and about 1.8 times higher in patients with episodic migraine (EM) or cluster headaches ($p < 0.05$), identifying a potential biomarker for primary headache disorders [13].

Treatment of migraine consists of abortive and preventive therapy [14, 15]. Mild attacks can be managed by acetaminophen, aspirin, and non-steroidal anti-inflammatory drugs (NSAIDs). Triptans are commonly used for more severe attacks. However, one-third of the patients fail triptans, many patients demonstrate poor tolerance, and the presence of cardiovascular co-morbidities is a contraindication [16]. For very severe episodes, administration of dopamine receptor agonists (e.g., prochlorperazine), dihydroergotamine (DHE), and/or intravenous NSAIDs (diclofenac or ketorolac) is recommended, especially when the attacks have surpassed the peripheral phase of activation [17]. In some patients, high flow oxygen may alleviate acute attacks of migraine [18].

Preventive daily treatment of migraine is recommended when migraine episodes exceed 6–8 headache days per month or what is tolerable to the patient, if the patient has to use abortive medications more than 8–9 times per month, or if headache-related disability is significant [19]. Beta-blockers such as propranolol or metoprolol, topiramate, amitriptyline, and divalproex sodium (DVPX) are commonly recommended for preventive treatment of migraine [20]. Newer preventive measures include supraorbital percutaneous electrical stimulation (once daily for 20 min) [21] and transcranial magnetic stimulation [22]; both are now approved by the FDA for the treatment of chronic migraine. Finally, monoclonal antibodies targeted to CGRP and oxytocin nasal spray have both shown promise in relieving chronic migraine in phase 2 studies [23, 24], and are now being evaluated in phase 3 investigations.

Botulinum Toxin Treatment of Migraine Headaches

Botulinum toxins can reduce pain via a variety of peripheral and central mechanisms which reduce the phenomena of peripheral and central sensitizations integral to the pathophysiology of chronic pain syndromes [25]. On the peripheral side, onabotulinumtoxinA inhibits the release of pain peptides, substance P, bradykinin, CGRP, and glutamate from the dorsal root and trigeminal ganglia [26, 27]. Injection of BoNT-A into the ophthalmic division of the trigeminal nerve decreases TRPV1 immunoreactive neurons by reducing TRPV1 trafficking to the plasma membrane, an effect that persists for at least 14 days [28]. Luvisetto et al. have postulated that in the capsaicin model of pain, the reduction in pain with BoNT pretreatment may be due to its downregulation of TRPV1 responsiveness to capsaicin, a TRPV1 agonist [29]. In an acute model of peripherally generated pain (formalin model), injection of both type A and type B toxins into the rat's paw prior to formalin injection alleviates the secondary peak of pain (inflammatory peak) and reduces local inflammation and accumulation of glutamate [30, 31]. Local onabotulinumtoxinA (ona-A) injection impairs sympathetic transmission [32], thus interfering with maintenance of pain by decreasing sympathetic overactivity. Intramuscular injection of ona-A decreases the discharge of muscle spindles, a major sensory input to the spinal cord [33].

Over the past decade, evidence for central effects of BoNTs has accumulated in the literature from a variety of observations. In animal models of diabetic neuropathy, unilateral, peripheral injection of onabotulinumtoxinA alleviates limb pain bilaterally, indicating a central action [34]. Femtomolar concentrations of BoNT type A inhibit membrane sodium channels in rats in both central and peripheral neurons [35]. Following BoNT type A injection into the rat whisker pad, truncated SNAP-25 was detected in the dorsal horn of the trigeminal nucleus caudalis [36] and in the ipsilateral dorsal and ventral horns of the spinal cord and the spinal cord astrocytes following peripheral sciatic nerve injection [37, 38]. Notably, simultaneous administration of colchicine (which inhibits retrograde axonal transport) negates any antinociceptive effect as observed by rat behavior, highlighting the importance of axonal transport on the effects of BoNT type A.

Administration of BoNT-A directly to the C-meningeal nociceptors in the dura inhibits responses to mechanical stimulation, reverses mechanical hypersensitivity, and prevents the development of mechanical hypersensitivity [39]. Chemical stimulation of dura via application of an inflammatory soup leads to a substantial increase of glutamate in trigeminal nuclear caudalis, and electrophysiological recording from this nucleus demonstrates significant neuronal hypersensitivity. Based on this observation, Orinsky proposed that chemical stimulation of the dura during migraine leads to the communication of dural afferents with trigeminal afferents through axon–axon glutamate secretion, resulting in recruitment and stimulation of a large number of trigeminal afferents and central sensitization of the trigeminal system [40].

Botulinum Toxin Treatment of Chronic Migraine

Chronic migraine is defined as a headache with a frequency of 15 or more headache days per month (at least 8 migraine type), and lasting more than 4 h per day for more than 3 months [2]. A pioneering study of BoNT in episodic migraine [41] generated interest in the investigation of BoNT treatment efficacy in all forms of headaches. Results of subsequent studies of BoNT in episodic migraine and chronic daily headaches (CDH) (including a large number of patients with migraine) were for the most part negative, casting some doubt on the efficacy of BoNT therapy for headaches. However, concurrent positive observations with onabotulinumtoxinA, albeit in smaller populations, kept the door open for further studies. In a subset of 228 patients from a large Chronic Daily Headache trial (CDH) (with no subject on prophylactic headache medication), Dodick et al. found a statistically significant difference in pain relief among patients treated with onabotulinumtoxinA compared to placebo at successive time points over 3 months ($p = 0.004$, $p = 0.032$, and $p = 0.023$) [42]. Also, Freitag et al., in a double-blind placebo-controlled study, compared the effect of a fixed-dose (100 units), fixed-site (glabella, frontalis, temporal, trapezius, suboccipital) paradigm treatment with onabotulinumtoxinA (20 patients) with placebo (21 patients) in chronic migraine [43]. All patients with medication overuse were excluded. The primary outcome was the number of migraine episodes. Secondary outcomes consisted of the number of headache days and headache index (HI—a measure of both intensity and frequency). The authors found ona-A statistically superior to placebo for both primary ($p < 0.01$) and secondary outcomes (frequency of pain days: $p = 0.041$ at 4 weeks and $p = 0.046$ at 16 weeks, and HI: $p = 0.003$ at 16 weeks).

In the summer of 2010, the results of two Phase III Research Evaluating Migraine Prophylaxis Therapy (PREEMPT 1 and PREEMPT 2) trials, two class I multicenter studies assessing the efficacy of onabotulinumtoxinA in chronic migraine, were published [44, 45]. Each study assessed approximately 700 subjects, including comparable numbers of subjects with chronic migraine in the toxin and placebo groups, in a 24-week blind arm followed by a 32-week open arm. Both studies comprised of patients with a history of medication overuse. The primary outcome for PREEMPT 1 was the number of headache episodes, and for PREEMPT 2 the number of headache days, evaluated at 24 weeks. A number of secondary outcomes were also evaluated at the 24-week time point, including frequency of moderate/severe headache days and cumulative headache hours. Although PREEMPT 1 did not meet the primary outcome, it met its secondary outcomes. PREEMPT 2 met its primary outcome with a decrease in headache days by 9 in the ona-A compared to 6.7 in the placebo groups ($p < 0.001$). The pooled data from the two studies also showed a significant change from baseline in favor of ona-A regarding the primary and secondary outcome parameters [46]. The FDA considered headache days (used in PREEMPT 2) a better outcome measure than headache episodes (used in PREEMPT 1) for the study of chronic migraine. Consequently, onabotulinumtoxinA was approved for the treatment of chronic migraine in the UK, Canada, and the USA in

2010. Subsequent prospective real-life studies in large numbers of patients confirmed the efficacy of onabotulinumtoxinA in reducing headaches and improving the quality of life in chronic migraine [47].

Comparator Studies of BoNTs and Oral Agents in Chronic Migraine

Botulinum Toxin Versus Topiramate

Two double-blind, placebo-controlled studies, one single center (60 subjects) and one multicenter (59 subjects) compared the relative efficacy, tolerability, and safety of botulinum neurotoxin versus topiramate in chronic migraine [48, 49]. In both studies, the primary endpoint was the Physician Global Assessment. The secondary endpoints included a number of headache days, Headache Impact Test (HIT-6), and Migraine Disability Assessment (MIDAS) scores. In the first study, subjects had no history of medication overuse and received injections at time points 0 and 3 months. Subjects were followed for 9 months. Authors found similar efficacy for onabotulinumtoxinA and topiramate (40.9% and 42.9% respectively) noting at least a 50% reduction in headache days after 9 months. Although nearly all study participants reported at least one adverse effect (AE), more patients in the topiramate group permanently discontinued treatment due to side effects than those in the BoNT group (24.1% versus 7.7%).

The second study had a placebo arm that lasted 3 months, followed by a 14-week open trial [48]. Both therapeutic approaches were effective with no significant difference between the two groups. AEs were mild, and their rate of occurrence was similar in the two groups.

Botulinum Toxin Versus Divalproex Sodium (DVPX)

Blumenfeld et al. explored the efficacy and tolerability of BoNT and DVPX in patients with episodic or chronic migraine [50]. In a single-center, double-blind, prospective trial, 59 subjects received either BoNT plus oral placebo or placebo injections plus DVPX 250 mg twice daily. Subjects received injections at time 0 and at month 3, with evaluations at months 1, 3, 6, and 9. Outcome measures consisted of the reduction in a number of headache days, responder rate (percentage of patients with a ≥50% reduction in attack frequency per month), maximum headache severity, and overall headache index (related to a combination of headache frequency and severity). Patients in both groups demonstrated significant improvements in headache frequency and severity as measured by headache days per month, responder rates, Headache Index scores, MIDAS, and HIT-6 scores. Adverse effects occurred more commonly in patients who took DVPX (DVPX 75.8%, BoNT-A 50%, $p = 0.04$), and these patients were more likely to discontinue treatment because of AEs (DVPX 27.6%, BoNT-A 3.3%, $p = 0.012$).

The Issue of Medication Overuse in Chronic Migraine

Silberstein et al. studied a subset of PREEMPT study cohort who had both medication overuse (MO) and chronic migraine (CM) [51]. Of the 1384 patients in the two PREEMPT studies, 65.3% met the criteria for medication overuse. At 24 weeks, the reduction of pain days in MO + CM subjects compared to the placebo group was significant (−8.2 versus −6.2, $p < 0.001$). MO + CM subjects also met many secondary endpoints: frequency of migraine days, frequency of moderate to severe headache days, cumulative headache hours on headache days, headache episodes, migraine episodes, and percentage of patients with severe HIT-6 scores (all $p < 0.05$). The subjects' triptan intake was significantly reduced after ona-A treatment ($p < 0.001$). The authors concluded that treatment with onabotulinumtoxinA is effective in patients with a history of medication overuse and chronic migraine.

Long-Term Efficacy, Safety, and Effects on Quality of Life

Aurora et al. studied the efficacy of botulinum toxin and changes in the quality of life in the PREEMPT study cohort after five cycles of treatment (week 56) [52]. The mean reduction in headache days, migraine days, and moderate to severe headache days was significantly more in the botulinum toxin group compared to placebo ($p < 0.05$). The quality of life, measured by a >5 point increase in HIT-6 scores, also improved by 44% at week 25 and 59% at week 56 in the botulinum toxin group.

In a more recent study, Silberstein et al. reported on the percent of patients with chronic migraine who responded to the onabotulinumtoxinA treatment cycle in the PREEMPT studies [53]. Of 688 patients who received ona-A, 49.3% described more than 50% improvement after the first cycle of treatment, and an additional 11.3% and 10.3% after the second and third cycles of treatment respectively (a total of 70.9% after the third cycle). These data further support that repeat injections in subsequent cycles increase the efficacy of onabotulinumtoxinA in chronic migraine.

Response of Imploding Versus Exploding Migraine to Botulinum Toxin Therapy

In imploding migraine headaches, patients describe experiencing pressure from outside the head (crushed, clamped, or stabbed by an external force). In exploding headaches, headaches are felt as pressure building inside of the head. Jakubowski et al., in a study of 63 patients with chronic migraine, found that 74% of responders had imploding headaches whereas 92% of non-responders described exploding headaches [54].

Techniques of Injection

Currently, onabotulinumtoxinA (Botox, Allergan Inc.) is the only form of BoNT approved by the FDA for the treatment of chronic migraine. A variety of approaches have been employed for the treatment of chronic migraine with onabotulinumtoxinA injections. Almost all investigators advocate the inclusion of the procerus, corrugator, frontalis, temporalis, occipitalis, and posterior cervical muscles as injection sites. Three of these methods which have proven efficacious in blinded studies are described below.

In one of the earliest publications of an injection scheme for BoNT therapy for migraine [55], authors advocated use of five injections (2.5 units) into each side of the frontalis muscle, two injections into each corrugator, and one injection into the procerus muscle at midline (Table 2 and Fig. 1a). A slight modification of this technique was used by Silberstein at Jefferson's Headache Center until 2009 [56]. A total dose of 130–160 units was delivered into 32 injection sites.

The PREEMPT study recommends two injections (5 units) into each side of the frontalis, four injections (5 units each) into each temporalis, three injections (5 units each) into each occipitalis, two 5 unit injections into upper cervical muscles (each side), and three 5 unit injections into the trapezius muscle on each side (Table 2 and Fig. 1b) [57]. This technique uses a total of 31 injection sites and 165 units with expansion to 195 units in special cases.

For the past 12 years, Jabbari and his colleagues at Yale have used a technique that employs fewer temporal injections (two, each 15 units), one occipital injection (5 units), three cervical injections (10 units each), and no shoulder trapezius injections (Table 2 and Fig. 1c). The rationale for fewer temporal injections is that the tendon of the temporalis muscle is large and can extend up to 45 mm vertically from the zygomatic arch [58]. Hence, the lower temporal injection site of PREEMPT (Fig. 1b) may be into the temporalis tendon and not into the muscle in many patients. Furthermore, in the cervical area, if one considers the possible contribution of cervical muscles in migraine, two 5 unit injections in the upper cervical region (PREEMPT) may not produce an optimal effect for such powerful muscles. The Yale technique has the advantage of using fewer injection sites (23 versus 31 in PREEMPT) while using comparable doses (185–195 units). The Yale technique has been evaluated by an open label and a small double-blind study. In the open investigation, 50 subjects with CM reported prospectively their level of satisfaction with BoNT treatment in the Patient Global Impression of Change (PGIC) [59]. After the first injection, 72% of the patient and after the third injection, 85% of the patients reported their chronic migraine as "much improved" (follow-up 2–8 years). Fifty percent of patients discontinued preventive medication and 61% of patients discontinued abortive medication by the 12th month of treatment. Of the 15 patients who had presented to the emergency room for the relief of a severe headache, 73% had no more visits to the emergency room within 1 year of starting treatment. No significant side effects were reported. More recently, the efficacy and safety of this technique was tested in a double-blind, parallel study followed by an open arm [60]. The

Table 2 Comparison of three techniques of ona-A treatment in CM: muscles, doses in units, and number of injections per side

Method	Procerus (midline)	Corrugator	Frontalis	Temporalis	Occipitalis	Splenius/paraspinalis	Trapezius	Masseter
Blumenfeld et al. 2003 [55]; Silberstein 2009 [56] (Fig. 1)	2.5–5 u	2.5 u × 2	2.5 u × 5	2.5–5 u × 4	2.5–5 u × 1	2.5–5 u × 1	2.5 u × 2	2.5–5 u × 1
PREEMPT 2010 [57] (Fig. 1)	5 u	5 u × 1	5 u × 2	5 u × 4	5 u × 3	5 u × 2	5 u × 3	–
Jabbari et al. (Yale) 2016 [60][a] (Fig. 1)	5 u	5 u × 1	5 u × 3	15 u × 2	10 u × 1	10 u × 3	–	–

[a]There are other neurologists at Yale who use the PREEMPT method for the treatment of migraine

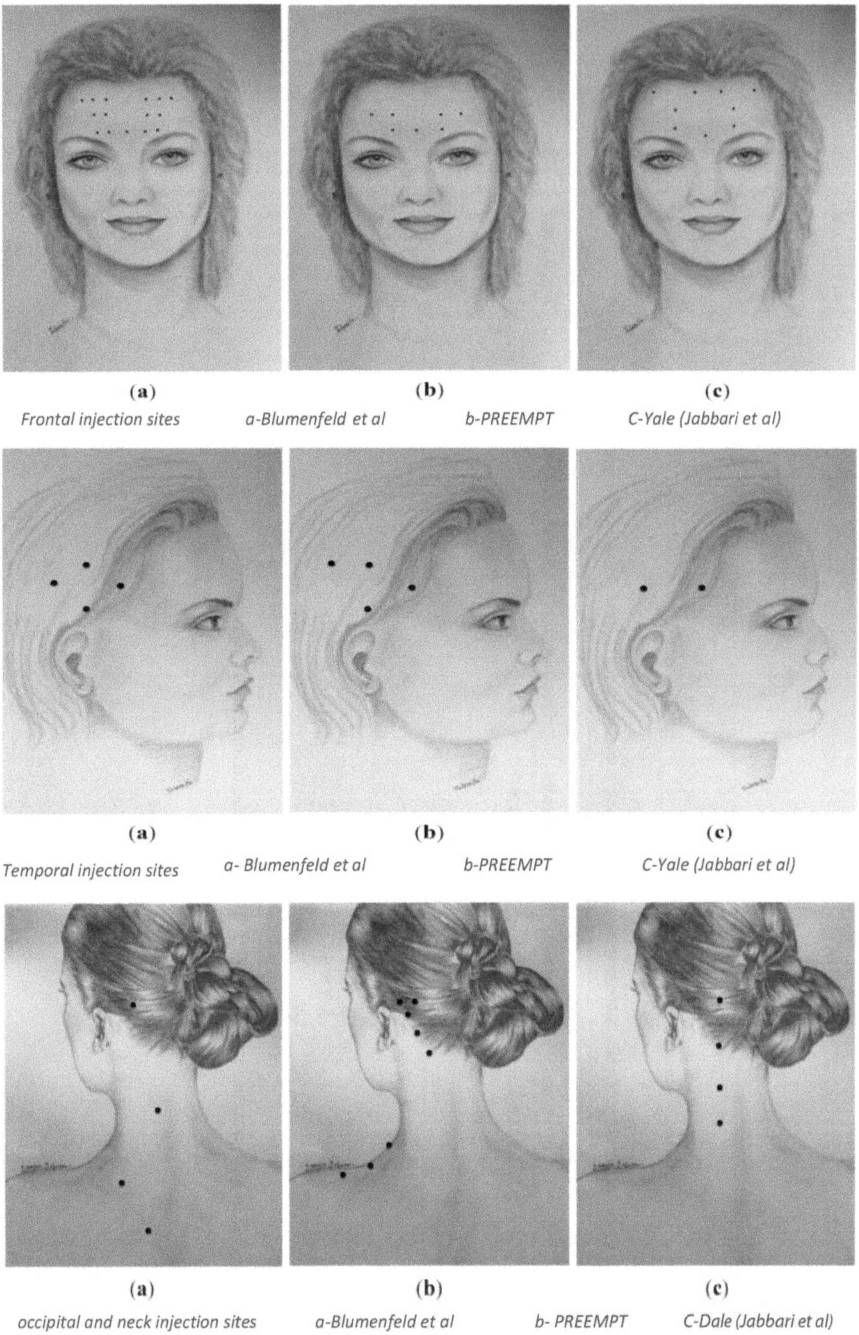

Fig. 1 Comparison of three injection methods used for the treatment of chronic migraine with onabotulinumtoxinA. The *top* row represents frontal injection, *middle* row temporal, and *lower* row low posterior (occipital and neck). In each row, the figure on the *left* represents the earlier method produced by Blumenfeld et al., the *middle* figure the one used in the PREEMPT study, and the *right-most* figure the Jabbari/Yale injection protocol. Drs. Tahereh Mousavi and Damoun Safarpour produced the drawing for these figures

blinded arm of the study included 25 subjects, of whom 17 continued in the open-label investigation. The reduction of pain days at 4 weeks (primary outcome) was significantly in favor of onabotulinumtoxinA (6.67 versus 1.20, $p = 0.0347$). With regards to PGIC, 9 of 11 and 3 of 10 patients reported satisfaction with onabotulinumtoxinA and placebo treatment, respectively ($p = 0.030$). In the open arm of the study at 4 weeks, 58.8% reported 50% or more reduction of pain and 88.2% of those treated with onabotulinumtoxinA demonstrated reduction of HIT scores compared to baseline. Table 2 compares the three aforementioned techniques regarding dose and injected muscles.

Episodic Migraine (EM)

In the year 2000, Silberstein et al. published the results of the first double-blind, placebo-controlled, prospective study (class II) investigating the efficacy of onabotulinumtoxinA (ona-A) in 123 patients with episodic migraine (<15 headaches per month) [41]. The study had 3 arms: ona-A 25 units, ona-A 75 units, and placebo. In the 25 unit group, ona A was injected into the procerus muscle (3 units) and bilaterally into corrugators (two on each side, 6 units), frontalis (two on each side, 6 units), and temporalis (one on each side, 6 units) muscles. In the 75 unit group, the dose injected into these sites was 9, 18, 18, and 8 units respectively. The primary efficacy outcome, a significant change from the baseline of migraine attacks, was not met. However, at 3 months, subjects who were injected with 25 units demonstrated significant reduction in headache frequency, headache intensity, and 50% reduction of headaches compared to baseline.

Another class II study of 60 subjects with EM that considered 50% or more reduction of migraine frequency as the primary outcome also failed to meet its primary endpoint [61]. Subsequently, two large class I studies were conducted with onabotulinumtoxinA on 238 and 418 subjects with EM [62, 63]. Both studies failed to meet their primary outcome measure—reduction of migraine frequency. The total dose applied in the aforementioned two studies was 25 and 100 units. Finally, two more class I studies were published which investigated the results of larger doses of onabotulinumtoxinA in episodic migraine [64, 65]. The first study [64] compared the effect of different doses of ona-A (75, 150, and 225 units) to placebo using the mean number of migraine days at day 180 as the primary outcome measure. All four groups (including the placebo group) improved with either ona-A or saline (the placebo) and there was no significant difference between ona-A subgroups and the placebo group. In the second study [65], authors compared the effect of ona-A (mean of 190.5 units) with placebo in 369 subjects. The primary endpoint, defined as the mean change in migraine episodes over 30 days prior to day 180, was not met. Although the study failed to meet the primary endpoint, a subgroup analysis of patients with 12–14 headache days per month showed significant improvement in the ona-A group versus placebo ($p = 0.04$).

Comment

The PREEMPT study data published in 2010 showed the efficacy of onabotulinumtoxinA in chronic migraine, a finding that agrees with the consensus view of experienced clinicians in this field. In the subsequent 6 years, efforts of PREEMPT investigators produced additional data from the large PREEMPT cohort, which demonstrated long-term safety and efficacy of onabotulinumtoxinA in chronic migraine and improved efficacy as well as the quality of life with repeated injections. The most recent report of the Guideline Development Subcommittee of the American Academy of Neurology (2016) [66] designated a level A (established) efficacy for onabotulinumtoxinA in chronic migraine regarding the reduction of headache days per month and a level B (probably effective) in improving the quality of life. A level C (ineffective) was given to onabotulinumtoxinA for episodic migraine.

Tension Headache

Tension-type headaches (TTH) are the most common type of primary headaches with an annual prevalence of approximately 38% [67]. Compared to migraine, tension headaches are more often bilateral, more often have scalp tenderness, and are less often associated with nausea and photophobia [68]. TTHs are not usually as severe as migraine, but severe episodes lead to loss of work days in 8–10% of the affected individuals. Chronic tension headaches (>15 per month) have the same prevalence as chronic migraine (2%) in the general population [69].

It is currently believed that TTHs result from a multifactorial process with contributions from psychological factors, muscle tension, and central processes. Diamond and Dalessio proposed a cascade of events in the pathophysiology of TTHs starting with peripheral muscle contractions that then polysynaptically activate thalamic and cortical neurons via a spinal reflex. Excitation of cortical neurons in turn leads to activation of the descending reticulospinal system, which causes increased muscle tone and muscle contraction through the gamma loop-muscle spindle activation [70].

The mainstays of treatment for episodic tension-type headaches are non-steroidal anti-inflammatory drugs; paracetamol may also be used. For chronic tension headaches, tricyclic antidepressants (especially amitriptyline) are recommended [69]. European guidelines also recommend administration of serotonin/norepinephrine reuptake inhibitors venlafaxine and mirtazapine [71].

Botulinum Toxin Treatment of Tension-Type Headaches

Seven prospective double-blind, placebo-controlled studies have investigated the efficacy of BoNTs in TTH [72–78]. Three studies were class I [75–77] and 4 were class II (Table 3) [72–74]. None but a small class II study met the study's primary

Table 3 Placebo-controlled botulinum toxin studies in tension-type headaches (TTH)

Author	BoNT	Class	Number of patients	Dose (units)	POM	Results	Comments and limitations
Schmidt et al. 2001 [72]	ona-A	II	60	20	WHYPI HD days	Negative	Low dose, limited injected areas
Rollnik et al. 2002 [73]	ona-A	II	21	200	VAS, HD days	Negative	Low dose, mixed chronic and episodic
Shulte-Muttler et al. 2004 [75]	abo-A	I	60	250	Area under curve	Negative	Low dose
Padberg et al. 2004 [74]	ona-A	II	40	100	VAS, HD days	Negative	Low dose, limited injected areas
Silberstein et al. 2008 [76]	ona-A	I	300	50, 100, 150	HD free days	Negative/ positive	POM too rigid
Straube et al. 2008 [77]	abo-A	I	120	210/420	HD free days	Negative	POM too rigid
Hamdy et al. 2009 [78]	ona-A	II	28	50	HD days, VAS, QoL	Positive	Small sample size

VAS visual analog scale, *POM* primary outcome measure, *WHYPI* West Haven Yale Pain Inventory, *HD* Headache, *QoL* quality of life

outcome measure [78]. However, there are major issues with interpretation of the results of these studies regarding the efficacy of BoNTs in TTHs. If one uses the PREEMPT studies of chronic migraine as a model for successful treatment of headache, none of the seven studies meet the dose/technique/primary outcome criteria of PREEMPT. All seven used doses smaller (and sometimes much smaller) than PREEMPT (which used 165–195 units of ona-A). All employed fewer numbers of injections. Three studies (Table 3) used reduction of pain days as the primary outcome (similar to PREEMPT 2), but all three had employed smaller doses and fewer numbers of injections. Interestingly, in a study of TTH by Silberstein et al. [76] the number of pain days (the outcome measure of PREEMPT 2)—which was not the primary outcome measure of their study—was significantly reduced in the toxin-injected group compared to the placebo group ($p = 0.03$). Recently, Harden et al. [79] studied subjects with TTH secondary to cervical myofascial disease with trigger points. Injection of ona-A into cervical trigger points decreased chronic TTH days in the ona-A group ($p = 0.03$), but had no effect on the pain intensity.

We strongly believe that the design of the reported clinical trials in TTHs is suboptimal and the final word on the efficacy of BoNTs in TTHs awaits conduction of a multicenter study using the technique, dosing, and primary outcome measures similar to a study design which has already shown efficacy in one form of severe headaches (migraine)—for example, that used in the PREEMPT or Yale studies.

Trigeminal Autonomic Cephalalgias [80]

Trigeminal autonomic cephalalgias (TAC) are pain disorders characterized by unilateral orbital, supraorbital, and/or temporal pain that may be stabbing or pulsating, associated with ipsilateral autonomic symptoms. The symptoms consist of conjunctival injection, lacrimation, edema, diaphoresis, miosis, ptosis, and nasal congestion. The subclassifications of these disorders are largely based on duration and frequency of attacks (Table 1). This group includes cluster headaches, paroxysmal hemicranias, short-lasting unilateral neuralgiform headache attacks with conjunctival injection and tearing (SUNCT), and short-lasting unilateral neuralgiform headache attacks with cranial, autonomic dysfunction (SUNA).

The autonomic dysfunction seen in TAC syndromes is thought to arise from the trigeminal-autonomic reflex. This reflex extends from the pain fibers of the trigeminal nerve through the trigeminal ganglion, descending to the brainstem and trigeminocervical complex, and resulting in activation and outflow of parasympathetic fibers [81]. The ipsilateral hypothalamus is the major central site for this reflex (Fig. 2) [80].

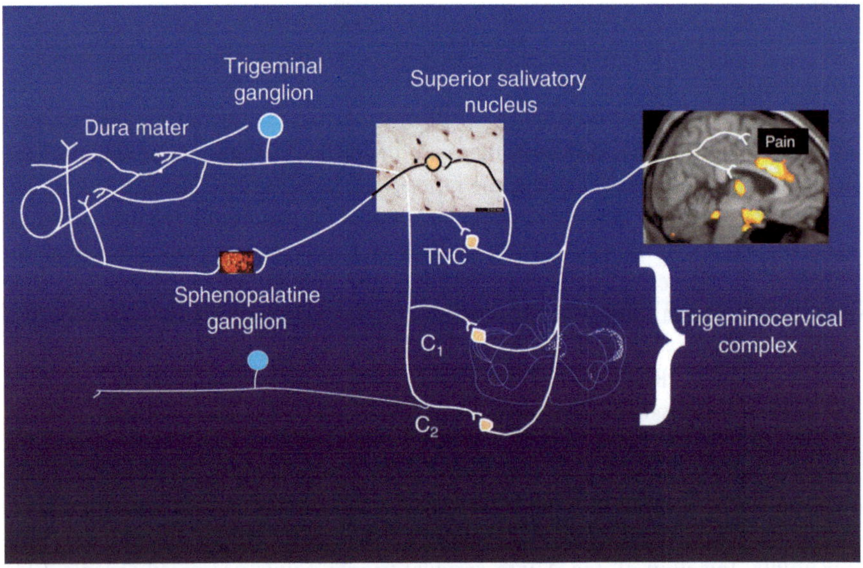

Fig. 2 The anatomy of trigeminal autonomic reflex. From Eller and Goadsby [80], printed from Oral Disease with permission from Wiley and Sons Publisher

First-line therapy for acute cluster headache includes 100% oxygen, at the rate of 6–12 l/min for at least 15 min using a non-rebreather mask, in combination with injectable triptans [82, 83]. Second-line treatments with less compelling data to support their use include ipsilateral intranasal lidocaine and DHE. Verapamil is the best studied prophylactic agent for cluster headaches, with proven efficacy in a randomized, placebo-controlled, double-blinded trial. The patient should start verapamil at a dose of 40–80 mg three times daily, with an increase of 80 mg every week to a target dose of 120 mg three times daily (360 mg per day, total). The main side effects are cardiac arrhythmias; patients should be followed with serial electrocardiograms (ECGs) during therapy. Lithium may be used separately or as an adjunct to verapamil, though the data are less compelling. Topiramate may also be useful for prophylaxis. Other prophylactic agents such as melatonin, valproate, gabapentin, levetiracetam, and baclofen have been tried, but with small sample sizes, and require further investigation [84]. Paroxysmal hemicrania and hemicrania continua (Table 1) respond well to indomethacin but gastrointestinal side effects sometimes limit its use. COX-2 inhibitors may be used as an alternative. Lamotrigine is a first-line drug for patients with SUNCT or SUNA [85].

In refractory cases, resectional and ablative surgeries and neurostimulation have been tried in cluster headache patients [84]. Trigeminal nerve root resection has caused many surgical complications, and has been replaced by gamma knife radiosurgery of the trigeminal and sphenopalatine ganglia. Results have been mixed, with high complication and pain recurrence rates. Occipital nerve and sphenopalatine ganglion stimulation are safer procedures that are gaining traction in refractory populations. As the hypothalamus is a major site in TACs' reflex arc, deep brain stimulation of this site has been explored with promising results. In a recent review of 69 patients (mostly cluster headaches), published in 2015, approximately 70% of patients reported >50% improvement of TAC over 2 years of follow-up [86]. Despite its effectiveness, morbidity and mortality associated with stimulation of this site is a cause for concern [85].

Botulinum Toxin Treatment of Trigeminal Autonomic Cephalalgias (TAC)

A limited number of case reports and open trials claim efficacy of facial and periocular injections of BoNTs in refractory cases of trigeminal autonomic cephalalgias. To date, there are no reports of any blinded and placebo-controlled clinical trials in this area.

Cluster Headaches (CH)

Sostak et al. [87], in an open-label investigation, studied the effect of onabotulinumtoxinA in 12 subjects with cluster headaches who failed preventive medications. Each patient was injected with a total of 50 units of onabotulinumtoxinA ipsilaterally into frontalis, temporalis, cervical splenius, and trapezius muscles. Three out of nine patients with chronic CH improved significantly after ona-A injections. In one subject, the attacks totally ceased for 18 months. None of the three patients with episodic CH improved, however.

Bratbak et al. [88] injected 25 units of onabotulinumtoxinA in each sphenopalatine ganglion of ten patients with refractory cluster headaches. The main efficacy outcome was the number of CH attacks, which dropped significantly at weeks 3 and 4 after injection ($p = 0.038$). One patient experienced a severe adverse effect—posterior epistaxis.

Hemicrania Continua (HC)

In an open label study, nine subjects with hemicrania continua, unresponsive to indomethacin and other treatments, were injected with onabotulinumtoxinA using the PREEMPT dose/design protocol [89]. Five patients who demonstrated 50% or more reduction of headache days were classified as responders. The median reduction of total headache days was 90% ($p = 0.026$), and for moderate to severe headache days, the reduction was 80% ($p = 0.012$). HIT-6 showed a median change of 12 points ($p = 0.069$). These results suggest the usefulness of onA treatment in HC.

SUNCT and SUNA

Significant improvement of SUNCT after injection of onabotulinumtoxinA has been reported in two case reports [89, 90]. Zabalza [89] treated a 55-year-old man with a 20-year history of severe orbital and periorbital pain associated with redness of the eye and rhinorrhea with the right periocular injection of onabotulinumtoxinA. Four sites were injected, each with 10 units. The patient had failed to respond to a long list of medications including lamotrigine and gabapentin. He was experiencing 20–30 episodes of pain each day with the intensity of 8–10 on a visual analog scale (VAS). After injections, the frequency of pain dropped down to 8–10 per week and the intensity was reduced to 2–3 on VAS. Improvement continued with quarterly injections over a follow-up period of 2.5 years.

Zhan et al. [90] reported a 12-year-old boy with severe episodes of pain affecting the left eye, left upper gums, and the left temporal area. The pain was refractory to the SUNCT conventional pharmacotherapeutic agents. The authors injected the left periocular region, left temporal, and left upper gum at multiple sites, 2.5–5 units/site for a total dose of 70 units. The pain was significantly diminished at day 4 and stopped at day 7 after BoNT injection. All SUNCT medications were discontinued at day 11. The child continued to do well over 17 months.

Comment

The recently published open studies and case observations describing the improvement of refractory TACs with onabotulinumtoxinA therapy are encouraging. Proof of efficacy of BoNT treatment for this form of headaches awaits conduction of clinical trials in a sizeable number of patients, but the low prevalence of TACs makes conduction of large clinical trials difficult. The optimal technique of injection and optimum dose remains to be determined which will most likely differ from those used in migraine due to the more localized nature of pain in trigeminal autonomic cephalalgias.

References

1. World Health Organization. The global burden of disease: 2004 update. Geneva, Switzerland: WHO Press; 2008. p. 31.
2. Headache Classification Subcommittee of the International Headache, S. The international classification of headache disorders: 2nd edition. Cephalalgia. 2004;24(Suppl 1):9–160.
3. Lipton RB, Bigal ME, Diamond M, Freitag F, Reed ML, Stewart WF, Group, A.A. Migraine prevalence, disease burden, and the need for preventive therapy. Neurology. 2007;68:343–349.
4. Lipton RB, Manack Adams A, Buse DC, Fanning KM, Reed ML, Headache A. Comparison of the Chronic Migraine Epidemiology and Outcomes (CaMEO) Study and American Migraine Prevalence and Prevention (AMPP) Study: demographics and headache-related disability. Headache. 2016;56:1280–9.
5. Goldberg LD. The cost of migraine and its treatment. Am J Manag Care. 2005;11:S62–7.
6. Ruggeri M. The cost effectiveness of botox in italian patients with chronic migraine. Neurol Sci. 2014;35(Suppl 1):45–7.
7. Cao Y, Welch KM, Aurora S, Vikingstad EM. Functional mri-bold of visually triggered headache in patients with migraine. Arch Neurol. 1999;56:548–54.
8. Waeber C, Moskowitz MA. Therapeutic implications of central and peripheral neurologic mechanisms in migraine. Neurology. 2003;61:S9–20.
9. Noseda R, Burstein R. Migraine pathophysiology: anatomy of the trigeminovascular pathway and associated neurological symptoms, csd, sensitization and modulation of pain. Pain 2013;154(Suppl 1):S44–S53.
10. Benemei S, De Cesaris F, Fusi C, Rossi E, Lupi C, Geppetti P. Trpa1 and other trp channels in migraine. J Headache Pain. 2013;14:71.
11. Del Fiacco M, Quartu M, Boi M, Serra MP, Melis T, Boccaletti R, Shevel E, Cianchetti C. Trpv1, cgrp and sp in scalp arteries of patients suffering from chronic migraine. J Neurol Neurosurg Psychiatry. 2015;86:393–397.
12. Burstein R, Collins B, Jakubowski M. Defeating migraine pain with triptans: a race against the development of cutaneous allodynia. Ann Neurol. 2004;55:19–26.
13. Cernuda-Morollon E, Larrosa D, Ramon C, Vega J, Martinez-Camblor P, Pascual J. Interictal increase of cgrp levels in peripheral blood as a biomarker for chronic migraine. Neurology. 2013;81:1191–6.
14. Silberstein SD. Treatment recommendations for migraine. Nat Clin Pract Neurol. 2008;4:482–9.
15. Diener HC, Holle D, Dodick D. Treatment of chronic migraine. Curr Pain Headache Rep. 2011;15:64–9.
16. Hoffmann J, Goadsby PJ. Emerging targets in migraine. CNS Drugs. 2014;28:11–7.
17. Gelfand AA, Goadsby PJ. A neurologist's guide to acute migraine therapy in the emergency room. Neurohospitalist. 2012;2:51–9.

18. Ozkurt B, Cinar O, Cevik E, Acar AY, Arslan D, Eyi EY, Jay L, Yamanel L, Madsen T. Efficacy of high-flow oxygen therapy in all types of headache: a prospective, randomized, placebo-controlled trial. Am J Emerg Med. 2012;30:1760–1764.
19. Silberstein SD. Preventive treatment of migraine: an overview. Cephalalgia. 1997;17:67–72.
20. Goadsby PJ. Therapeutic prospects for migraine: can paradise be regained? Ann Neurol. 2013;74:423–34.
21. Schoenen J, Vandersmissen B, Jeangette S, Herroelen L, Vandenheede M, Gerard P, Magis D. Migraine prevention with a supraorbital transcutaneous stimulator: a randomized controlled trial. Neurology. 2013;80:697–704.
22. Goadsby P. Decade in reviewmigraine: incredible progress for an era of better migraine care. Nat Rev Neurol. 2015;11:621–2.
23. Bigal ME, Dodick DW, Krymchantowski A.V, VanderPluym JH, Tepper SJ, Aycardi E, Loupe PS, Ma Y, Goadsby PJ. TEV-48125 for the preventive treatment of chronic migraine: efficacy at early time points. Neurology. 2016;87:41–48.
24. Sun H, Dodick DW, Silberstein S, Goadsby PJ, Reuter U, Ashina M, Saper J, Cady R, Chon Y, Dietrich J, Lenz R. Safety and efficacy of AMG 334 for prevention of episodic migraine: a randomized, double-blind, placebo-controlled, phase 2 trial. Lancet Neurol. 2016;15:382–390.
25. Aoki KR. Review of a proposed mechanism for the antinociceptive action of botulinum toxin type A. Neurotoxicology. 2006;26:785–93.
26. Meng J, Wang J, Lawrence G, Dolly JO. Synaptobrevin i mediates exocytosis of cgrp from sensory neurons and inhibition by botulinum toxins reflects their anti-nociceptive potential. J Cell Sci. 2007;120:2864–74.
27. Lucioni A, Bales GT, Lotan TL, McGehee DS, Cook SP, Rapp DE. Botulinum toxin type a inhibits sensory neuropeptide release in rat bladder models of acute injury and chronic inflammation. BJU Int. 2008;101:366–70.
28. Shimizu T, Shibata M, Toriumi H, Iwashita T, Funakubo M, Sato H, Kuroi T, Ebine T, Koizumi K, Suzuki N. Reduction of trpv1 expression in the trigeminal system by botulinum neurotoxin type-a. Neurobiol Dis. 2012;48:367–378.
29. Luvisetto S, Vacca V, Cianchetti C. Analgesic effects of botulinum neurotoxin type a in a model of allyl isothiocyanate- and capsaicin-induced pain in mice. Toxicon. 2015;94:23–8.
30. Cui M, Khanijou S, Rubino J, Aoki KR. Subcutaneous administration of botulinum toxin a reduces formalin-induced pain. Pain. 2004;107:125–33.
31. Marino MJ, Terashima T, Steinauer JJ, Eddinger KA, Yaksh TL, Xu Q. Botulinum toxin B in the sensory afferent: transmitter release, spinal activation, and pain behavior. Pain. 2014;155:674–84.
32. Rand MJ, Whaler BC. Impairment of sympathetic transmission by botulinum toxin. Nature. 1965;206:588–91.
33. Filippi GM, Errico P, Santarelli R, Bagolini B, Manni E. Botulinum a toxin effects on rat jaw muscle spindles. Acta Otolaryngol. 1993;113:400–4.
34. Bach-Rojecky L, Salkovic-Petrisic M, Lackovic Z. Botulinum toxin type a reduces pain supersensitivity in experimental diabetic neuropathy: bilateral effect after unilateral injection. Eur J Pharmacol. 2010;633:10–4.
35. Shin MC, Wakita, M, Xie, DJ, Yamaga T, Iwata S, Torii Y, Harakawa T, Ginnaga A, Kozaki S, Akaike N. Inhibition of membrane Na+ channels by A type botulinum toxin at femtomolar concentrations in central and peripheral neurons. J Pharmacol Sci. 2012;118:33–42.
36. Matak I, Bach-Rojecky L, Filipovic B, Lackovic Z. Behavioral and immunohistochemical evidence for central antinociceptive activity of botulinum toxin a. Neuroscience. 2011;186:201–7.
37. Matak I, Riederer P, Lackovic Z. Botulinum toxin's axonal transport from periphery to the spinal cord. Neurochem Int. 2012;61:236–9.
38. Marinelli S, Vacca V, Ricordy R, Uggenti C, Tata, AM, Luvisetto S, Pavone F. The analgesic effect on neuropathic pain of retrogradely transported botulinum neurotoxin a involves schwann cells and astrocytes. PLoS One. 2012;7:e47977.

39. Burstein R, Zhang X, Levy D, Aoki KR, Brin MF. Selective inhibition of meningeal nociceptors by botulinum neurotoxin type a: therapeutic implications for migraine and other pains. Cephalalgia. 2014;34:853–69.
40. Orinsky M, Poso-Rosich P, Luo J, Hayman S, Silberstein SD. Botulinum toxin a blocks sensitization of neurons in trigeminal nucleus caudalis. Cephalalgia. 2004;24:781.
41. Silberstein S, Mathew N, Saper J, Jenkins S. Botulinum toxin type a as a migraine preventive treatment. For the botox migraine clinical research group. Headache. 2000;40:445–50.
42. Dodick D, Mauskop A, Elkind AH, DeGryse R, Brin MF, Silberstein S, Group, B.C.S. Botulinum toxin type a for the prophylaxis of chronic daily headache: a subgroup analysis of patients not receiving other prophylactic medications: a randomized double-blind, placebo-controlled study. Headache. 2005;45:315–324.
43. Freitag FG, Diamond S, Diamond M, Urban G. Botulinum toxin type a in the treatment of chronic migraine without medication overuse. Headache. 2008;48:201–9.
44. Aurora SK, Dodick DW, Turkel CC, DeGryse RE, Silberstein SD, Lipton RB, Diener HC, Brin MF, Group, P.C.M.S. Onabotulinumtoxina for treatment of chronic migraine: results from the double-blind, randomized, placebo-controlled phase of the preempt 1 trial. Cephalalgia. 2010;30:793–803.
45. Diener HC, Dodick DW, Aurora SK, Turkel CC, DeGryse RE, Lipton RB, Silberstein SD, Brin MF, Group, P.C.M.S. Onabotulinumtoxina for treatment of chronic migraine: results from the double-blind, randomized, placebo-controlled phase of the preempt 2 trial. Cephalalgia. 2010;30:804–814.
46. Dodick DW, Turkel CC, DeGryse RE, Aurora SK, Silberstein SD, Lipton RB, Diener HC, Brin MF, Group, P.C.M.S. Onabotulinumtoxina for treatment of chronic migraine: pooled results from the double-blind, randomized, placebo-controlled phases of the preempt clinical program. Headache. 2010;50:921–936.
47. Khalil M, Zafar HW, Quarshie V, Ahmed F. Prospective analysis of the use of onabotulinumtoxinA (BOTOX) in the treatment of chronic migraine; real-life data in 254 patients from Hull, U.K. J Headache Pain. 2014;15:54.
48. Mathew NT, Jaffri SF. A double-blind comparison of onabotulinumtoxina (botox) and topiramate (topamax) for the prophylactic treatment of chronic migraine: a pilot study. Headache. 2009;49:1466–78.
49. Cady RK, Schreiber CP, Porter JA, Blumenfeld AM, Farmer KU. A multi-center double-blind pilot comparison of onabotulinumtoxina and topiramate for the prophylactic treatment of chronic migraine. Headache. 2011;51:21–32.
50. Blumenfeld AM, Schim JD, Chippendale TJ. Botulinum toxin type a and divalproex sodium for prophylactic treatment of episodic or chronic migraine. Headache. 2008;48:210–20.
51. Silberstein S.D, Blumenfeld AM, Cady RK, Turner IM, Lipton RB, Diener HC, Aurora SK, Sirimanne M, DeGryse RE, Turkel CC, et al.. Onabotulinumtoxina for treatment of chronic migraine: preempt 24-week pooled subgroup analysis of patients who had acute headache medication overuse at baseline. J Neurol Sci. 2013;331:48–56.
52. Aurora SK, Dodick DW, Diener HC, DeGryse RE, Turkel CC, Lipton RB, Silberstein SD. Onabotulinumtoxina for chronic migraine: efficacy, safety, and tolerability in patients who received all five treatment cycles in the preempt clinical program. Acta Neurol Scand. 2014;129:61–70.
53. Silberstein SD, Dodick DW, Aurora SK, Diener HC, DeGryse, RE, Lipton, RB, Turkel CC. Percent of patients with chronic migraine who responded per onabotulinumtoxinA treatment cycle: PREEMPT. J Neurol Neurosurg Psychiatry. 2015;86:996–1001.
54. Jakubowski M, McAllister PJ, Bajwa ZH, Ward TN, Smith P, Burstein R. Exploding vs. imploding headache in migraine prophylaxis with Botulinum Toxin A. Pain. 2006;125:286–95.
55. Blumenfeld AM, Binder W, Silberstein SD, Blitzer A. Procedures for administering botulinum toxin type a for migraine and tension-type headache. Headache. 2003;43:884–91.
56. Silberstein SD. Botulinum toxin in headache management. Botulinum toxin: therapeutic clinical practice and science. 1st ed. Philadelphia, PA: Saunders, Elsevier; 2009. p. 218.

57. Blumenfeld A, Silberstein SD, Dodick DW, Aurora SK, Turkel CC, Binder WJ. Method of injection of onabotulinumtoxinA for chronic migraine: a safe, well-tolerated, and effective treatment paradigm based on the PREEMPT clinical program. Headache. 2010;50:1406–18.
58. Choi YJ, Lee WJ, Lee HJ, Lee KW, Kim HJ, Hu KS. Effective botulinum toxin guide for treatment of temporal headache. Toxins. 2016;8:265.
59. Schaefer SM, Gottschalk C, Jabbari B. Treatment of chronic migraine with focus on botulinum toxins. Toxins. 2015;7:2615–28.
60. Richardson D, Jabbari B. Botulinum toxin treatment of chronic migraine: a double blind study with a novel technique employing fewer injections. Poster 124th American Academy of Neurology annual meeting, Vancouver, Canada, April 19, 2016.
61. Evers S, Vollmer-Haase J, Schwaag S, Rahmann A, Husstedt IW, Frese A. Botulinum toxin A in the prophylactic treatment of migraine--a randomized, double-blind, placebo-controlled study. Cephalalgia. 2004;24:838–43.
62. Elkind AH, O'Carroll P, Blumenfeld A, DeGryse R, Dimitrova R, BoNTA-024-026-036 Study Group. A series of three sequential, randomized, controlled studies of repeated treatments with botulinum toxin type A for migraine prophylaxis. J Pain. 2006;7:688–96.
63. Saper JR, Mathew NT, Loder EW, DeGryse R, VanDenburgh AM, BoNTA-009 Study Group. A double-blind, randomized, placebo-controlled comparison of botulinum toxin type a injection sites and doses in the prevention of episodic migraine. Pain Med. 2007;8:478–85.
64. Relja M, Poole AC, Schoenen J, Pascual J, Lei X, Thompson C. A multicentre, double- blind, randomized, placebo-controlled, parallel group study of multiple treatments of botulinum toxin type A (BoNTA) for the prophylaxis of episodic migraine headaches. Cephalalgia. 2007;27:492–503.
65. Aurora SK, Gawel M, Brandes JL, Pokta S, Vandenburgh AM, BOTOX North American Episodic Migraine Study Group. Botulinum toxin type A prophylactic treatment of episodic migraine: a randomized, double-blind, placebo-controlled exploratory study. Headache. 2007;47:486–99.
66. Simpson DM, Hallett M, Ashman EJ, Comella CL, Green MW, Gronseth GS, Armstrong, MJ, Gloss D, Potrebic S, Jankovic J, Karp BP, Naumann M, So YT, Yablon SA. Practice guideline update summary: botulinum neurotoxin for the treatment ofblepharospasm, cervical dystonia, adult spasticity, and headache: report of the Guideline Development Subcommittee of the American Academy of Neurology. Neurology. 2016;86:1818–26.
67. Schwartz BS, Stewart WF, Simon D, Lipton RB. Epidemiology of tension-type headache. JAMA. 1998;279:381–3.
68. Jensen R, Rasmussen BK. Muscular disorders in tension-type headache. Cephalalgia. 1996;16:97–103.
69. Freitag F. Managing and treating tension-type headache. Med Clin North Am. 2013;97:281–92.
70. Diamond S, Dalessio DJ. Muscle contraction headache. In: Diamond D, Dalessio DJ, editors. The practicing physician's approach to headache. 4th ed. Baltimore, MD: Williams and Wilkins; 1986. p. 99–113.
71. Bendtsen L, Evers S, Linde M, Mitsikostas DD, Sandrini G, Schoenen J. FNS guideline on the treatment of tension-type headache—report of an EFNS task force. Eur J Neurol. 2010;17:1318–25.
72. Schmitt WJ, Slowey E, Fravi N, Weber S, Burgunder JM. Effect of botulinum toxin A injections in the treatment of chronic tension-type headache: a double-blind, placebo-controlled trial. Headache. 2001;41:658–64.
73. Rollnik JD, Dengler R. Botulinum toxin (DYSPORT) in tension-type headaches. Acta Neurochir Suppl. 2002;79:123–6.
74. Padberg M, de Bruijn SF, de Haan RJ, Tavy DL. Treatment of chronic tension-type headache with botulinum toxin: a double-blind, placebo-controlled clinical trial. Cephalalgia. 2004;24:675–80.
75. Schulte-Mattler WJ, Krack P, BoNTTH Study Group. Treatment of chronic tension-type headache with botulinum toxin A: a randomized, double-blind, placebo-controlled multicenter study. Pain. 2004;109:110–4.

76. Silberstein SD, Göbel H, Jensen R, Elkind AH, Degryse R, Walcott JM, Turkel C. Botulinum toxin type A in the prophylactic treatment of chronic tension-type headache: a multicentre, double-blind, randomized, placebo-controlled, parallel-group study. Cephalalgia. 2006;26:790–800.
77. Straube A, Empl M, Ceballos-Baumann A, Tölle T, Stefenelli U, Pfaffenrath V. Dysport Tension-Type Headache Study Group. Pericranial injection of botulinum toxin type A (Dysport) for tension-type headache—a multicentre, double-blind, randomized, placebo-controlled study. Eur J Neurol. 2008;15:205–13.
78. Hamdy SM, Samir H, El-Sayed M, Adel N, Hasan R. Botulinum toxin: could it be an 'effective treatment for chronic tension-type headache? J Headache Pain. 2009;10:27–34.
79. Harden RN, Cottrill J, Gagnon CM, Smitherman TA, Weinland SR, Tann B, Joseph P, Lee TS, Houle TT. Botulinum toxin a in the treatment of chronic tension-type headache with cervical myofascial trigger points: a randomized, double-blind, placebo-controlled pilot study. Headache. 2009;49:732–43.
80. Eller M, Goadsby PJ. Trigeminal autonomic cephalalgias. Oral Dis. 2016;22:1–8.
81. Ailani JA. Practical approach to autonomic dysfunction in patients with headache. Curr Neurol Neurosci rep. 2016;16:41.
82. Petersen AS, Barloese MC, Jensen RH. Oxygen treatment of cluster headache: a review. Cephalalgia. 2014;34:1079–87.
83. Obermann M, Holle D, Naegel S, Burmeister J, Diener HC. Pharmacotherapy options forcluster headache. Expert Opin Pharmacother. 2015;16:1177–84.
84. Miller S, Matharu M. Trigeminal autonomic cephalalgias: beyond the conventional treatments. Curr Pain Headache Rep. 2014;18:438.
85. Goadsby PJ. Trigeminal autonomic cephalalgias. Continuum. 2012;18:883–95.
86. Leone M., Proietti Cecchini A. Deep brain stimulation in headache. Cephalalgia 2015; 36(12):1143–1148.
87. Sostak P, Krause P, Förderreuther S, Reinisch V, Straube A. Botulinum toxin type-A therapy in cluster headache: an open study. J Headache Pain. 2007;8:236–41.
88. Bratbak DF, Nordgård S, Stovner LJ, Linde M, Folvik M, Bugten V, Tronvik E. Pilot study of sphenopalatine injection of onabotulinumtoxinA for the treatment of intractable chronic cluster headache. Cephalalgia. 2016;36:503–509.
89. Zabalza RJ. Sustained response to botulinum toxin in SUNCT syndrome. Cephalalgia. 2012;32:869–72.
90. Zhang Y, Zhang H, Lian, YJ, Ma YQ, Xie NC, Cheng X, Zhang L. Botulinum Toxin A for the treatment of a child with SUNCT syndrome. Pain Res Manag. 2016;2016, 8016065 [Epub ahead of print].

Botulinum Toxin Treatment of Neuropathic Pain

Shivam Om Mittal and Bahman Jabbari

Introduction

Neuropathic pain (NP) is a common form of human pain, caused by a lesion or disease of the somatosensory system [1]. The disturbance or damage responsible for pain can have a peripheral (peripheral nerve, plexus or root) or central (spinal cord, brain stem, or thalamus) site. Affected patients often describe the pain as burning, jabbing, or searing, and have allodynia (touch perceived as pain), hyperalgesia (enhanced pain after exposure to painful stimuli), and hyperesthesia or dysesthesia (enhanced or altered sensations to touch).

Damage to the peripheral nervous system leads to irritation of peripheral nerve endings and accumulation of nociceptive agents (calcitonin gene-related peptide, substance P, glutamate, bradykinin, and others). The accumulation of pain modulators and the ensuing focal inflammation lowers the sensory threshold of peripheral nerve endings to nociceptive stimuli (peripheral sensitization). Peripheral sensitization increases the barrage of nociceptive volleys into the spinal cord and sensitizes the sensory spinal cord neurons (central sensitization). Sustained peripheral and central sensitization lead to chronicity of pain [2].

Botulinum toxins have seven major serotypes (A to G) from which types A and B are approved for human use. The molecular structure of the botulinum toxins and their mechanisms of action through SNARE proteins is described in detail in Chap. 1 of this book (see Rossetto). A sizeable volume of emerging literature indicates that botulinum toxins inhibit the release of pain modulators and transmitters in cell culture, animal pain models, and asymptomatic human volunteers [3, 4].

S.O. Mittal, M.D.
Department of Neurology, Mayo Clinic, Rochester, MN, USA
e-mail: shivamommittal@gmail.com

B. Jabbari, M.D. (✉)
Department of Neurology, Yale University School of Medicine, New Haven, CT, USA
e-mail: bahman.jabbari@yale.edu

B. Jabbari (ed.), *Botulinum Toxin Treatment in Clinical Medicine*,
DOI 10.1007/978-3-319-56038-0_10

In the cell culture studies, application of botulinum toxin A inhibits the release of glutamate, calcitonin gene-related peptide (CGRP), and other pain transmitters from dorsal root ganglia sensory neurons, trigeminal sensory neurons, and trigeminal satellite cultured cells after cleaving the SNARE proteins [5–9]. BoNT-A in molar concentration inhibits the function of membrane sodium channels in the peripheral and sensory neurons [10].

In animal pain models, BoNTs have alleviated the neuropathic pain through a number of mechanisms (Fig. 1): Injection of botulinum toxins A and B into the rat's paw a few days before formalin injection reduces local accumulation of glutamate, local inflammation, and alleviates pain behavior [11, 12]. There is evidence that the injected toxin travels to the spinal cord and inhibits the release of substance P from spinal neurons along with a reduction of cFos expression at the spinal cord level [12]. In the ischemic pain model secondary to sciatic ligation, injection of BoNT-A into the ipsilateral paw (rat) reduces upregulated nociceptive interleukins and increases the anti-nociceptive interleukins along with amelioration of the animal's pain behavior (paw licking) [13]. Intramuscular injection of BoNT-A in rats diminishes muscle spindle discharge [14] and sympathetic transmission [15], factors which can enhance central sensitization.

Eight examples of peripheral neuropathic pain (PNP) for which prospective and controlled data are available on BoNT efficacy are discussed in this chapter; these include

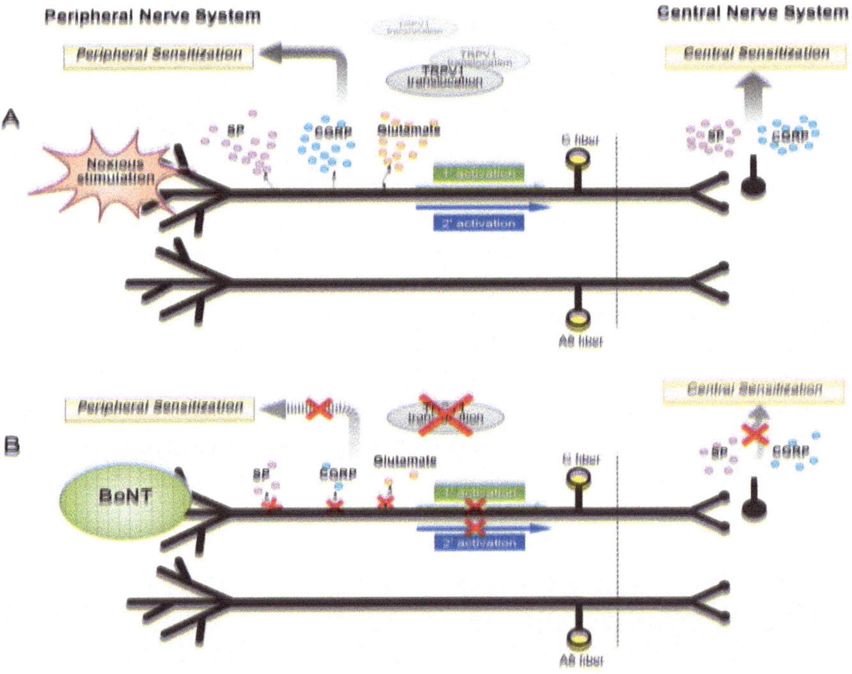

Fig. 1 Mechanisms of neuropathic pain and modes of action of botulinum toxins (From Oh and Chung, Toxins 2015 with permission) SP- Substance P, CGRP-Calcitonin gene-related peptide, BoNT-Botulinum neuro toxin

post-herpetic neuralgia, post-traumatic neuralgia, trigeminal neuralgia, painful diabetic neuropathy, complex regional pain syndrome, carpal tunnel syndrome, phantom pain, and central neuropathic pain. Case reports are provided from the authors' experience.

The level of efficacy for BoNTs is defined according to the guidelines of the Therapeutics and Assessment Subcommittee of the American Academy of Neurology (AAN) [16, 17]. Hence, level A evidence (effective or not effective) requires two class I studies. For level B evidence (probably effective/ineffective), one class I or two class II studies are needed while one class II study denotes level C (possibly effective/ineffective) evidence. Level U indicates undetermined efficacy. The Yale medical library's search system which encompasses a number of search programs including Pub Med and Ovid was used for literature search.

In pain medicine, only chronic migraine is so far an approved FDA indication for botulinum toxin treatment (see Chap. 9). All other areas of pain are currently considered off-label, although for several of them the literature strongly suggests efficacy. The four FDA-approved neurotoxins (three A and one B) are generally considered safe in the recommended doses. Nonetheless, it is prudent before administering any BoNT, to obtain a signed acknowledgment from the patient about having reviewed the list of potentially serious, albeit rare side effects.

Post-herpetic Neuralgia (PHN)

Dorsal root ganglia and cranial nerves are common sites of reactivation of varicella-zoster (VZ) virus which then can spread to the sensory nerves and corresponding dermatomes. Adult Zoster infection often affects elderly, diabetic, and immunocompromised patients. Pathology involves substantial loss of epidermal nerve fibers (small unmyelinated) and the subepidermal plexus [18]. In one study, during the acute phase, cerebrospinal fluid showed inflammatory cells in 61% of the patients and magnetic resonance imaging demonstrated signal changes in the spinal cord and brain stem in 56%. [19] Antiviral therapy lowers the risk of developing PHN [20]; varicella-zoster vaccination reduces development of PHN by 66.5% between ages 60 and 80 [21].

The typical PHN usually persists beyond 3 months after the zoster infection. The incidence of post-herpetic neuralgia increases with age: 5% for individuals younger than 60, 10% between 60 and 69, and 20% for age 80 or older [22]. Older age, severity of the initial acute pain, and presence of larger fiber neuropathy (A-beta fibers with loss of vibration) increase the risk of PHN [23, 24].

Treatment

Patients with PHN have a poor quality of life due to severe bouts of pain in the distribution of affected dermatomes [25]. A variety of oral and topical medications are advocated for the treatment of PHN [26, 27]. Non-steroidal analgesics, gabapentin, pregabalin, and tricyclic agents are among the first line of drugs, used alone or in combination. The starting dose of gabapentin can be 100–300 mg at night and, if needed, it can be increased slowly to up to 900 mg three times daily. Pregabalin may be started with 25–75 mg at night and increased slowly to 300 mg twice daily. In more severe forms, tramadol 50–100 mg daily as a starting dose (not to exceed 600 mg daily) may help [28].

In the most severe cases, oxycodone 5 mg every 4 h, increased by 5 mg four times daily every 2 days (as tolerated) may be used. In the case of chronic use, the long-acting formulation of oxycodone used every 12 h is recommended. Administration of corticosteroids and chronic application of anesthetic patches (lidocaine and others) are other modes of treatment. Although the exact percentage of patients who fail modern analgesic treatment for PHN is not known, failures are not uncommon—challenging the clinicians. Polytherapy is also a problem in elderly patients who are more prone to develop PHN. There is, hence, a need for newer modes of treatment with fewer side-effect profiles and low or no interactions with commonly used analgesics.

BoNT Studies in Post-herpetic Neuralgia

A recent meta-analysis of this subject identified six studies on the efficacy of BoNTs in post-herpetic and trigeminal neuralgia, five without evidence of significant bias [29]. The pooled results showed a difference in post-treatment pain intensity of −3.009 (95% confidence interval − 4.566 to −1.453; $P < 0.001$) in favor of BoNT-A compared with placebo in managing TN or PHN.

To date, two double-blind studies (Class I) [30, 31] have assessed the efficacy of BoNTs in post-herpetic neuralgia.

Xiao et al. [31] evaluated pain relief by visual analog scale (VAS) at 1, 7, and 90 days after subcutaneous injection of BoNT-A in 60 patients with PHN. The quality of life was assessed by improvement in sleep hours. Patients were randomized and assigned blindly into three groups: BoNT-A, lidocaine, and placebo (20 in each group). The baseline level of pain and sleep disturbance was comparable between the three groups. The location of herpetic skin lesions was orofacial ($n = 11$), cervical and upper extremity ($n = 14$), thoracic ($n = 18$), and lumbar and lower limbs ($n = 17$).

The injecting solution was prepared by mixing 100 units of the Type A toxin (Chinese toxin form Lanzhou Institute) with 2 cc of preservative-free saline (5 units/cc). Injections were subcutaneous, grid-like, 1 cm apart, and into the region of tactile allodynia. Patients in the BoNT group had significantly better pain relief compared to the two groups on lidocaine and saline ($P < 0.01$). BoNT analgesic response began at days 3–5, peaked at 1 week, and continued for 3 months. The improvement of sleep from BoNT was also superior to lidocaine and placebo groups ($P < 0.05$). Patients in the BoNT group also used significantly less opioids (22% vs. 52% and 66%). Side effects consisted only of mild pain at the site of injections.

Apalla et al. [30] conducted a prospective, double-blind, parallel study comparing the effect of BoNT-A (ona-A) to placebo in 30 adult subjects with PHN. In the

BoNT-A group, the toxin was diluted with 4 cc of normal saline and injected subcutaneously via a 30-gauge needle in a "chessboard manner." The dose per injection site was 5 units. A total of 100 units was used. The severity of pain was assessed by VAS (0–10) at baseline, and then daily for the first 2 weeks, then every 2 weeks until the 12th week and every 4 weeks until the 24th week. The primary outcome was 50% or more reduction in VAS score measured at week 4 compared to baseline. The secondary outcome was an improvement of the quality of sleep evaluated by a 5-point questionnaire (very bad to very good) recorded at the same timeframes. Persistence of improved VAS scores beyond the first 4 weeks was also considered a secondary outcome. Significant VAS improvement was reported at 4 weeks and over subsequent weeks (for the toxin group, $P < 0.001$). Patients in BoNT also demonstrated significant improvement in the quality of sleep and reduction of sleep scores along the same timelines.

Retrospective observations in a small number of patients reported significant pain relief after BoNT administration in patients with PHN supporting blinded observations [32, 33]. The study of Ranoux et al. [34] which demonstrated the efficacy of ona-A in neuropathic pain (rated class I by AAN subcommittee) also included four patients with PHN. The specifics of these four patients, however, were not provided.

Patient Report

A 62-year-old female was referred to the Yale Botulinum Toxin Treatment Clinic for the management of severe pain behind the left ear which had started 2 years earlier. A few weeks after the pain onset, typical herpetic skin lesions appeared. Treatment with Acyclovir gradually improved the skin lesions but did not alter the pain which grew in intensity. More severe bouts of pain often ended in disabling headaches. The pain was described as jabbing and stabbing, resulted in the loss of sleep and prompted marked apprehension in anticipation of the next bout. Treatment with gabapentin, pregabalin, and oxycodone was not helpful. The pain was often scored as 10 of 10 on a visual analog scale and described as "unbearable."

On examination, residual scars of zoster infection were seen behind the right ear. A total of 60 units of ona-A was injected in a grid-like pattern behind the left ear subcutaneously at 20 points (3 units/point) using a 30-gauge needle (Fig. 2). The dilution was 100 units per 2 cc. The patient reported a sharp drop in pain frequency and intensity (VAS down from 10 to 3) 5 days after the injections. The pain then disappeared at week 2 post-injection and gradually reappeared at 2.5 months. Over the next 3 years following the first treatment, the patient received injections every 3 months. Each treatment resulted in significant reduction in pain. During the third year, injections lasted for 6 months or longer with the returning pain reported as subtle (1–2 in VAS scale). She was very pleased with the outcome when last seen 4 years after the first BoNT treatment.

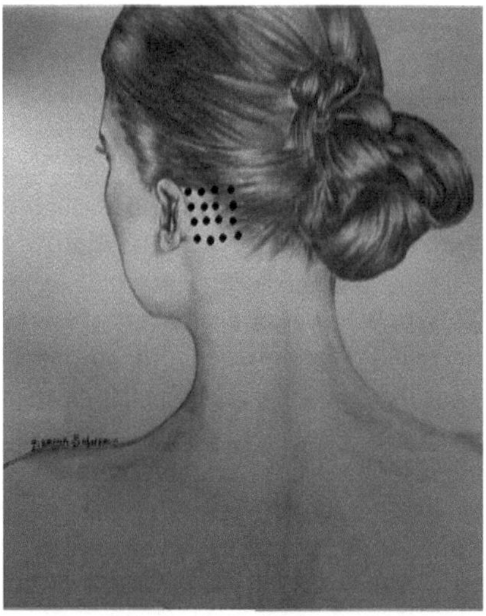

Fig. 2 Pattern of botulinum toxin injection in a patient with post-herpetic neuralgia behind the left ear. Drawing from Damoun Safarpour M.D.

Comment

BoNT-A treatment of post-herpetic neuralgia possesses level A efficacy (effective) based on the two randomized class I studies. The role of BoNTs other than ona-A needs to be further investigated for the management of PHN. One of the two authors of this chapter (BJ) has treated seven patients suffering from PHN with subcutaneous ona-A injections. The dose ranged from 60 to 200 units based on the extent of the involved skin. The treatment was very effective in five patients (example: case 1). Of the two remaining patients, one had extensive zoster infection over the left chest, and another, a 91-year-old man demonstrated diffuse hemicranial residual scalp lesions; neither one reported pain relief after BoNT injections. Failure of some patients with PHN to respond to BoNT treatment may be related to extensive pathology possibly extending to the CNS.

Trigeminal Neuralgia (TN)

Trigeminal neuralgia is characterized by bouts of severe pain described as jabbing, stabbing, and shock-like, usually affecting one side of the face. In most cases, the pain lasts seconds but durations up to 2 min are also observed. Bouts of pain may occur multiple times a day and disable the patient. Facial movements, eating, speaking, chewing, and shaving often exacerbate the pain. Many patients have local trigger points in the face that upon touching provoke severe pain. The incidence of TN has been reported as 4/100,000 in the US with the onset in most patients observed between ages 50 and 70 [35, 36]. Antiepileptic drugs such as carbamazepine, oxcarbazepine, gabapentin, lamotrigine, and GABAergic medications such as baclofen

(30–60 mg) may provide relief. In one blinded study, a combination of carbamazepine and baclofen proved more effective, than either of the two alone [37]. Unfortunately, pharmacological failures are not uncommon. In recalcitrant cases, surgical microvascular decompression and Gamma knife surgery may alleviate the pain [38]. Surgery is not devoid of side effects which may be substantial to include ataxia, brain stem damage, and cranial nerve palsies.

Pathophysiology: Cultured trigeminal neurons, within days, release large amounts of CGRP, a major inflammatory pain mediator and adding onaA to the cultured trigeminal neurons results in marked reduction of CGRP release from stimulated trigeminal neurons [6]. In acute infraorbital nerve injury model that causes significant local allodynia in the rat, subcutaneous injection of ona-A improved allodynia and reduced release of pain mediators from disconnected trigeminal neurons [39]. The introduction of A/E chimera of BoNT (which specifically targets sensory neurons) to the trigeminal cell culture inhibits CGRP release by subduing the function of transient receptor potential vanilloid 1 (TRPV1) [8]. TRPV1, a cation channel, which promotes the release of CGRP, is highly expressed in a large number of trigeminal neurons. Subcutaneous injection of 0.25 and 0.5 ng/kg of ona-A into the rat's face markedly reduces the expression of TRPV1 in the trigeminal neurons within 2 days [40].

Matak et al. [41] promote the view that the analgesic effect of the BoNT-A in experimental trigeminal neuralgia of rats (formalin injection into the whiskers) results in a large part from a direct central effect of the toxin. In this model, after BoNT-A administration truncated SNAP25 was detected in the sensory trigeminal nucleus in the medulla. The analgesic effect of the toxin was blocked by injection of colchicine into the trigeminal ganglia which block and prevents the toxin from reaching the CNS.

Botulinum Toxin Treatment of Trigeminal Neuralgia

Three double-blind and one prospective single-blind clinical trial have assessed the efficacy of BoNT treatment in trigeminal neuralgia.

Wu et al. [42] enrolled 42 patients with trigeminal neuralgia in a 13-week, randomized, parallel design, double-blind, placebo-controlled study. Forty patients, 21 in the BoNT and 19 in the saline (placebo) group, completed the study. BoNT type A (Chinese brand from Lanshou Institute) was diluted in 1 cc of normal saline and injected with a 16 mm long needle, either between the epidermis and dermis or submucosal in the areas affected by pain. Subjects in the BoNT group received up to 75 units and a comparable volume was administered to the subjects in the saline group. Patients remained on the same dose of their medications (carbamazepine, gabapentin, and pregabalin) during the study. The primary outcome was a significant change in pain frequency and intensity (VAS) compared to the placebo. Secondary outcomes were the patient global impression of change (PGIC) and proportion of responders defined as 50% or more compared to baseline. Both primary outcome and all the secondary outcomes improved significantly in the BoNT group compared to the placebo ($P < 0.001$). Side effects were noted in the subjects who received BoNT; seven subjects developed mild facial asymmetry which disappeared after 7 weeks and three developed local facial swelling which subsided in a week.

Two years later, the same group of authors [43] conducted another blinded study in trigeminal neuralgia comparing specifically the effect of 25 units of BoNT type A with 75 units. Both doses compared to placebo significantly reduced the pain as early as week 1, and the effect was sustained until week 8 throughout the study. There was no significant difference in efficacy between the two dose groups. Patient Global Impression of Change (PGIC) was significant in the treatment group (67% in 25 U group and 76% in 75 U group) compared to the placebo group (32%). The authors concluded that the low dose of 25 units is sufficient to significantly alleviate the pain of TN. Higher doses are not necessarily better and could cause more side effects (facial weakness). Zuniga et al. [44] conducted a double-blind, randomized, placebo-controlled study where 20 subjects received ona-A and 16 subjects received placebo. The dose of ona-A was 50 U subcutaneously with and extra 10 U into the masseter muscle if there was involvement of mandibular branch of the trigeminal nerve. At 2 months, mean VAS showed a trend toward improvement in the ona-A group compared to the placebo group ($P = 0.07$). At 3 months after the injection, significant improvement in VAS was seen in the ona-A group ($P = 0.01$).

In the single-blinded study of Shehata et al. [45], 20 subjects with TN were randomized into BoNT and placebo groups. In the BoNT group, subjects received subcutaneous injections of 40–60 units of ona-A into 8–12 points (5 units per point) in the face. The primary outcome was a decrease in pain intensity at 12 weeks measured by VAS compared to the placebo. At 12 weeks, the ona-A group demonstrated a reduction of 6.5 points VAS compared to three points in the placebo group ($P = 0.0001$). As a secondary outcome, the quality of life also improved significantly and more patients in the BoNT could reduce the number of their pain medications. In a 14-month longitudinal study, repeated injections of ona-A in 88 subjects with TN maintained pain relief, improvement in anxiety, depression, sleep, and the quality of life [46].

Patient Report

A 41-year-old woman was referred to the Yale Botulinum Neurotoxin Treatment Clinic for consideration of BoNT therapy of a disabling trigeminal neuralgia. Twenty years earlier, following a car accident, she began to experience severe left-sided face pain and headaches. The pain was dull and deep at first but gradually transformed into bouts of sharp and jabbing pain lasting 15–20 s. Many factors provoked pain especially exposure to the cold environment. She reported several trigger points close to the nose and corner of the mouth, making application of makeup difficult. In "bad days," pain affected the region around the left eye and made it "twitch."

Over the years, the patient had tried multiple medications for the pain including beta blockers, antiepileptic drugs, calcium channel blockers, non-steroidal anti-inflammatory drugs, oxycodone, and acupuncture which offered no significant relief. She had had three surgical procedures in the past: decompression surgery via retro-mastoid craniotomy for relieving pressure upon the trigeminal nerve, exploration for possible cerebello-pontine angle pathology (second surgery), and cortical stimulation for the pain relief. None of the three procedures relieved her pain. The patient described constant daily background facial pain with superimposed bouts of sharp pain. Past medical, family, and social history disclosed no issues of concern.

On examination, several trigger points were identified on the left side of the face close to the nose and corner of the mouth. A total of 30 units of ona-A was injected subcutaneously in 20 sites (1.5 units per site) into the V2 distribution. In addition, she received another 10 units (4 points) into the left frontalis (2.5 units, four sites) and 5 units into the anterior temporal region (2.5 units, two points).

After 2 weeks, the patient reported a marked reduction in the severity of pain (VAS 9 changed to 2) and in the frequency of sharp pains (90% reduction). This response lasted for 5 months at which time the severity of pain returned and required another injection that produced a similar effect. No side effects were reported. The patient described her experience as very satisfactory in the patient global impression of change.

Comment

The efficacy of BoNT treatment for trigeminal neuralgia is supported by two class I studies [43, 47], providing level A evidence (effective). Much remains to be established regarding the optimal type of toxin, technique, dose, and the number of injections. In our experience, a dose of 25–40 units, injected into 15–20 sites is effective and devoid of serious side effects. Transient facial weakness remains a side effect but due to subcutaneous nature of the toxin and low dose per site, it is mild and transient. At the Yale Botulinum Toxin Treatment Clinic, we have treated six patients with 25–40 units of ona-A toxin for trigeminal neuralgia. Five of six reported significant pain relief. Only one developed mild and transient facial weakness.

Post-traumatic Neuralgia

Pathophysiology: Peripheral trauma triggers a cascade of events which involve nociceptor receptor sites, peripheral nerve endings, dorsal root ganglia (DRGs), spinal cord neurons, and central sensory neurons. Pain mediators (glutamate, substance P) accumulate in the damaged nerve endings. New sprouts develop with increased density of sodium channels [48], which via increased nociceptive excitability generate ectopic discharges. New sprouts show increased sensitivity to cytokines, prostaglandins, and catecholamine. This peripheral sensitization increases the volume of nociceptive volleys which enter dorsal root ganglia and spinal cord. Histologic changes which develop after peripheral trauma in DRG and spinal cord indicate increased neural excitation. In DRG, there is an overgrowth of sympathetic nerves and abnormal linkage of A and C fibers [49]. In the spinal cord, dark cells appear in dorsal horns which presumably represent dying inhibitory neurons of glycinergic and GABAergic types [50, 51]. The demise of inhibitory neurons leads to enhanced excitation of central neurons. It has also been shown that after peripheral injury, many large alpha/beta afferents (usually ending in Rexed lamina III) grow and penetrate more superficial levels (Rexed lamina II and I of dorsal horn) and gain access to low threshold, pain afferents [52].

Treatment

Medical treatment consists mainly of administration of analgesic agents previously defined under post-herpetic and trigeminal neuralgia. Additional treatments include nerve block by single injection or infusion, transcutaneous electrical nerve stimulation (TENS), peripheral nerve stimulation (PNS), or spinal cord (dorsal horn) stimulation which increases GABA release.

BoNT Treatment of Post-traumatic Neuralgia

Ranoux et al. [34] screened 61 consecutive patients of whom 29 met the criteria of neuropathic pain and eligibility for BoNT treatment. Nineteen patients were women. Twenty-five patients had post-traumatic neuralgia and four patients had post-herpetic neuralgia. In the post-traumatic group, 18 patients had surgical trauma and seven non-surgical trauma to single nerves. The patients were enrolled in a randomized, prospective double-blind, parallel design study. The primary outcome was a self-reported level of pain over a 24-h period on an 11-point scale of brief pain inventory (0–10) from a diary. Pain level was assessed at baseline and at 4 and 12 weeks. Secondary outcomes included degrees of brush allodynia, mechanical sensation and pain threshold, thermal sensations and pain threshold as well as neuropathic pain symptom inventory; all assessed at the aforementioned time points.

A neurologist, not involved in the study, administered intradermal BoNTA (ona-A) solution at points 1.5 cm apart. The dilution was 100 units in 4 cc of preservative-free saline. The mean number of injections was 20 + 8.3. The dose ranged from 20 to 190 units. In the BoNT group, patients noticed an improvement in pain intensity from the second week ($P = 0.02$) with persistent results until the 14th week ($P = 0.03$). The average pain intensity assessed at each visit improved in the toxin group (0.007). Allodynia to brush also improved significantly and pain threshold to cold was decreased in the BoNT group. Injections were painful, but no patient reported any side effects.

The same group of authors recently published another randomized, double-blind study in a larger group of 46 subjects with post-traumatic neuralgia [53]. In this study, the primary outcome was the efficacy of two successive administrations of ona-A or placebo, delivered at week 1 and week 12. The subjects were followed for 24 weeks with four visits. Subjects reported the intensity of pain on a numerical scale of 1–11 weekly. The percentage of pain relief in the toxin group was 26.4% versus 10.6% for the placebo ($P = 0.008$). Pain frequency and sleep were also improved ($P = 0.001$ and $P = 0.02$) in the toxin group.

Patient Report

A 56-year-old woman was referred to the Yale Movement Disorder Clinic for the evaluation of severe post-traumatic neuralgia. Twelve years earlier, her car was forcefully rear ended after she braked hard to avoid hitting a car in front of her. The accident heavily bruised her right ankle and the lateral aspect of her right foot. The foot and ankle continued to ache and an area of intense allodynia developed over the lateral malleolus extending up to the lower leg. Multiple medications failed to improve either the pain or the local allodynia. The most recent medications included gabapentin, pregabalin, tramadol, capsaicin ointment, and diclofenac gel. In patient's words: "the physical, emotional and psychological impact of my chronic pain defies description"; "Every night, I have to take Tylenol, Advil, and Ambien and apply ankle soak, topical pain cream, and heat wrap in order to be able to sleep. With all this, many nights I am unable to sleep due to pain"; "Even the pressure of sheets would cause the pain to flare up. "Sleeping on my side is impossible."

On examination, muscle strength was normal, but foot movements were slow and intensified the ankle pain. A large area of allodynia and hyperesthesia was present including the lateral aspect of the right foot extending 10 cm above the right ankle. The most intense allodynic region was over the lateral malleolus with extension to 5 cm above it (Fig. 3).

Ona-A was injected subcutaneously into the dorsolateral aspect of the right foot (total 50 units at 20 sites in a grid pattern) including the region of lateral malleolus. The patient reported 30% reduction of pain (7 on VAS scale) after the first injection and 90% decrease after the second injection (VAS 1–2) 6 months later. In patient's words: "the effect after the second injection was astounding. I stopped taking gabapentin and using pain wrap at night. I can now wear boots for the first time in 12 years!" An examination 3 months after the second injection showed a marked reduction of allodynia which was now limited to a small area above the lateral malleolus. Over the next 3 years, the patient received similar injections every 6–9 months. When the pain returned, the intensity remained low and, for the most part, was tolerable (VAS level 2–3).

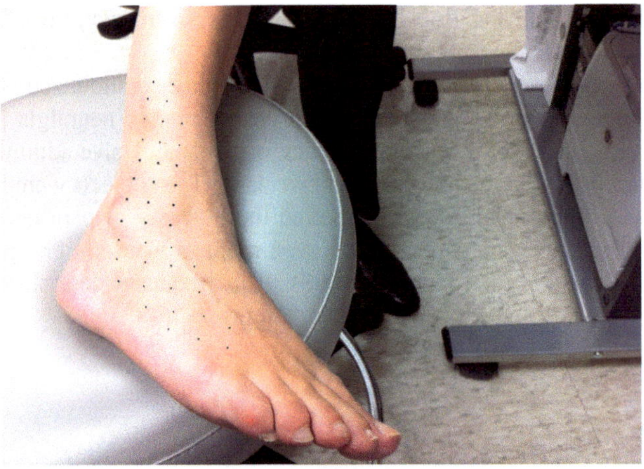

Fig. 3 Region of right foot allodynia (*darker dots* denote areas of higher sensitivity) in the patient with post-traumatic neuropathic pain with points of BoNT injection

Clinical Comment: The level of evidence for the efficacy of ona-A for PTN is A (effective) based on two class I studies. The case presented above is an example of PTN with severe allodynia showing a remarkable response to ona-A after two treatments. Some patients with PTN may later develop complex regional pain syndrome (CRPS), a condition which is more difficult to treat. An important question to consider is whether or not an early treatment of PTN with BoNTs can reduce the risk of developing CRPS.

Complex Regional Pain Syndrome

Complex regional pain syndrome (CRPS) often evolves from post-traumatic neuralgia. For reasons, which are yet poorly understood, a traumatized limb affected by somatic pain gradually develops additional autonomic and trophic dysfunction. In CRPS I, the causative factor does not damage or disrupt the nerve, whereas, in CRPS II peripheral nerve is damaged. Causalgia, first described in detail by Weir Mitchell among soldiers with traumatized limbs during the American Civil War, belongs to the CRPS II category [54]. CRPS-related pain has a burning and jabbing quality and the affected limb has areas of allodynia and hyperesthesia. Autonomic dysfunctions take a variety of pattern including coldness or warmth of the limb with hyper- or hypohydrosis. Skin atrophy, hair loss, and nail deformity are among trophic changes [55]. In some patients, motor symptoms such as finger, hand, and arm dystonia and tremor develop and cause further discomfort. Symptoms may extend to the proximal part of the limb and cause pain and dystonia of the arm and shoulder muscles. In severe cases, loss of vascular supply threatens the development of gangrene and may necessitate limb amputation.

Pathophysiology

For years, primary dysfunction of the sympathetic system was held responsible for the development of CRPS. This view is now modified in favor of neuroinflammation and deranged autoimmunity with small C-fiber damage playing a pivotal role. Damage to C-fibers could lead to neurogenic inflammation, ectopic firing, vasodilation (via axon reflex), and/or hypoxic/ischemic injury [56, 57]. Evidence exists that, in some patients, neural inflammation extends to the spinal cord. In one patient with longstanding CRPS, tissue examination of the dorsal horn demonstrated significant activation of microglia and astrocytes with neuronal loss [58].

Conventional Treatment

Treatment of CRPS is difficult and geared to a relief of pain and modification of the course of the disease. Treatment of pain with tricyclic antidepressants, calcium channel blockers including gabapentin and pregabalin, serotonin/norepinephrine reuptake inhibitors, and locally delivered anesthetics is partially effective. Intranasal calcitonin (100–400 units) may relieve pain in some patients. In a blinded study, intravenous infusion of ketamine (NMDA antagonist) effectively reduced pain in 16 of 20 patients with a follow-up of 6 months [59]. However, the recommended dose of 100 mg for 4 h/day for 10 days can be associated with significant hepatotoxicity requiring close liver function monitoring. A small double-blind cross-over study of 12 patients suggested the efficacy of intravenous immunoglobulin (IVIG) [60]. In general, CRPS is considered a very difficult condition to treat.

BoNT Treatment of CRPS

Argoff et al. [61] reported pain relief and improvement of skin color and local edema in 11 patients with CRPS after intramuscular injection of ona-A. In agreement with his observation, a single case report described marked reduction of allodynia after subcutaneous injection of ona-A in a patient with CRPS and dorsal hand allodynia [62].

In contrast, in a blinded, controlled, parallel study, Safarpour et al. [63] found no statistically significant difference between ona-A and placebo in eight patients with severe CPRS allodynia. The authors also reported the failure of ona-A in an open trial of an additional six CRPS patients. In another publication, however, these same authors reported significant improvement of proximal pain, proximal and distal dystonia, and shooting arm pain in two patients with CPRS after intramuscular injection of ona-A into several painful proximal muscles (deltoid, trapezius, levator scapulae, supraspinatus, upper thoracic paraspinal, and flexor digitorum superficialis) with a total dose of 300 units [64]. In one of these patients, concurrent exquisite dorsal hand allodynia also gradually improved after 2 years of repeated proximal intramuscular injections. A retrospective report of 37 patients by Kharkar et al. [65] also indicated an improvement of CRPS after intramuscular injection of shoulder girdle muscles.

Comment

The role of BoNT treatment in CRPS is evolving and, at this point, the level of efficacy is U (undetermined) due to lack of class I and II studies. The encouraging reports of open observations need to be examined by larger controlled studies. On the technical side, patients with severe allodynia (advanced CRPS) tolerate injections poorly. Three important questions to be addressed in the future studies are:

1. Is a combined subcutaneous and intramuscular injection more effective than subcutaneous or intradermal injection alone?
2. Can early and aggressive treatment with BoNTs slow down the dismal course of CRPS?
3. Are proximal injections combined with distal injections more effective than distal injections alone?

Metabolic and Drug-Induced Painful Peripheral Neuropathies

A large number of metabolic derangements and medications affect the peripheral nerves. In some, pain is a major symptom. The focus of this section is on painful diabetic neuropathy, the only metabolic neuropathy for which blinded, placebo-controlled clinical trial results with BoNT treatment is available.

Diabetic Neuropathy

Among metabolic disorders, diabetic neuropathy (DN) can be considered a model of metabolic neuropathic pain. The prevalence of painful neuropathy is 25–26% in type 2 diabetes versus 16% reported for type 1 which occurs among the younger individuals [66, 67]. In the examination, loss of different sensory modalities can coexist with areas of hyperesthesia and allodynia. Chronic pain of diabetic neuropathy can incite anxiety and depression impairing the quality of life due to psychosocial distress and disrupted sleep.

Pathophysiology

For many years, hyperglycemia was considered the reason for the development of pain in DN. Recent data suggest hypoinsulinism and abnormal insulin signaling as a more relevant factor [68]. The pain of diabetic neuropathy has been attributed to dysfunction of sodium channels, and non-selective calcium channels linked to transient receptor potential receptor (TRP) and receptors for nerve growth factors which are all expressed highly in DRG neurons. More recently, CaV3.2 T-type voltage-gated calcium channels (T-channels) have been identified as key players in the sensitized (hyperexcitable) state of nociceptive sensory neurons (nociceptors) in response to hyperglycemia and regarded as the basis for painful symptoms of diabetic neuropathy [69].

Treatment of Painful Diabetic Neuropathy (PDN)

The treatment strategy focuses on modifying the mechanisms which cause neuropathic pain. Per American Academy of Neurology guidelines, pregabalin is established as effective for PDN (Level A) [70]. Venlafaxine, duloxetine, amitriptyline, gabapentin, valproate, opioids (morphine sulfate, tramadol, and oxycodone-controlled release), and capsaicin are probably effective for PDN (Level B) [70]. A palliative role for erythropoietin analogs, angiotensin II type 2 receptor, voltage-gated sodium channel antagonists, and lipo-prostaglandin E3 agents has been suggested by earlier observations and is now being further explored by blinded studies [71, 72].

BoNT Treatment in Diabetic Neuropathy

Two placebo-controlled, blinded studies have investigated the efficacy of ona-A in painful diabetic neuropathy.

Yuan et al. [73] conducted a double-blind cross-over study in 18 patients injecting ona-A or saline intradermally into the hypersthetic and allodynic foot regions (4 units/site in case of ona-A). The pain reduction, measured by VAS was significant in favor of ona-A at 1, 4, 8, and 12 weeks ($P < 0.05$). Ona-A administration improved sleep at 1 week (using the Chinese version of the Pittsburg sleep quality index-CPSQI) ($P < 0.05$). The quality of life assessed by SF36 also improved in more patients in the ona-A group compared to the placebo group, but the difference was not statistically significant. Chen et al. [74] published the results of the secondary outcomes of this study (sensory perception and mechanical pain threshold) in a separate communication 5 years later. At weeks 1, 4, 8, and 12, both tactile perception and mechanical pain decreased markedly in ona-A group compared to baseline ($P < 0.05$ at all-time points).

Ghasemi et al. [75], in a double-blind, placebo-controlled, parallel study, assessed the efficacy of abobotulinumtoxinA (abo-A) in 40 patients (20 toxin and 20 placebo) with painful diabetic neuropathy. Abo-A was injected into the dorsum of the foot intradermally at 12 points using a 3 × 4 grid pattern. The dose per site was 8–10 units and the total dose per subject was 100 units. Primary outcomes of the study were changes in a visual analog scale and a neuropathic pain scale in 3 weeks. There was a significant reduction of burning pain, sharp pain, sensitivity to brush and pins in the abo-A group compared to the placebo group ($P < 0.05$). Thirty percent in the abo-A group and zero percent in the placebo (saline) group reported no pain at 3 weeks ($P = 0.01$).

Comment

The level of evidence for the efficacy of BoNT-A in painful diabetic neuropathy is B (probably effective) based on one class I and one class II study. Larger studies with different toxins are needed to support these results.

Painful Neuropathy Related to Drugs and Chemotherapeutic Agents

There are no controlled studies assessing the efficacy of BoNTs in drug-induced and chemotherapy-related painful neuropathies. One of the authors of this chapter (BJ) has treated two patients with chemotherapy-induced peripheral neuropathy with severe allodynia of dorsum of the foot and distal lower leg. OnabotulinumtoxinA, 30 and 40 units, was injected into the area of allodynia. Both patients reported significant improvement of foot pain and allodynia within 2 weeks.

Comment

Randomized and placebo-controlled studies are needed for assessment of the efficacy and utility of BoNT treatment in painful neuropathy related to chemotherapeutic agents. It is noteworthy that these patients are often on polypharmacy which makes the introduction of additional pain medications unwelcome.

Residual Limb Pain and Phantom Pain

Serious limb injuries are becoming a major surgical and medical challenge due to the increasing number of military conflicts. Such injuries could lead to a variety of chronic pain syndromes. In the US, by the year 2050, the number of patients affected by this type of pain may exceed three million [76]. Pain associated with loss of a limb can be a pain in the stump (residual limb pain: RLP) or felt in the region of the lost limb (phantom limb pain: PLP). The reported incidence of RLP after amputation is 22–43% and for PLP is 66% [77, 78]. The possible mechanism and pathophysiology of phantom pain has been discussed in detail in a recent review by Hsu et al. [79].

Pharmacological Treatment

Based on several high-quality studies, Cochrane review of the literature [80] concluded that morphine, gabapentin, and ketamine demonstrate trends toward short-term analgesic efficacy in PLP while memantine and amitriptyline were ineffective. No data on the long-term efficacy of conventional analgesic drugs are available. The role of calcitonin, anesthetics, and dextromethorphan requires further clarification. Since long-term efficacy of drugs against PLP is low (less than 5% in one large review) [81], exploration of novel therapeutic approaches is necessary.

BoNT Treatment of RLP and PLP

Two clinical observations, each on a small number of patients, claimed BoNT administration into stump muscles improves phantom pain. In one study [82], 2500–5000 units of rimabotulinum toxinB (rima-B) was injected into the arm and leg stumps of four patients (two injections into each limb). Injections were performed at multiple trigger points. All patients reported improvement in stump pain, PLP attacks, and improvement of local allodynia. One patient noted significant improvement of sleep. Improvements lasted for “many weeks.” In one patient, a 12-month follow-up showed almost total pain relief. In another study [83], authors described a significant improvement of phantom pain in three patients (two with accident injury and one with landmine injury) after EMG-guided administration of abo-A (up to 500 units) into the stump muscles. All three patients reported level 3 (on a 0–3 scale) improvement on the global clinical scale as well as substantial pain improvement on VAS. Pain relief lasted 11 months. Patients were able to reduce their pain medications after BoNT treatment.

Unfortunately, these positive observations did not bear out in a prospective, parallel design, blinded study (class III, no placebo) which compared the effect of ona-A with that of combined lidocaine/methylprednisolone therapy [42]. Investigators injected a total of 250–300 units of ona-A or 10 mg depomedrol in 1% lidocaine in up to 6 tender points of 14 patients with RLP and PLP. There was no significant effect on phantom pain from any of the two agents. Both agents, however, significantly improved RLP and pain tolerance. Effect of ona-A on RLP and pain tolerability was stronger than that of lidocaine/depomedrol injection ($P = 0.002$ versus $P = 0.06$ and $P = 0.01$ versus 0.07, respectively). The relief of RLP in both groups lasted for 6 months.

Comment

Phantom pain is a fascinating area for BoNT research. Efficacy, if confirmed, would imply that peripheral administration of BoNTs can influence allodynia caused by central pain. The class III study cited above and open observations suggest an efficacy of ona-A for RLP. At this time, the level of efficacy of BoNT is U (undetermined) for both RLP and PLP due to lack of high quality, class I or II studies.

Carpal Tunnel Syndrome

One class I study (randomized and blinded) and one class IV (retrospective) have reported on the safety and efficacy of BoNTs in carpal tunnel syndrome. In the study of Breuer et al. [84], investigators injected 2500 units of rima-B into the hypothenar muscles and compared the results with saline (placebo injection). Both injections improved pain but there was no difference between the toxin and placebo at weeks 1, 5, 9, and 13. In another study [85], prospective, but open-label, intracarpal injection of abo-A (60 units) improved the severity of pain, measured by VAS at 1, 2, and 3 months in three of five patients. The degree of improvement, however, was statistically insignificant. No muscle weakness was noted. These data indicate that injection of rima-B into the hypothenar muscles is probably not effective in the carpal tunnel syndrome (one class A study).

Occipital Neuralgia

Two retrospective case series (Class IV), each comprised of six patients, reported on the efficacy of BoNTS in occipital neuralgia. In one study [86], authors injected 50 units of ona-A into the region of pain and measured the outcome with VAS and Pain Disability Index (PDI). Four weeks after injection, five of six patients demonstrated significant improvement of VAS (mean VAS of 8 changed to 2) and PDI (mean value of 50 changed to 19). Compared to the anesthetic bupivacaine, the effect of ona-A injection lasted significantly longer (16 weeks versus 2 weeks). In the second study [87], the investigators injected 50 units of ona-A along the line traversing between greater and lesser occipital nerves. The outcome was measured by VAS, pain-free days, and several scales for the quality of life. Both VAS and quality of life improved significantly after ona-A treatment. Improvement of quality of life occurred at week 6 and continued over the subsequent weeks until week 12.

Central Neuropathic Pain

The data on the treatment of central neuropathic pain with botulinum toxins are scant. Jabbari et al. [88] first described two patients in whom subcutaneous injection of ona-A into the affected dermatomes improved the neuropathic pain secondary to spinal cord pathology. One of the two patients is presented in some detail below.

Case Report

A 55-year-old female complained of severe burning pain over the elbows, upper forearms, and the medial aspects of both lower arms for 6 years. The pain which affected more the left side was described as "excruciating" with an intense burning quality "as if hot charcoal was applied directly to the skin." Minimal contact with this region, particularly near the left elbow, consistently resulted in worsening of pain. Medications, including tricyclic antidepressants, anticonvulsants, nonsteroidal anti-inflammatory drugs, and opioids failed to improve pain. In her last visit before BoNT treatment, she stated, "life is becoming unbearable," "I cannot live like this."

The patient's history was significant for the onset of progressive weakness of both legs and loss of sensation in lower limbs 7 years ago. Six years prior to presentation, she underwent partial resection of an intramedullary spinal cord angioma at C7-T1. Her pain had begun a few months prior to the surgical intervention but intensified significantly after surgery.

During the examination, the patient held her arms in constant abduction to avoid garments touching the inner part of the forearms. There was marked hyperalgesia and allodynia throughout the T1 and part of the T2 dermatomes, with exquisite sensitivity to touch about the elbows (left > right) (Fig. 4). The level of pain was rated at 8–10 on the visual analog scale (VAS). A magnetic resonance imaging (MRI) of the cervical and thoracic cord demonstrated a residual angioma at the C7 and T1 levels. Intradermal injection of 100 units of ona-A, divided in 25 sites and over the left T1 and T2 dermatomes, resulted in significant improvement of spontaneous pain and skin sensitivity. At day 7, post-injection, the intensity of spontaneous pain in VAS was 2–3 and frequency of recurring pains dropped by 80%. Rubbing of garments against the left elbow no longer caused pain, and tapping the skin over the left elbow produced only mild discomfort. The analgesic effect of ona-A lasted for approximately 3 months. Over the next 3 years, treatment with botulinum toxin A at 4-month intervals provided similar pain relief. Eventually, the pain lessened to such a degree that she elected to discontinue treatments.

In 2016, Han et al. [89], published the results of a double-blind, placebo-controlled parallel study on 40 patients (20 toxin and 20 saline) with neuropathic pain secondary to spinal cord injury. The primary outcome was a reduction in the severity of pain measured by VAS (0–100 scale). A total of 200 units of botulinum toxin A (Daihan pharmaceutical in Seoul, South Korea) was injected into 40 sites in

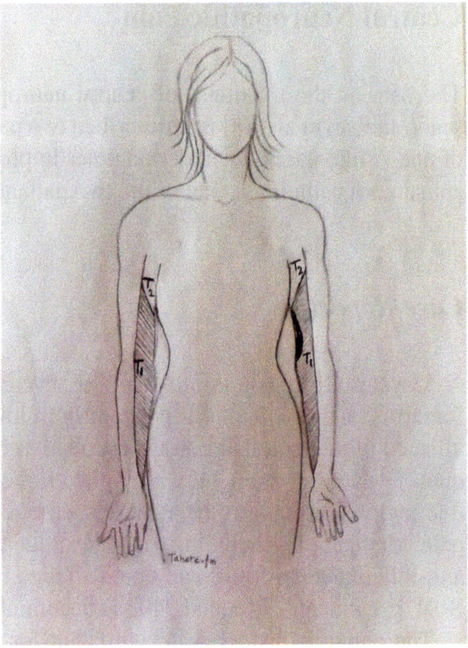

Fig. 4 Regions of allodynia (hatched—T1 segment) in the patient with central NP secondary to C8-T1 spinal cord hemangioma. The most intense region of skin sensitivity is at the region of the elbow on the left side (*darkest area*). Drawing from Tahereh Mousavi M.D.

the region of neuropathic pain. At 4 and 8 weeks after injection, the VAS score for pain was significantly reduced by 18.6 ± 16.8 and 21.3 ± 26.8, respectively, in the BoNT group, whereas it was reduced by 2.6 ± 14.6 and 0.3 ± 19.5, respectively, in the placebo group ($P < 0.05$). No motor side effects were noted. The authors concluded that injection of BoNT-A improves pain and allodynia secondary to spinal cord injury.

Conclusion

Neuropathic pain is one of the most disabling forms of human pain. Many patients with NP pain fail conventional analgesic medications. The data on type A toxin (mostly with ona-A) are encouraging and indicate efficacy in post-herpetic neuralgia, trigeminal neuralgia, and post-traumatic neuralgia. There is evidence for probable efficacy (level B) for painful diabetic neuropathy and central neuropathic pain of spinal cord origin (level B, one class I or two class II studies). Blinded and placebo-controlled trials are necessary to assess the efficacy of BoNTs in other forms of neuropathic pain: drug-induced neuropathies, complex regional pain syndrome, phantom pain, carpal tunnel syndrome, and occipital neuralgia. Much remains to be learned about the optimal dose and technique of injection as well as difference between various BoNTs in the treatment of human neuropathic pain.

Acknowledgments Drs Tahere Mousavi and Damoun Safarpour provided drawings for Figs. 2 and 4, respectively.

References

1. Treede R-D. Peripheral and central mechanisms of neuropathic pain. In: Simpson DM, McArthur JC, Dworkin RH, editors. Mechanisms, diagnosis and treatment. Oxford: Oxford University Press (OUP); 2012.
2. Aoki KR, Francis J. Updates on the antinociceptive mechanism hypothesis of botulinum toxin A. Parkinsonism Relat Disord. 2011;17:S28–33.
3. Oh H-M, Chung M. Botulinum toxin for neuropathic pain: a review of the literature. Toxins. 2015;7:3127–54.
4. Pellett S, Yaksh T, Ramachandran R. Current status and future directions of Botulinum neurotoxins for targeting pain processing. Toxins. 2015;7:4519–63.
5. Dolly JO, O'Connell MA. Neurotherapeutics to inhibit exocytosis from sensory neurons for the control of chronic pain. Curr Opin Pharmacol. 2012;12:100–8.
6. Durham PL, Cady R, Cady R. Regulation of calcitonin Gene-related peptide secretion from trigeminal nerve cells by Botulinum toxin type a: implications for migraine therapy. Headache. 2004;44:35–43.
7. Edvinsson J, Warfvinge K, Edvinsson L. Modulation of inflammatory mediators in the trigeminal ganglion by botulinum neurotoxin type A: an organ culture study. J Headache Pain. 2015;16:555.
8. Meng J, Wang J, Lawrence G, Dolly JO. Synaptobrevin I mediates exocytosis of CGRP from sensory neurons and inhibition by botulinum toxins reflects their anti-nociceptive potential. J Cell Sci. 2007;120:2864–74.
9. Silva LBD, Poulsen JN, Arendt-Nielsen L, Gazerani P. Botulinum neurotoxin type A modulates vesicular release of glutamate from satellite glial cells. J Cell Mol Med. 2015;19:1900–9.
10. Shin M-C, Wakita M, Xie D-J, Yamaga T, Iwata S, Torii Y, Harakawa T, Ginnaga A, Kozaki S, Akaike N. Inhibition of membrane Na+ channels by A type Botulinum toxin at Femtomolar concentrations in central and peripheral neurons. J Pharmacol Sci. 2012;118:33–42.
11. Cui M, Khanijou S, Rubino J, Aoki KR. Subcutaneous administration of botulinum toxin A reduces formalin-induced pain. Pain. 2004;107:125–33.
12. Marino MJ, Terashima T, Steinauer JJ, Eddinger KA, Yaksh TL, Xu Q. Botulinum toxin B in the sensory afferent: transmitter release, spinal activation, and pain behavior. Pain. 2014;155:674–84.
13. Zychowska M, Rojewska E, Makuch W, Luvisetto S, Pavone F, Marinelli S, Przewlocka B, Mika J. Participation of pro- and anti-nociceptive interleukins in botulinum toxin A-induced analgesia in a rat model of neuropathic pain. Eur J Pharmacol. 2016;791:377–88.
14. Filippi GM, Errico P, Santarelli R, Bagolini B, Manni E. Botulinum A toxin effects on rat jaw muscle spindles. Acta Otolaryngol. 1993;113:400–4.
15. Rand MJ, Whaler BC. Impairment of sympathetic transmission by Botulinum toxin. Nature. 1965;206:588–91.
16. French J, Gronseth G. Invited article: lost in a jungle of evidence: we need a compass. Neurology. 2008;71:1634–8.
17. Gronseth G, French J. Invited article: practice parameters and technology assessments: what they are, what they are not, and why you should care. Neurology. 2008;71:1639–43.
18. Oaklander AL. The density of remaining nerve endings in human skin with and without postherpetic neuralgia after shingles. Pain. 2001;92:139–45.
19. Haanpää M1, Dastidar P, Weinberg A, Levin M, Miettinen A, Lapinlampi A, Laippala P, Nurmikko T. CSF and MRI findings in patients with acute herpes zoster. Neurology. 1998;51:1405–11.

20. Wood MJ, Kay R, Dworkin RH, Soong SJ, Whitley RJ. Oral Acyclovir therapy accelerates pain resolution in patients with herpes zoster: a meta-analysis of placebo-controlled trials. Clin Infect dis. 1996;22:341–7.
21. Oxman MN, Levin MJ, Johnson GR, Schmader KE, Straus SE, Gelb LD, Arbeit RD, Simberkoff MS, Gershon AA, Davis LE, Weinberg A, Boardman KD, Williams HM, Zhang JH, Peduzzi PN, Beisel CE, Morrison VA, Guatelli JC, Brooks PA, Kauffman CA, Pachucki CT, Neuzil KM, Betts RF, Wright PF, Griffin MR, Brunell P, Soto NE, Marques AR, Keay SK, Goodman RP, Cotton DJ, Gnann JW, Loutit J, Holodniy M, Keitel WA, Crawford GE, Yeh SS, Lobo Z, Toney JF, Greenberg RN, Keller PM, Harbecke R, Hayward AR, Irwin MR, Kyriakides TC, Chan CY, Chan ISF, Wang WWB, Annunziato PW, Silber JL. A vaccine to prevent herpes zoster and Postherpetic neuralgia in older adults. N Engl J Med. 2005;352:2271–84.
22. Yawn BP, Saddier P, Wollan PC, Sauver JLS, Kurland MJ, Sy LS. A population-based study of the incidence and complication rates of herpes zoster before zoster vaccine introduction. Mayo Clin Proc. 2007;82:1341–9.
23. Baron R, Haendler G, Schulte H. Afferent large fiber polyneuropathy predicts the development of postherpetic neuralgia. Pain. 1997;73:231–8.
24. Thyregod HG, Rowbotham MC, Peters M, Possehn J, Berro M, Petersen KL. Natural history of pain following herpes zoster. Pain. 2007;128:148–56.
25. Oster G, Harding G, Dukes E, Edelsberg J, Cleary PD. Pain, medication use, and health-related quality of life in older persons with postherpetic neuralgia: results from a population-based survey. J Pain. 2005;6:356–63.
26. Cohen S, Hsu E. Postamputation pain: epidemiology, mechanisms, and treatment. J Pain Res. 2013;6:121–36.
27. Jeon YH. Herpes zoster and postherpetic neuralgia: practical consideration for prevention and treatment. Korean J Pain. 2015;28:177.
28. Beiteke U, Bigge S, Reichenberger C, Gralow I. Pain and pain management in dermatology. J Dtsch Dermatol Ges. 2015;13:967–87.
29. Shackleton T, Ram S, Black M, Ryder J, Clark GT, Enciso R. The efficacy of botulinum toxin for the treatment of trigeminal and postherpetic neuralgia: a systematic review with meta-analyses. Oral Surg Oral Med Oral Pathol Oral Radiol. 2016;122:61–71.
30. Apalla Z, Sotiriou E, Lallas A, Lazaridou E, Ioannides D. Botulinum toxin A in Postherpetic neuralgia. Clin J Pain. 2013;29:857–64.
31. Xiao L, Mackey S, Hui H, Xong D, Zhang Q, Zhang D. Subcutaneous injection of Botulinum toxin A is beneficial in Postherpetic neuralgia. Pain Med. 2010;11:1827–33.
32. Liu H-T, Tsai S-K, Kao M-C, Hu JS. Botulinum toxin A relieved neuropathic pain in a case of post-herpetic neuralgia. Pain Med. 2006;7:89–91.
33. Sotiriou E, Apalla Z, Panagiotidou D, Ioannidis D. Severe post-herpetic neuralgia successfully treated with botulinum toxin A: three case reports. Acta Derm Venereol. 2009;89:214–5.
34. Ranoux D, Attal N, Morain F, Bouhassira D. Botulinum toxin type a induces direct analgesic effects in chronic neuropathic pain. Ann Neurol. 2008;64:274–83.
35. Katusic S, Beard CM, Bergstralth E, Kurland LT. Incidence and clinical features of trigeminal neuralgia, Rochester, Minnesota, 1945-1984. Ann Neurol. 1990;27:89–95.
36. Yoshimasu F, Kurland LT, Elveback LR. Tic douloureux in Rochester, Minnesota, 1945-1969. Neurology. 1972;22:952.
37. Fromm GH, Terrence CF, Chattha AS. Baclofen in the treatment of trigeminal neuralgia: double-blind study and long-term follow-up. Ann Neurol. 1984;15:240–4.
38. Baschnagel AM, Cartier JL, Dreyer J, Chen PY, Pieper DR, Olson RE, Krauss DJ, Maitz AH, Grills IS. Trigeminal neuralgia pain relief after gamma knife stereotactic radiosurgery. Clin Neurol Neurosurg. 2014;117:107–11.
39. Kitamura Y, Matsuka Y, Spigelman I, Ishihara Y, Yamamoto Y, Sonoyama W, Kamioka H, Yamashiro T, Kuboki T, Oguma K. Corrigendum to "botulinum toxin type A (150 kDa) decreases exaggerated neurotransmitter release from trigeminal ganglion neurons and relieves

neuropathy behaviors induced by infraorbital nerve constriction" [Neuroscience 159 (2009) 1422–1429]. Neuroscience. 2009;161:950.
40. Shimizu T, Shibata M, Toriumi H, Iwashita T, Funakubo M, Sato H, Kuroi T, Ebine T, koizumi K, Suzuki N. Reduction of TRPV1 expression in the trigeminal system by botulinum neurotoxin type-A. Neurobiol Dis. 2012;48:367–78.
41. Matak I, Bach-Rojecky L, Filipović B, Lacković Z. Behavioral and immunohistochemical evidence for central antinociceptive activity of botulinum toxin a. Neuroscience. 2011;186:201–7.
42. Wu H, Sultana R, Taylor KB, Szabo A. A prospective randomized double-blinded pilot study to examine the effect of Botulinum toxin type A injection versus lidocaine/depomedrol injection on residual and phantom limb pain. Clin J Pain. 2012b;28:108–12.
43. Zhang H, Lian Y, Ma Y, Chen Y, He C, Xie N, Wu C. Two doses of botulinum toxin type A for the treatment of trigeminal neuralgia: observation of therapeutic effect from a randomized, double-blind, placebo-controlled trial. J Headache Pain. 2014a;15:65.
44. Zúñiga C, Piedimonte F, Díaz S, Micheli F. Acute treatment of trigeminal neuralgia with Onabotulinum toxin A. Clin Neuropharmacol. 2013;36:146–50.
45. Shehata HS, El-Tamawy MS, Shalaby NM, Ramzy G. Botulinum toxin-type A: could it be an effective treatment option in intractable trigeminal neuralgia? J Headache Pain. 2013;14:92.
46. Li S, Lian Y-J, Chen Y, Zhang H-F, Ma Y-Q, He C-H, Wu C-J, Xie N-C, Zheng Y-K, Zhang Y. Therapeutic effect of Botulinum toxin-A in 88 patients with trigeminal neuralgia with 14-month follow-up. J Headache Pain. 2014;15:43.
47. Wu CJ, Lian YJ, Zheng YK, Zhang HF, Chen Y, Xie NC, Wang LJ. Botulinum toxin type A for the treatment of trigeminal neuralgia: results from a randomized, double-blind, placebo-controlled trial. Cephalalgia. 2012a;32:443–50.
48. Katz J, Seltzer ZE. Transition from acute to chronic postsurgical pain: risk factors and protective factors. Expert Rev Neurother. 2009;9:723–44.
49. Mclachlan EM, Jänig W, Devor M, Michaelis M. Peripheral nerve injury triggers noradrenergic sprouting within dorsal root ganglia. Nature. 1993;363:543–6.
50. Garrison CJ, Dougherty PM, Kajander KC, Carlton SM. Staining of glial fibrillary acidic protein (GFAP) in lumbar spinal cord increases following a sciatic nerve constriction injury. Brain Res. 1991;565:1–7.
51. Todd AJ, Sullivan AC. Light microscope study of the coexistence of GABA-like and glycine-like immunoreactivities in the spinal cord of the rat. J Comp Neurol. 1990;296:496–505.
52. Yaksh TL, Chaplan SR. Physiology and pharmacology of neuropathic pain. Anesthesiol Clin North Am. 1997;15:335–52.
53. Attal N, de Andrade DC, Adam F, Ranoux D, Teixeira MJ, Galhardoni R, Raicher I, Üçeyler N, Sommer C, Bouhassira D. Safety and efficacy of repeated injections of botulinum toxin A in peripheral neuropathic pain (BOTNEP): a randomised, double-blind, placebo-controlled trial. Lancet Neurol. 2016;15(6):555–65.
54. Casale R, Atzeni F, Masala IF, Sarzi-Puttini P. The words of pain in complex regional pain syndrome. Best Pract Res Clin Rheumatol. 2015;29:71–6.
55. Harden RN, Oaklander AL, Burton AW, Perez RSGM, Richardson K, Swan M, Barthel J, Costa B, Graciosa JR, Bruehl S. Complex regional pain syndrome: practical diagnostic and treatment guidelines, 4th edition. Pain Med. 2013;14:180–229.
56. Coderre TJ, Xanthos DN, Francis L, Bennett GJ. Chronic post-ischemia pain (CPIP): a novel animal model of complex regional pain syndrome-type I (CRPS-I; reflex sympathetic dystrophy) produced by prolonged hindpaw ischemia and reperfusion in the rat. Pain. 2004;112:94–105.
57. Weber M, Birklein F, Neundörfer B, Schmelz M. Facilitated neurogenic inflammation in complex regional pain syndrome. Pain. 2001;91:251–7.
58. del Valle L, Schwartzman RJ, Alexander G. Spinal cord histopathological alterations in a patient with longstanding complex regional pain syndrome. Brain Behav Immun. 2009;23:85–91.

59. Schwartzman RJ, Alexander GM, Grothusen JR, Paylor T, Reichenberger E, Perreault M. Outpatient intravenous ketamine for the treatment of complex regional pain syndrome: a double-blind placebo controlled study. Pain. 2009;147:107–15.
60. Goebel A. Intravenous immunoglobulin treatment of the complex regional pain syndrome. Ann Intern med. 2010;152:152.
61. Argoff CE. A focused review on the use of Botulinum toxins for neuropathic pain. Clin J Pain. 2002;18:S177–81.
62. Birthi P, Sloan P, Salles S. Subcutaneous Botulinum toxin A for the treatment of refractory complex regional pain syndrome. PM & R. 2012;4:446–9.
63. Safarpour D, Salardini A, Richardson D, Jabbari B. Botulinum toxin A for treatment of Allodynia of complex regional pain syndrome: a Pilot study. Pain Med. 2010;11:1411–4.
64. Safarpour D, Jabbari B. Botulinum toxin A (Botox) for treatment of proximal myofascial pain in complex regional pain syndrome: two cases. Pain Med. 2010;11:1415–8.
65. Kharkar S, Ambady P, Yedatore V, Schwartzman RJ. Intramuscular botulinum toxin A (BtxA) in complex regional pain syndrome. Pain Physician. 2011;14:311–6.
66. Barrett AM, Lucero MA, Le T, Robinson RL, Dworkin RH, Chappell AS. Epidemiology, public health burden, and treatment of diabetic peripheral neuropathic pain: a review. Pain Med. 2007;8:S50–62.
67. Boulton AJM. Diabetic neuropathy: classification, measurement and treatment. Curr Opin Endocrinol Diabetes Obes. 2007;14:141–5.
68. Romanovsky D, Cruz NF, Dienel GA, Dobretsov M. Mechanical hyperalgesia correlates with insulin deficiency in normoglycemic streptozotocin-treated rats. Neurobiol Dis. 2006;24:384–94.
69. Orestes P, Osuru HP, Mcintire WE, Jacus MO, Salajegheh R, Jagodic MM, Choe W, Lee J, Lee SS, Rose KE, Poiro N, Digruccio MR, Krishnan K, Covey DF, Lee JH, Barrett PQ, Jevtovic-Todorovic V, Todorovic SM. Reversal of neuropathic pain in diabetes by targeting glycosylation of Cav3.2 T-type calcium channels. Diabetes. 2013;62:3828–38.
70. Bril V, England J, Franklin GM, Backonja M, Cohen J, del Toro D, Feldman E, Iverson DJ, Perkins B, Russell JW, Zochodne D. Evidence-based guideline: treatment of painful diabetic neuropathy: report of the American Academy of Neurology, the American Association of Neuromuscular and Electrodiagnostic Medicine, and the American Academy of Physical Medicine and Rehabilitation. PM R. 2011;3:345–52. 352.e1–21
71. Hong L, Zhang J, Shen J. Clinical efficacy of different doses of lipo-prostaglandin E1 in the treatment of painful diabetic peripheral neuropathy. J Diabetes Complicat. 2015;29:1283–6.
72. Javed S, Alam U, Malik RA. Burning through the pain: treatments for diabetic neuropathy. Diabetes Obes Metab. 2015;17:1115–25.
73. Yuan RY, Sheu JJ, Yu JM, Chen WT, Tseng IJ, Chang HH, Hu CJ. Botulinum toxin for diabetic neuropathic pain: a randomized double-blind crossover trial. Neurology. 2009;72:1473–8.
74. Chen W-T, Yuan R-Y, Chiang S-C, Sheu J-J, Yu J-M, Tseng I-J, Yang S-K, Chang H-H, Hu C-J. OnabotulinumtoxinA improves tactile and mechanical pain perception in painful diabetic polyneuropathy. Clin J Pain. 2013;29:305–10.
75. Ghasemi M, Ansari M, Basiri K, Shaigannejad V. The effects of intradermal botulinum toxin type a injections on pain symptoms of patients with diabetic neuropathy. J Res Med Sci. 2014;19:106–11.
76. Ziegler-Graham K, Mackenzie EJ, Ephraim PL, Travison TG, Brookmeyer R. Estimating the prevalence of limb loss in the United States: 2005 to 2050. Arch Phys Med Rehabil. 2008;89:422–9.
77. Carlen PL, Wall PD, Nadvorna H, Steinbach T. Phantom limbs and related phenomena in recent traumatic amputations. Neurology. 1978;28:211.
78. Jensen TS, Krebs B, Nielsen J, Rasmussen P. Phantom limb, phantom pain and stump pain in amputees during the first 6 months following limb amputation. Pain. 1983;17:243–56.
79. Hsu E, Cohen SP. Postamputation pain: epidemiology, mechanisms, and treatment. J Pain Res. 2013;6:121–36.

80. Alviar MJM, Hale T, Dungca M. Pharmacologic interventions for treating phantom limb pain. Cochrane Database of Systematic Reviews. Wiley-Blackwell; 2011.
81. Sherman RA, Sherman CJ, Parker L. Chronic phantom and stump pain among American veterans: results of a survey. Pain. 1984;18:83–95.
82. Kern U, Martin C, Scheicher S, Müller H. Effects of Botulinum toxin type B on stump pain and involuntary movements of the stump. Am J Phys Med Rehabil. 2004;83:396–9.
83. Jin L, Kollewe K, Krampfl K, Dengler R, Mohammadi B. Treatment of phantom limb pain with botulinum toxin type A. Pain Med. 2009;10:300–3.
84. Breuer B, Sperber K, Wallenstein S, Kiprovski K, Calapa A, Snow B, Pappagallo M. Clinically significant placebo analgesic response in a Pilot trial of Botulinum B in patients with hand pain and carpal tunnel syndrome. Pain Med. 2006;7:16–24.
85. Tsai C-P, Liu C-Y, Lin K-P, Wang K-C. Efficacy of Botulinum toxin type A in the relief of carpal tunnel syndrome. Clin Drug Investig. 2006;26:511–5.
86. Kapural L, Stillman M, Kapural M, Mcintyre P, Guirgius M, Mekhail N. Botulinum toxin occipital nerve block for the treatment of severe occipital neuralgia: a case series. Pain Pract. 2007;7:337–40.
87. Taylor M, Silva S, Cottrell C. Botulinum toxin type-A (BOTOX®) in the treatment of occipital neuralgia: a pilot study. Headache. 2008;48:1476–81.
88. Jabbari B, Maher N, Difazio MP. Botulinum toxin A improved burning pain and allodynia in two patients with spinal cord pathology. Pain Med. 2003;4:206–10.
89. Han Z-A, Song DH, Oh H-M, Chung ME. Botulinum toxin type A for neuropathic pain in patients with spinal cord injury. Ann Neurol. 2016;79:569–78.

The Role of Botulinum Toxins in Treatment of Brain and Spinal Cord Injury Symptoms

Taraneh Hashemi-Zonouz and Bahman Jabbari

Traumatic brain injury (TBI) occurs as a result of blunt or penetrating head trauma and presents with a broad spectrum of symptoms and disabilities [1, 2]. TBIs constitute a major cause of death and critical public health around the world. The severity of TBI correlates with a significant social and financial burden with more than $1 billion dollars per year spending on hospitalizations [3]. The overall prevalence of TBIs for individuals between 0 and 25 years is 31–44% [4–6]. An increasing rate of road traffic injuries has resulted in rising numbers of traumatic brain injuries [7–9]. Annually, approximately 1.7 million people experienced some degree of TBI in the United States and 1.4 million of these injuries result in hospitalizations, 52,000 deaths, and 124,000 disabilities [1, 10]. Improved management of acute TBI has decreased the fatality rate, but has also caused a concomitant increase in the number of patients living with TBI-related disabilities [11]. Falls are the most common cause of TBI-related emergency department visits, while TBI-related deaths are mostly due to motor-vehicle accidents [12, 13].

This chapter discusses three symptoms of post-traumatic brain injury—spasticity, pain (including headaches), and post-traumatic movement disorders with a potential for improvement by botulinum toxin treatment.

T. Hashemi-Zonouz, M.D. (✉)
Radiology and Biomedical Imaging, Yale University, New Haven, CT, USA
e-mail: Taraneh.hashemi-zonouz@yale.edu; Taran.hz@gmail.com

B. Jabbari, M.D., FAAN
Department of Neurology, Yale University, New Haven, CT, USA
e-mail: bahman.jabbari@yale.edu

B. Jabbari (ed.), *Botulinum Toxin Treatment in Clinical Medicine*,
DOI 10.1007/978-3-319-56038-0_11

Spasticity

Spasticity is defined as a motor disorder characterized by a velocity-dependent increase in tonic stretch reflexes with exaggerated tendon jerks, resulting from hyperexcitability of the stretch reflex, as one component of the upper motor neuron syndrome [14]. The exact pathophysiology of spasticity is still unclear. Jean-Michael Gracies discussed the likely and unlikely mechanisms responsible for development of spasticity in a recent comprehensive review [15, 16]. Decreased reciprocal Ia inhibition (which inhibits alpha motor neurons via a disynaptic interneuron) decreased non-reciprocal Ib inhibition and hyperexcitability of small group II afferents (originating from muscle spindle secondary endings) have been noted as possible mechanisms. The acute effects of TBI include paresis and short-term immobilization, whereas chronic effects result from plastic rearrangements in the CNS as the result of CNS injury, chronic disuse, or both. Changes in muscle innervation and reflex arch cause spasticity, spastic dystonia, and spastic co-contractions. Chronic spasticity and muscle disuse lead to contractures, which is often associated with significant disability. The TBI Model Systems National Database identified 75,000–100,000 annual cases of severe spasticity in U.S. [17], of which as high as 85% may develop contractures.

Although mild spasticity may not require treatment, moderate to severe spasticity often interferes with the individual's daily function [18, 19] and requires treatment. Treatment is aimed at reducing muscle tone, improving function and quality of life as well as preventing development of contractures. The currently available treatments for spasticity include: (1) pharmacological therapy combined with physical therapy and rehabilitation. Among pharmacological agents, baclofen, tizanidine, and diazepam are commonly used either as a single agent or in combination. Unfortunately, most patients with severe spasticity require high doses of these medications, which cause disturbing side effects such as sedation, mental changes, and dizziness. (2) For severe focal spasticity, injection of neurolytic nerve blocker phenol and/or anesthetic nerve blocks such as procaine and lidocaine are recommended [17, 20]. (3) In disabling spasticity, baclofen pump is helpful and can markedly reduce the spasticity [21]. Insertion of the baclofen pump, however, requires a dedicated setting and special expertise. Overdosing and withdrawal symptoms occur and can lead to serious side effects such as seizures and suppressed level of consciousness. (4) Corrective orthopedic surgery.

Botulinum Toxin Therapy

Over the past ten years, treatment of stroke-related spasticity with BoNT injections has been studied by several high-quality clinical trials [15, 22]. The positive results of these studies led to approval of botulinum toxin therapy for upper limb spasticity by FDA in 2010 and 2015 (extended approval for including additional muscles) and for lower limb spasticity in 2016.

The literature on clinical trials of botulinum toxin therapy in spasticity caused by traumatic brain injury is limited to eight publications (Table 1). Five studies have a double blind-parallel design, one is double blind-crossover and two are open label. All five double blind-parallel studies have a mixed cohort, mostly stroke with TBI subjects comprising a much smaller proportion in the cohort. One small double blind and crossover and two small open label clinical trials are conducted exclusively on subjects with traumatic brain injury (Table 1).

The largest study conducted by Gracies et al. [23] assessed the efficacy of two doses of abobotulinum toxinA in a cohort consisting of 238 subjects with stroke and 23 subjects with TBI. This study showed that both low and high doses of aboA reduce muscle tone significantly and significantly improved the scores of Patient Global Assessment (PGA) (P's < 0.05). The patient Disability Assessment Scale (DAS) also improved, but the values did not reach statistical significance (0.07). The study of Barbaud et al. [24], which was conducted on 23 patients with TBI (double blind crossover), demonstrated that injection of 1000 units of aboA significantly improves spasticity, range of movement of ankle invertors and extenders as well as improving, to some extent, the gait velocity (Table 1). Significant improvement of the range of motion was also noted in another study that used 20–40 units of onaA per spastic muscles [25]. The study of Simpson et al. [26] compared the effect of onaA injections (maximum 500 units) in the upper extremity muscles of patients with TBI and stroke with the effect of tizanidine and placebo. OnaA was significantly better than tizanidine and placebo in reducing the muscle tone as well as improving the DAS score. Regarding side effects, one study mentioned that 10 out of 238 subjects experienced mild transient weakness after aboA injection (three in low-dose and seven in high-dose group) [23]. Transient local swelling and local pain at the site of injection were noted in two other patients [24, 25].

Comment

Using the guidelines of the American Academy of Neurology [27], the clinical trials using type A botulinum neurotoxin (aboA and onaA) for spasticity caused by TBI indicate efficacy (level B evidence) in reducing muscle tone, improving the range of motion, and attaining positive scores in physician global assessment (PGA) (one Class I and three class II studies). For rimaB, the level of evidence in C (possibly effective) is based on one class II study. One problem with the larger studies is that the number of TBI patients in the mixed cohort is too small. Assessment of disability and quality of life requires conduction of studies geared to specific evaluations in these areas of concerns.

Table 1 Clinical trials with BoNTs in patients with spasticity caused by Traumatic Brain Injury (TBI)

Author(s)	Study design	N and diagnosis	Limb	Toxin	Dose (U)	Result
Gracies et al. 2015 [23]	Double blind, parallel	238: Stroke 215 TBI 23	Upper	aboA	500, 1000	Mean change in MAS −0.3, −1.2, and −1.4 for placebo, 500 and 1000 toxin groups, respectively ($P < 0.0001$). Mean change in PGA score: 0.6, 1.4, and 1.8 for placebo, 500 and 1000 groups ($P = 0.0003$), ($P = 0.0001$). DAS reduction −0.5, −0.7, −07, placebo, 500 and 1000 groups (0.077) SE: mild transient hand weakness, 3 and 7 pts
Fietzek et al. 2014 [28]	Double blind, parallel	52: Stroke 35 Hypoxia 11 TBI 6	Lower	onaA	230–460	At week 12, MAS scores improved significantly in the onaA group compared to placebo ($P = 0.01$) SE: None
Gracies et al. 2014 [29]	Double blind, parallel	24: Stroke 19 TBI 5	Upper	rimaB	5000, 10,000, 15,000 Into each elbow flexor	Both doses improved elbow extension +8.3° ($P = 0.28$). Higher dose improved subject-perceived stiffness ($P = 0.05$). Subjective global self-assessment on pain, stiffness, and function also improved ($P = 0.17$) SE: None
Simpson et al. 2009 [26]	Double blind, parallel Comparator AboA/ tizanidine/ placebo	60: Stroke 49 TBI 11	Upper	onaA	500 (Max dose). All: 50 U into wrist flexors and extensors	Greater tone reduction in Ashworth scale with onaA compared to tizanidine or placebo ($P < 0.001$ and $P < 0.02$). Greater improvement in the cosmesis domain of DAS at week 6 ($P < 0.01$) SE: No focal weakness with onaA. SE higher with tizanidine (onaA and placebo the same)

(continued)

Table 1 (continued)

Author(s)	Study design	N and diagnosis	Limb	Toxin	Dose (U)	Result
Smith et al. 2000 [30]	Double blind, parallel	23: Stroke 21 TBI 2	Upper	aboA	500, 1000, 1500	Significant reduction of spasticity in MAS; significant increase in passive range of movements at the wrist, modest improvement at the elbow; significant improvement in patient global assessment (PGA); no change in upper limb disability scale
Pavesi et al. 1998 [31]	Open label	6: All TBI	Upper	onaA	90–100	Ashworth scale improved. One patient by 3°, two patients by 2°, and one patient by 1°. Three patients showed functional improvement (one writing, one using utensils, one dressing) SE: None
Burbaud et al. 1996 [24]	Double blind, crossover	23: All TBI	Lower	aboA	1000	Subjective improvement of foot spasticity ($P = 0.004$). Ankle invertor and extensors improved in MAS ($P = 0.001$ and 0.002). Modest improvement of gait velocity ($P = 0.071$) Less effective if spasticity had longer duration ($P = 0.008$) SE: transient local pain
Yablon et al. 1996 [25]	Open label	21: All TBI	Upper	onaA	20–40 per muscle	Mean passive range of motion improved 42.92° and 36.2° at 4 and 8 weeks ($P < 0.001$). Mean MAS rating improved 1.5 and 1.47 ($P = 0.01$ and 0.02) SE: one patient local swelling

OnaA botulinumtoxinA (Botox), *aboA* botulinumtoxinA (Dysport), *rimaB* rimabotulinumtoxinB (My bloc), *MAS* modified Ashworth scale, *DAS* disability assessment scale, *PGA* patient global assessment, *SE* side effects, *N* = number of patients

Pain in Post-traumatic Brain Injury

TBI-related pain and painful muscle spasm can be either neuropathic due to dysfunction of the nervous system or nociceptive as a result of damage to the musculoskeletal or visceral systems. A combination of both is also possible, depending on the extent and the level of the lesion. Furthermore, physiological and psychological factors may complicate pain sensation [32]. In the early phases of severe brain injury, affected individuals may experience very rigid and painful body postures. The strong subjective component of pain in TBI may complicate the design of effective drug therapies. Pain can arise from the brain, spinal cord, or even peripheral structures [33, 34]. TBI patients with severe spasticity often have pain associated with spasticity and, in carefully selected patients, release of muscle contractures can relief the pain [35]. A comprehensive review of RCTs published on the subject of chronic pain in TBI disclosed a prevalence of 51.5 among civilians and 43.1 among veterans [36]. Pain was more prevalent in patients with mild and moderate brain injury, although the reason for it was not clear.

Spasticity and contractures, common symptoms of chronic TBI, are often associated with pain. Jabbari reviewed the reported literature on the effect of botulinum toxin therapy on spasticity-associated pain regardless of the etiology [37]. Five of nine clinical trials reported significant improvement of pain, while four did not. The positive studies were more recent and used better pain scales. The effect of BoNT therapy on the pain associated with TBI-related spasticity needs exploration. Of the eight studies cited above (Table 1), only one [29] mentioned improvement of pain in three patients. However, it is not known whether three patients had TBI or stroke (mixed cohort).

Post-traumatic Headache (PTM)

Post-traumatic headache (PTH) is described as the headache that develops within 1 week after head trauma or within 1 week after regaining consciousness [38]. Approximately, 2% of the US population is disabled by post-traumatic headaches [37]. Headache is reported in nearly 93% of athletes after sports-related concussion [39]. Approximately, 81% of US service members report post-traumatic headaches [40, 41]. The most common patterns of PTH are migraine or probable migraine and tension-type headaches; migraine-type headaches are more prevalent [42]. PTH frequently has a persistent nature, which challenges its treatment. Besides analgesics and physical therapy, patients may benefit from a comprehensive psychological and cognitive therapy [38].

Botulinum toxin therapy is a major line of treatment for chronic migraine. The treatment improves migraine intensity and frequency and patients' quality of life. Long-term follow-up has proved its efficacy over several years and the safe profile of BoNT therapy in chronic migraine (for more detail in this subject, see Chap. 9 of this book). Yerry et al. [43] reported the result of botulinum toxin therapy with onabotulinumtoxinA in 64 service members suffering from post-traumatic chronic migraine in a real-time retrospective consecutive case series. Blast injury was the most common type of trauma and was the cause in 56% of the patients. The mean age of the patients in the cohort was 31 years. The mean time from injury to the first onaA injections was 10.8 months. The injection protocol was the one recommended by the PREEMPT study group for treatment of chronic migraine [44]. After a single injection, 64% of the patients reported significant improvement of headaches. Two patients withdrew from the study due to side effects. The positive results of this study in PTM are encouraging. Proof of efficacy of BoNT treatment in post-traumatic migraine requires confirmation by controlled studies.

Post-traumatic Brain Injury and Involuntary Movement Disorders.

The history of botulinum toxin therapy began in the area of movement disorders and movement disorders continue to be major indications for this form of treatment [45]. Traumatic brain injury, similar to other forms of brain injury, can cause a variety of movement disorders such as dystonia, tremor, chorea, ballism, and tics [46]. Krauss et al. [47], followed 221 patients with severe traumatic head injury (Glascow score of <8) for 5 years and found that 50 patients (22.6%) developed involuntary movement disorders. The movements were transient in 10.4% and persistent in 12.2%. Forty-two patients (19%) had tremors which in 12 of them (5.4%) had a low frequency (2.5–4 Hz) and were disabling. Nine patients (4.1%) had dystonia which developed with a latency of 2 months to 2 years and seven (3.2%) had other movement disorders. In a later study, the same authors found a prevalence of 10.1% for involuntary movements in a cohort of 158 patients with mild to moderate head injury. Persistent movement was noted in 2.6% of this cohort [48].

Treatment with BoNTs is rarely reported for movement disorders caused by traumatic brain injury. Kemp et al. [49] reported a 42 year-old man who following a motor bike accident sustained a severe TBI. Six months later, he developed involuntary, action-induced dystonic posturing of the left leg, which interfered with ambulation. When attempted to ambulate, the left foot assumed a dorsiflexion posture and the whole leg extended. Injection onabotulinumtoxinA (Botox) into the left quadriceps (200 units) and left gastrocnemius (50 medial, 25 lateral) resulted in marked improvement of involuntary movement and helped ambulation. The case described below is from our experience with a patient who suffered from post-traumatic hemibalismus.

Case Report

A 74-year-old man, within days following a car accident, developed continuous ballistic movements of the left side, more prominent in the left upper extremity. A computerized tomography scan demonstrated an area of intracerebral hemorrhage affecting the left globus pallidus. His examination showed mild left hemiparesis and hyperreflexia. The left upper limb displayed high amplitude continuous movements consisting of forceful flexion and extension of the elbow, adduction/abduction of the left arm, left shoulder elevation, and wrist extension. Treatment with baclofen, diazepam, anticholinergic, and muscle relaxants was not helpful. The patient was exhausted 3 days after the onset of the movements. OnabotulinumtoxinA was injected into the following muscles on the left side: trapezius, triceps, biceps, and pectoralis each 100 units; Deltoid 50 units. Forty-eight hours following treatment with onaA, patient's movement showed marked reduction in amplitude and intensity. The treatment enables him to rest and sleep and get through the acute phase of the movements. The patient's examination 3 months later showed mild left hemi-chorea and a subtle left hemiparesis.

Traumatic Spinal Cord Injury

The National Spinal Cord Injury Statistics Center report in 2014 gives an estimate of 273, 000 cases of traumatic SCI in the US and an incidence of 12,000/year for traumatic SCI [50]. Traumatic spinal cord injury is the cause of a variety of major health problems. High-quality clinical trials have shown that treatment with BoNTs is efficacious in spasticity, bladder dysfunction, and pain disorders in a variety of medical conditions. Patients with traumatic spinal cord injury also often suffer from these three disorders. This section discusses the role of botulinum toxin therapy for management of spasticity, bladder dysfunction, and pain in traumatic SCI. In one report, 85% of the patients with severe spasticity caused by SCI demonstrated notable improvement with baclofen pump and 65% of them have shown reduction of muscle spasm frequency [51]. Treatment with the pump, however, needs special setting and technical expertise to avoid overdosing and dealing with withdrawal issues.

Spasticity

Spasticity affects approximately 70% of the patients with spinal cord injury and can be the cause of significant disability [52]. Holtz et al. followed 465 patients with spinal cord injury for 10 years through a prospective registry [53]. After trauma, 65% of the patients demonstrated some degree of spasticity. Spasticity was "problematic" and interfered with functioning in 35% of the patients. At 1-, 2-, and 5-year period after spinal cord trauma, 27%, 24%, and 20% of the patients, respectively, reported significant interruption in daily activities by spasticity. Mild spasticity may not require treatment. Moderate or severe spastic limbs, however, interfere with motor function and, in case of lower limbs, with ambulation.

Botulinum toxin treatment of Spasticity resulting from traumatic SCI. The literature on this area is surprisingly scarce compared to treatment of spasticity with

BoNTs in traumatic brain injury. No high-quality clinical trials exist. There are a number of retrospective and prospective open label observations with reports in small number of patients (Table 2). These studies collectively suggest that BoNTs improve spasticity of traumatic spinal cord injury and the quality of life in the affected patients, a conclusion that is also supported by a handful of case reports.

Bladder Problems in Traumatic SCI

Micturition is controlled by sacral (S2-S4) center (SC) and pontine micturition center (PMC) with participation of cerebral cortex [57]. However, trauma or lesions in other spinal cord regions can also interfere with micturition via involvement of

Table 2 Clinical trials assessing the efficacy of BoNTs in spasticity caused by traumatic SCI

Author(s)	Design	*N*	Toxin	Dose	Injection	Results
Opera et al. 2007 [54]	Pros Open Label	8	onaA	100–400	Hip adductors knee flexors Foot flexors	Three weeks after injection: Decreased MAS ($P < 0.001$) and pain in VAS ($P < 0.02$) Increased RFI ($P < 0.003$) and MRMI ($P < 0.003$)
Marciniak et al. 2008 [55]	Retros Open Label	28	onaA	50–500	Large number of proximal and distal flexors and extensors	Improvement of upper limb function (78%) Improvement of hygiene (67%) Improvement of ambulation (56%)
Bernuz et al. 2012 [56]	Pros Open Label	15	onaA	200	Rectus femoris	Three weeks after injection: Increase gait velocity, swing phase and Stride length ($P < 001$). MTD angle and grade improvement ($P < 0.05$) Reduced walking discomfort
Spiegel et al. 2014 [50]	Pros Open Label	9	onaA	800–2000	Six muscles in lower limbs	At 2 weeks, significant reduction of spasticity (two points or more on Ashworth scale) in six of nine patients Five of nine patients reported significant functional improvement (Transfers, getting in and out of wheelchair, etc.)

Pros prospective, *Retros* retrospective, *MST* Modified Tandieu Scale, *MAS*: modified Ashworth Scale, *MRMI* modified Rivermead mobility index, *RFI* functional index descending motor and autonomic fibers. Traumatic spinal cord injury causes a variety of voiding problems including overactive and underactive bladder and voiding problems related to detrusor and sphincter muscle communication. Neurogenic detrusor overactivity (NDO) and detrusor-sphincter dys-synergia (DSD) are common complications of traumatic spinal cord injury. Both conditions can cause disturbing symptoms such as urinary urgency, incontinence and intermittent urinary retention as well as predisposing the patients to urinary tract to infection. Anticholinergic drugs are commonly used to alleviate the symptoms of NDO, but are often poorly tolerated in the older patients. The symptoms of NDO, OAB (idiopathic overactive bladder), and DSD are described in more detail in Chap. 4 of this book entitled Applications of Botulinum Toxin in the Urinary Tract.

Treatment of Bladder Problems Caused by Traumatic SCI with BoNTs

Most studies conducted to prove the efficacy of BoNTs in NDO have been in cohorts that comprise more than one etiology. In each large study cohort, however, a substantial number consists of patients with traumatic SCI (Table 3). These investigations demonstrate several important points: (1) The evidence-based data from these studies justifies assignment of level A efficacy [27] (effective due to two or more class I studies) for BoNT therapy to NDO caused by traumatic SCI. (2) The efficacy of BoNTs on the NDO of SCI is comparable with the onaA effect upon the NDO caused by other etiologies (i.e., multiple sclerosis). In other words, BONT therapy improves NDO regardless of etiology. (3) The effect of BoNTs on the NDO of SCI is independent of anticholinergic therapy. The FDA based on the results of multicenter studies approved the use of onabotulinum toxin A for treatment of NDO in 2011 and for treatment of idiopathic overactive bladder (OAB) in 2013.

A recent retrospective review of 211 patients comparing the results of 750 units of aboA with 200 units of onaA injected into detrusor muscle for NDO claims a higher rate of success with aboA (66% versus 41%) in patients with spinal cord injury. This finding requires verification by future controlled studies [58].

The optimal technique of injection is still a matter of debate. The FDA's approved dose for onaA treatment of NDO is a total of 200 units into 30 injection sites, sparing the bladder's trigon. However, some authorities in the field prefer trigon injection due to the abundance of nerve fibers in this area [59]. Emerging data also suggests that smaller doses between 100 and 150 may be sufficient at least in some cases of NDO and, in case of abobotulinumtoxinA treatment, recent data in both human and animals suggest that 15 injection sites are sufficient to produce desirable effects [60, 61].

Table 3 Major clinical studies launched to assess the role of botulinum toxin therapy on NDO of patients with traumatic brain injury

Authors	Design	*N*	Type	Toxin	Dose (unit)	Results
Denys et al. 2016 [61]	Double blind placebo-controlled	47 SCI and MS SCI?	NDO	aboA	750 U Detrusor 15 injections 30 injections	Maximum cystometric capacity, maximum detrusor pressure and volume at first contraction improved the Dysport groups compared with placebo ($P < 0.05$). 15 injection sites as effective as 30 Quality of life improved
Hui et al. 2016 [69]	Single blind comparator	91 SCI	NDO	onaA	1–200 into detrusor 2–1600 into detrusor + 40 into trigon	At 12 weeks the group with combined injection did better on QoL scale, mean urinary incontinence episodes, complete dryness (mean voiding volume (159.72 vs. 139.07 ml, $P = 0.02$)), VFIDC with improvement of the duration of first detrusor contraction and the number of patients with detrusor contraction—All *P* values <0.05
Sussman et al. 2013 [70]	Double blind placebo-controlled	183 SCI and MS	NDO	onaA	200 Detrusor 300 Detrusor	Both groups faired significantly more than placebo at 6 and 12 weeks in regard to several quality of life measures: I-QOL, HRQoL, 16-item modified Overactive Bladder-Patient Satisfaction with Treatment Questionnaire (OAB-PSTQ), Patient Global Assessment ($P < 0.05$)

(continued)

Table 3 (continued)

Authors	Design	*N*	Type	Toxin	Dose (unit)	Results
Reitz et al. 2004 [76] European	Retrospective Multicenter	200 SCI and MS 165 SCI	NDO	onaA	300 Detrusor	Increased mean bladder capacity and mean bladder compliance ($P < 0.001$), increased mean reflex volume ($P < 0.01$), decreased mean voiding pressure ($P < 0.001$). Patient reduced anticholinergic, some even stopped
Cruz et al. 2011 [74]	Double blind placebo-controlled	275 SCI and MS 121 SCI	NDO	onaA	200 300 Placebo	UI episodes decreased in toxin groups ($P < 0.01$) Quality of life measured by I-QoL significantly improved in toxin groups at week 6 Side effects—urinary infection and retention
Ginsberg et al. 2012 [73]	Double blind placebo-controlled	414 189 SCI	NDO	onaA	200 300 Placebo	Reduced UI frequency, improved incontinence quality of life score, prolonged median time to patient retreatment request ($P < 0.001$)
Ginsberg et al. 2013 [71]	Pooled data on two double blind studies	691 SCI and MS 310 SCI	NDO	onaA	200 300 Placebo	Toxin group 50% or more reduction in UI episodes. Maximum detrusor pressure, maximum cytometric capacity, detrusor contraction and quality of life all improved in the toxin group. No difference between 200 and 300 dose

(continued)

Table 3 (continued)

Authors	Design	*N*	Type	Toxin	Dose (unit)	Results
Chancellor et al. 2013 [72]	Double blind placebo-controlled	417 189 SCI	NDO	onaA	200 300 Placebo	Focus on quality of life—Measures of I-QoL, patient satisfaction with treatment questionnaire (OAB-PSTQ and Patient Global Assessment (PGA)) all significantly better in toxin groups compared to placebo ($P < 0.001$)
Herschrom et al. 2011 [75]	Double blind placebo-controlled	57 SCI and MS	NDO	onaA	300 Placebo	At week 6, marked reduction of UI and improvement of quality of life

I-QoL incontinence quality of life, *HRQoL* health-related quality of life, *OAB-PSTQ* 16-item modified overactive bladder-patient satisfaction with treatment questionnaire, *UI* urinary frequency, *NDO* neurogenic detrusor overactivity, *N* number

Detrusor-Sphincter Dys-synergia

In this condition, co-contraction of detrusor and sphincter muscles interferes with normal urination. It can be simply classified as intermittent or continuous depending on the pattern of sphincter's EMG activity [62]. Chronic DSD has a potential to cause renal failure, hence early treatment is advisable. Approximately 20–25% of patients with multiple sclerosis develop DSD, but the true incidence of DSD in traumatic SCI (although suspected to be high) is not known.

A few uncontrolled studies have suggested the efficacy of BoNT injection into the urethral sphincter for DSD caused by traumatic spinal cord injury (Table 4). The preliminary data on the effect of urethral injection of onabotulinum toxin A for DSD in traumatic SCI is promising, but proof of efficacy requires data from placebo-controlled studies.

Pain After Traumatic Spinal Cord Injury

Chronic pain is a common finding after spinal cord injury. In a recent study of 537 patients with traumatic spinal cord injury, 76% of the subjects reported chronic pain and in 60% pain was identified as neuropathic pain. The pain was characterized as severe in 28.1% of the patients. In the same cohort, 71% of the patients demonstrated spasticity in the examination [63].

The two major categories of pain after cord injury consist of neuropathic and nociceptive types. The former occurs following specific damage to neural tissue and

Table 4 Clinical trials on the efficacy of intraurethral sphincter injections of onabotulinum toxinA (onaA) for DSD caused by traumatic SCI

Author	Design	*N*	Toxin	Dose	Result—improvement	Side effect
Schurch et al. 1996 [77]	Open label	24	onaA	100 U	21 of 24 patients demonstrated significant improvement of symptoms. Effects lasted 3–9 months	Side efects never occurred
De Seze et al. 2002 [78]	Randomized, DB—onaA versus Lidocaine	13	onaA	100 U	onaA group showed significant decrease in PRUV and MAUP at days 7 and 30 compared to lidocaine (*P* values <0.01 and <0.04), respectively No improvement of MVP	Transitory exacerbation of preexisting urinary incontinence for 2 weeks (one patient)
Kuo 2008 [79]	Open label	50	onaA	100 U	78% satisfaction with treatment Voiding detrusor pressure ($P = 0.016$) Maximum flow rate ($P = 0.047$) Post-void residual volume ($P = 0.025$) IL-O-7 Score ($P = 0.025$)	Increase in incontinence

PRUV post-voiding residual urine volume, *MUP* maximum urethral pressure, *MVP* maximum voiding pressure, *onaA* onaboulinumtoxinA (Botox)

somatosensory system, whereas the latter arises from the musculoskeletal damage. Neuropathic pain often has a burning or searing quality and includes dermatomal allodynia. The pain can manifest above the level of injury, at the level of injury, or below the level of injury [64]. Pain at the level of injury is often associated with signs and symptoms of nerve root injury.

A recent review [65] of pharmacologic of treatment of NP after spinal cord injury identified 35 clinical trials in this area. According to this review, the evidence-based information justifies level 1 efficacy (high) for lidocaine, tramadol, gabapentin, and pregabaline for treatment of neuropathic pain after spinal cord injury, while a level 2 evidence is assigned to lomotrigine. There is level 1 evidence that amitriptyline and venlafaxine are effective in reducing NP, but only in patients with depression. There is level 1 evidence that mexelitine, levetiracetam, trazadone, and duloxetine are not effective in NP caused by traumatic SCI. The evidence for efficacy of cannabinoids for NP occurring after traumatic SCI is controversial.

In 1994, we have reported a women with intramedullary hemangioma at C7 level who suffered from severe neuropathic pain and disabling T1 dermatome allodynia

[66]. Injection of onaA into the allodynic dermatomes resulted in marked improvement of the pain and allodynia (see more detailed description of this case in Chap. 9, under central neuropathic pain). Han et al. [67] first reported significant improvement of neuropathic pain after spinal cord injury in a 51 year-old man who had suffered from C3 AIS B (American Spinal Cord Injury Association scale B) tetraplegia. Authors injected 10 units of onabotulinumtoxinA subcutaneously into the ten most painful areas of each sole. In 2016, the same group of authors reported on a randomized double blind, placebo-controlled study which investigated the effect of subcutaneous onabotulinumtoxinA injection in 40 patients with neuropathic pain after traumatic spinal cord injury [68]. Authors injected 200 units of onaA into the painful areas in a grid-like pattern and evaluated the response at 4 and 8 weeks with VAS, McGill pain questionnaire, and the WHO version of brief quality of life assessment (WHOQoL-BREF). At 4 and 8 weeks after injection, the VAS score for pain was significantly reduced by 18.6 ± 16.8 and 21.3 ± 26.8, respectively, in the toxin groups, whereas it was reduced by 2.6 ± 14.6 and 0.3 ± 19.5, respectively, in the placebo group ($P < 0.002$ and $P < 0.005$). A pain relief of >20% occurred in 55% and 45% (4 and 8 weeks) of the toxin group compared to 15% and 10% of the placebo group. Physical health domain of the WHOQOL-BREF also improved in the onaA group ($P = 0.052$).

Pain in traumatic SCI can also be associated with spasticity. In a retrospective study of 28 patients with traumatic spinal cord injury and spasticity, Marciniak et al. reported that treatment of spasticity with onabotulinumtoxinA improved the pain associated with spasticity in 81% of the patients [55].

Conclusions of the Section on Traumatic SCI

The efficacy of botulinum therapy (with onaA) in the neurogenic detrusor over activity (NDO) caused by SCI has been established via high-quality clinical trials. Further refinement of the technique of injection will provide better yield and more comfort to the patients. Subcutaneous injection of onabotulinum toxin A probably relieves the neuropathic pain caused by spinal cord injury (one class I study), but more RCTs are needed since the magnitude of response was modest (20%) in that single class I trial [68]. The positive findings regarding treatment of spasticity of SCI with BoNTs are all from class VI (retrospective) studies (Table 2); hence, the proof of efficacy should await availability of data from high-quality RCTs.

References

1. Lagbas C, et al. Traumatic brain injury related hospitalization and mortality in California. Biomed Res Int. 2013;2013:143092.
2. Thurman DJ, et al. Traumatic brain injury in the United States: a public health perspective. J Head Trauma Rehabil. 1999;14(6):602–15.

3. Schneier AJ, et al. Incidence of pediatric traumatic brain injury and associated hospital resource utilization in the United States. Pediatrics. 2006;118(2):483–92.
4. McKinlay A, et al. Prevalence of traumatic brain injury among children, adolescents and young adults: prospective evidence from a birth cohort. Brain Inj. 2008;22(2):175–81.
5. Segalowitz SJ, Brown D. Mild head injury as a source of developmental disabilities. J Learn Disabil. 1991;24(9):551–9.
6. Body C, Leathem J. Incidence and aetiology of head injury in a New Zealand adolescent sample. Brain Inj. 1996;10(8):567–74.
7. Roozenbeek B, Maas AIR, Menon DK. Changing patterns in the epidemiology of traumatic brain injury. Nat Rev Neurol. 2013;9(4):231–6.
8. Patel A, et al. Quality of the development of traumatic brain injury clinical practice guidelines: a systematic review. PLoS One. 2016;11(9):e0161554.
9. Song SY, et al. Analysis of mortality and epidemiology in 2617 cases of traumatic brain injury: Korean Neuro-Trauma Data Bank System 2010–2014. J Korean Neurosurg Soc. 2016;59(5):485–91.
10. Faul M, et al. Traumatic brain injury in the United States. Atlanta, GA: National Center for Injury Prevention and Control, Centers for disease Control and Prevention; 2010.
11. Marshall LF. Head injury: recent past, present, and future. Neurosurgery. 2000;47(3):546–61.
12. Coronado VG, et al. Surveillance for traumatic brain injury-related deaths: United States, 1997–2007. US Department of Health and Human Services, Centers for Disease Control and Prevention: Atlanta; 2011.
13. Coronado VG, et al. Trends in traumatic brain injury in the US and the public health response: 1995–2009. J Saf Res. 2012;43(4):299–307.
14. Gracies JM. Pathophysiology of spastic paresis. I: paresis and soft tissue changes. Muscle Nerve. 2005;31(5):535–51.
15. Moeini-Naghani I, Hashemi-Zonouz T, Jabbari B. Botulinum toxin treatment of spasticity in adults and children. Semin Neurol. 2016;36(1):64–72.
16. Gracies JM. Pathophysiology of spastic paresis. II: emergence of muscle overactivity. Muscle Nerve. 2005;31(5):552–71.
17. Schindler-Ivens S, Shields RK. Low frequency depression of H-reflexes in humans with acute and chronic spinal-cord injury. Exp Brain Res. 2000;133(2):233–41.
18. Heckman CJ, Gorassini MA, Bennett DJ. Persistent inward currents in motoneuron dendrites: implications for motor output. Muscle Nerve. 2005;31(2):135–56.
19. Kitzman P. Alteration in axial motoneuronal morphology in the spinal cord injured spastic rat. Exp Neurol. 2005;192(1):100–8.
20. Bose P, Hou J, Thompson FJ. Traumatic brain injury (TBI)-induced spasticity: neurobiology, treatment, and rehabilitation. In: Kobeissy FH, editor. Brain neurotrauma: molecular, neuropsychological, and rehabilitation aspects. Boca Raton, FL: CRC Press/Taylor & Francis; 2015.
21. Bose P, et al. Effects of acute intrathecal baclofen in an animal model of TBI-induced spasticity, cognitive, and balance disabilities. J Neurotrauma. 2013;30(13):1177–91.
22. Brown EA, Schütz SG, Simpson DM. Botulinum toxin for neuropathic pain and spasticity: an overview. Pain. 2014;4(2):129–51.
23. Gracies J-M, et al. Safety and efficacy of abobotulinumtoxinA for hemiparesis in adults with upper limb spasticity after stroke or traumatic brain injury: a double-blind randomised controlled trial. Lancet Neurol. 2015;14(10):992–1001.
24. Burbaud P, et al. A randomised, double blind, placebo controlled trial of botulinum toxin in the treatment of spastic foot in hemiparetic patients. J Neurol Neurosurg Psychiatry. 1996;61(3):265–9.
25. Yablon SA, et al. Botulinum toxin in severe upper extremity spasticity among patients with traumatic brain injury an open-labeled trial. Neurology. 1996;47(4):939–44.
26. Simpson DM, et al. Botulinum neurotoxin versus tizanidine in upper limb spasticity: a placebo-controlled study. J Neurol Neurosurg Psychiatry. 2009;80(4):380–5.
27. Gronseth G, French J. Invited article: practice parameters and technology assessments what they are, what they are not, and why you should care. Neurology. 2008;71(20):1639–43.

28. Fietzek U, et al. Early botulinum toxin treatment for spastic pes equinovarus—a randomized double-blind placebo-controlled study. Eur J Neurol. 2014;21(8):1089–95.
29. Gracies J-M, et al. Botulinum toxin type B in the spastic arm: a randomized, double-blind, placebo-controlled, preliminary study. Arch Phys Med Rehabil. 2014;95(7):1303–11.
30. Smith S, et al. A double-blind placebo-controlled study of botulinum toxin in upper limb spasticity after stroke or head injury. Clin Rehabil. 2000;14(1):5–13.
31. Pavesi G, et al. Botulinum toxin type A in the treatment of upper limb spasticity among patients with traumatic brain injury. J Neurol Neurosurg Psychiatry. 1998;64(3):419.
32. Siddall PJ, Finnerup NB. Pain following spinal cord injury. Handb Clin Neurol. 2006;81:689–703.
33. Pertovaara A. The noradrenergic pain regulation system: a potential target for pain therapy. Eur J Pharmacol. 2013;716(1):2–7.
34. Lemmens S, et al. Alpha-Adrenoceptor modulation in central nervous system trauma: pain, spasms, and paralysis—an unlucky triad. Med Res Rev. 2015;35(4):653–77.
35. Namdari S, et al. Shoulder tenotomies to improve passive motion and relieve pain in patients with spastic hemiplegia after upper motor neuron injury. J Shoulder Elb Surg. 2011;20(5):802–6.
36. Nampiaparampil DE. Prevalence of chronic pain after traumatic brain injury: a systematic review. JAMA. 2008;300(6):711–9.
37. Jabbari B. Botulinum toxin treatment of pain disorders. New York: Springer; 2015.
38. Lew HL, et al. Characteristics and treatment of headache after traumatic brain injury: a focused review. Am J Phys Med Rehabil. 2006;85(7):619–27.
39. Lenaerts ME. Post-traumatic headache: from classification challenges to biological underpinnings. Cephalalgia. 2008;28(1 suppl):12–5.
40. Seifert T. Post-traumatic headache therapy in the athlete. Curr Pain Headache Rep. 2016;20(6):1–9.
41. Holtkamp MD, Grimes J, Ling G. Concussion in the military: an evidence-base review of mTBI in US military personnel focused on posttraumatic headache. Curr Pain Headache Rep. 2016;20(6):1–6.
42. Theeler BJ, Flynn FG, Erickson JC. Headaches after concussion in US soldiers returning from Iraq or Afghanistan. Headache. 2010;50(8):1262–72.
43. Yerry JA, Kuehn D, Finkel AG. Onabotulinum toxin a for the treatment of headache in service members with a history of mild traumatic brain injury: a cohort study. Headache. 2015;55(3):395–406.
44. Blumenfeld A, et al. Method of injection of OnabotulinumtoxinA for chronic migraine: a safe, well-tolerated, and effective treatment paradigm based on the PREEMPT clinical program. Headache. 2010;50(9):1406–18.
45. Jabbari B. History of botulinum toxin treatment in movement disorders. Tremor Other Hyperkinet Mov. 2016;6:394.
46. Krause T, et al. Dantrolene—a review of its pharmacology, therapeutic use and new developments. Anaesthesia. 2004;59(4):364–73.
47. Krauss JK, Trankle R, Kopp K-H. Post-traumatic movement disorders in survivors of severe head injury. Neurology. 1996;47(6):1488–92.
48. Krauss JK, Tränkle R, Kopp KH. Posttraumatic movement disorders after moderate or mild head injury. Mov Disord. 1997;12(3):428–31.
49. Kemp S, et al. Delayed-onset focal dystonia of the leg secondary to traumatic brain injury. J Clin Neurosci. 2012;19(6):916–7.
50. Spiegl UJ et al. Antispastic therapy with botulinum toxin type A in patients with traumatic spinal cord lesion. GMS Interdiscip Plast Reconstr Surg DGPW 2014;3:Doc14.
51. Dario A, Tomei G. A benefit-risk assessment of baclofen in severe spinal spasticity. Drug Saf. 2004;27(11):799–818.
52. Gorgey AS, et al. Relationship of spasticity to soft tissue body composition and the metabolic profile in persons with chronic motor complete spinal cord injury. J Spinal Cord med. 2010;33(1):6–15.

53. Holtz KA, et al. The prevalence and effect of problematic spasticity following traumatic spinal cord injury. Arch Phys med Rehabil. 2016;98(6):1132–8.
54. Opara J, Hordyńska E, Swoboda A. Effectiveness of botulinum toxin A in the treatment of spasticity of the lower extremities in adults-preliminary report. Ortop Traumatol Rehabil. 2006;9(3):277–85.
55. Marciniak C, Rader L, Gagnon C. The use of botulinum toxin for spasticity after spinal cord injury. Am J Phys Med Rehabil. 2008;87(4):312–7. quiz 318–20, 329
56. Bernuz B, et al. Botulinum toxin effect on voluntary and stretch reflex-related torque produced by the quadriceps an isokinetic pilot study. Neurorehabil Neural Repair. 2012;26(5):542–7.
57. Goldmark E, Niver B, Ginsberg DA. Neurogenic bladder: from diagnosis to management. Curr Urol Rep. 2014;15(10):1–8.
58. Peyronnet B, et al. Intradetrusor injections of onabotulinum toxin A (Botox®) 300 U or 200 U versus abobotulinum toxin a (Dysport®) 750 U in the management of neurogenic detrusor overactivity: a case control study. Neurourol Urodyn. 2017;36(3):734–9.
59. Smith CP, Chancellor MB. Botulinum toxin to treat neurogenic bladder. Semin Neurol. 2016;36(1):5–9.
60. Denys P, et al. Efficacy and safety of two administration modes of an intra-detrusor injection of 750 units dysport®(abobotulinumtoxinA) in patients suffering from refractory neurogenic detrusor overactivity (NDO): a randomised placebo-controlled phase IIa study. Neurourol Urodyn. 2016;36(2):457–62.
61. Huynh Le Maux A, et al. Does reduction of number of Intradetrusor injection sites of aboBoNTA (Dysport®) impact efficacy and safety in a rat model of neurogenic detrusor Overactivity? Toxins. 2015;7(12):5462–71.
62. Stoffel JT. Detrusor sphincter dyssynergia: a review of physiology, diagnosis, and treatment strategies. Transl Androl Urol. 2016;5(1):127.
63. Andresen SR, et al. Pain, spasticity and quality of life in individuals with traumatic spinal cord injury in Denmark. Spinal Cord. 2016;54(11):973–9.
64. Bryce TN, et al. International spinal cord injury pain (ISCIP) classification: part 2. Initial validation using vignettes. Spinal Cord. 2012;50(6):404–12.
65. Teasell RW, et al. A systematic review of pharmacologic treatments of pain after spinal cord injury. Arch Phys Med Rehabil. 2010;91(5):816–31.
66. Jabbari B, Maher N, Difazio MP. Botulinum toxin A improved burning pain and allodynia in two patients with spinal cord pathology. Pain Med. 2003;4(2):206–10.
67. Han ZA, Song DH, Chung ME. Effect of subcutaneous injection of botulinum toxin A on spinal cord injury-associated neuropathic pain. Spinal Cord. 2014;52:S5–6.
68. Han ZA, et al. Botulinum toxin type A for neuropathic pain in patients with spinal cord injury. Ann Neurol. 2016;79(4):569–78.
69. Hui C, Keji X, Chonghe J, Ping T, Rubiao O, Jianweng Z, Xiangrong D, Liling Z, Maping H, Qingqing L, Qiuling L, Jiebing H, Tanghai H. Combined detrusor-trigone BTX-A injections for urinary incontinence secondary to neurogenic detrusor overactivity. Spinal Cord. 2015;54(1):46–50.
70. Sussman D, Patel V, Del Popolo G, Lam W, Globe D, Pommerville P. Treatment satisfaction and improvement in health-related quality of life with onabotulinumtoxinA in patients with urinary incontinence due to neurogenic detrusor overactivity. Neurourol Urodyn. 2013;32(3):242–9.
71. Ginsberg D, Cruz F, Herschorn S, Gousse A, Keppenne V, Aliotta P, Sievert KD, Brin MF, Jenkins B, Thompson C, Lam W, Heesakkers J, Haag-Molkenteller C. Onabotulinumtoxin A is effective in patients with urinary incontinence due to neurogenic detrusor activity regardless of concomitant anticholinergic use or neurologic etiology. Adv Ther. 2013;30(9):819–33.
72. Chancellor MB, Patel V, Leng WW, Shenot PJ, Lam W, Globe DR, Loeb AL, Chapple CR. Onabotulinumtoxin A improves quality of life in patients with neurogenic detrusor overactivity. Neurology. 2013;81(9):841–8.
73. Ginsberg D, Gousse A, Keppenne V, Sievert K-D, Thompson C, Lam W, Brin MF, Jenkins B, Haag-Molkenteller C. Phase 3 efficacy and tolerability study of onabotulinumtoxina for urinary incontinence from neurogenic detrusor overactivity. J Urol. 2012;187(6):2131–9.

74. Cruz F, Herschorn S, Aliotta P, Brin M, Thompson C, Lam W, Daniell G, Heesakkers J, Haag-Molkenteller C. Efficacy and safety of onabotulinumtoxina in patients with urinary incontinence due to neurogenic detrusor overactivity: a randomised, double-blind, placebo-controlled trial. Eur Urol. 2011;60(4):742–50.
75. Zwibel HL, Smrtka J. Improving quality of life in multiple sclerosis: an unmet need. Am J Manag Care. 2011;17:S139–45.
76. Reitz A, Stöhrer M, Kramer G, Del Popolo G, Chartier-Kastler E, Pannek J, Burgdörfer H, Göcking K, Madersbacher H, Schumacher S, Richter R, von Tobel J, Schurch B. European experience of 200 cases treated with botulinum-A toxin injections into the detrusor muscle for urinary incontinence due to neurogenic detrusor overactivity. Eur Urol. 2004;45(4):510–5.
77. Schurch B, Hauri D, Rodic B, Curt A, Meyer M, Rossier AB. Botulinum-A toxin as a treatment of detruosor-sphincter dyssynergia: a prospective study in 24 spinal cord injury patients. J Urol. 1996;155(3):1023–9.
78. de Sze M, Petit H, Gallien P, de Sze M-P, Joseph P-A, Mazaux J-M, Barat M. Botulinum A toxin and detrusor sphincter dyssynergia: a double-blind lidocaine-controlled study in 13 patients with spinal cord disease. Eur Urol. 2002;42(1):56–62.
79. Kuo H-C. Satisfaction with urethral injection of botulinum toxin A for detrusor sphincter dyssynergia in patients with spinal cordlesion. Neurourol Urodyn. 2008;27(8):793–6.

Botulinum Toxin Treatment in Cerebrovascular Disease

Iman Moeini-Naghani and Bahman Jabbari

Introduction

Approximately 800,000 strokes occur annually in the United States, causing nearly 130,000 deaths each year [1–3]. Among adults aged 35–44, the incidence of stroke is 30–120 in 100,000 per year, while for those aged 65–74, the incidence rises to 670–970 in 100,000 per year [4]. The chance of having a stroke nearly doubles for each decade of life after age 55 [5]. Approximately 87% of strokes among adults are ischemic infarctions, 10% are primary hemorrhages, and 3% are subarachnoid hemorrhage. The most common risk factors for stroke among adults include hypertension, hyperlipidemia, smoking, physical inactivity, diabetes, heart rhythm disorders, and chronic kidney disease.

According to the American Heart Association, the mean lifetime cost of ischemic stroke is approximately $140,048 per person in the United States [6]. In 2008, the cost of lost productivity ($15.5 billion) was nearly equivalent to the direct cost of treating stroke ($18.8 billion) [7]. The total direct and indirect annual costs related to stroke in the USA are currently estimated at between $36.5 and $65 billion [6, 8], an amount that is expected to exceed $180 billion by 2030 [6, 9]. A substantial amount of informal caregiving is required for the stroke-related morbidity in elderly and it is one of the largest cost components for stroke in the US [10, 11].

Neurological symptoms of stroke are many and their full discussion is beyond the scope of this chapter. The focus of this chapter is on those symptoms that are potentially amenable to botulinum toxin therapy which include post-stroke spasticity, pain, involuntary movements, and sialorrhea.

I. Moeini-Naghani, M.D. (✉) • B. Jabbari, M.D.
Department of Neurology, Yale University, New Haven, CT 06520, USA
e-mail: Iman.naghani@gmail.com; Bahman.jabbari@yale.edu

B. Jabbari (ed.), *Botulinum Toxin Treatment in Clinical Medicine*,
DOI 10.1007/978-3-319-56038-0_12

Stroke and Spasticity

The significant sequels of post-stroke spasticity include the following: impaired dexterity; development of muscle spasms; loss of balance; and pain. These sequels are often associated with major functional impairment, lower quality of life, and increased caregiver burden. After a stroke, the upper motor neuron syndrome occurs as a result of damage to the pyramidal tract and its accompanying parapyramidal corticoreticulospinal fibers. Clinically, it may present with hyperkinesia (e.g., unwanted involuntary movements, such as spasms and action-induced spastic dystonia) and hypokinesia (e.g., impaired active/passive movements associated with spasticity) [12]. Spasticity may evolve early in the post-stroke period, with an incidence of ~19% within 3 months of the stroke [13] and >33% within 12 months [14, 15]. The most widely affected muscles in the initial 1–2 weeks and at 3 months following stroke are anti-gravity muscles; furthermore, the severity of upper limb spasticity increases over time [16]. A study of lower limbs post-stroke reported a similar finding with 88% of study participants developed spasticity within 2 weeks of stroke [17]. The following three measures are often employed to assess the nature and severity of spasticity; modified Ashworth Scale (the clinical scoring method assessing the severity of spasticity), the quantity and patterns of electrical muscle activity during the passive movement (neurophysiological method), and the resistance encountered during passive stretching (biomechanical method) [18].

The treatment of spasticity can be complex and relies on a multidisciplinary approach. Specific functional objectives in the management of spasticity include strategies aimed at increasing mobility and range of motion. Not all patients with spasticity need pharmacological treatment. Physical therapy and occupational therapy are commonly used, conservative approaches that are targeted at improving daily activities by reducing muscle tone and enhancing range of motion (ROM). In more severe cases, treatment is aimed at reducing muscle tone, improving function, and preventing complications [19]. A large number of pharmacological agents are currently used for the treatment of spasticity (Table 1) [19]. For severe spasticity—especially when it involves the lower limbs—baclofen pump is helpful, but the procedure requires special setting and trained personnel. Although these drugs are effective and, in many cases, reduce muscle tone and improve the quality of life, side effects (sedation, dizziness, confusion) and drug interactions are common and especially bothersome in children and the elderly [19–25]. Hence, a new therapeutic modality with limited side effects and a low level of drug interaction would be welcome in this field.

Botulinum Toxins in Management of Stroke-Related Spasticity

Botulinum neurotoxins (BoNT) block the presynaptic cholinergic nerve endings by preventing the release of acetylcholine from presynaptic vesicles [26]. There are seven serotypes of this toxin designated as A, B, C, D, E, F, and G. They all prevent

Table 1 Pharmacological treatment of spasticity

Medication	Mechanism of action	Typical dose	Side effects
Benzodiazepines	Facilitate the postsynaptic action of GABA	Diazepam: 2–10 mg; 3–4 times/day	Drowsiness, sedation, ataxia, hypotension
		Clonazepam: 0.5–1.0 mg at bedtime	
Imidazolines (Clonidine, Tizanidine)	α2 adrenergic agonist	Tizanidine:	Sedation, hypotension, hepatotoxicity (Tizanidine)
		Initial dose: 4 mg orally every 6–8 h	
		Maximum dose: three doses in 24 h; 12 mg/dose; 36 mg/day	
		Clonidine:	
		Starting dose: 0.1 mg twice/day	
		Maximum dose: 2.4 mg/day	
Baclofen	Binds to $GABA_B$ receptor and causes membrane hyperpolarization and restriction of calcium influx to presynaptic nerve terminals, which results in reduced muscle contraction	Initial dose: 5 mg 3/day. This dose may be increased by 15 mg/day increments every 3 day	Confusion, drowsiness, nausea, muscle weakness
		Maximum dose: 80 mg/day divided into three or four doses	
Dantrolene	Inhibits the ryanodine receptor and reduces the release of calcium into the sarcoplasmic reticulum of muscles	Initial dose: 25 mg once daily	Hepatotoxicity, drowsiness, weakness, fatigue, malaise
		Maximum dose: 100 mg 3 times/day	

acetylcholine release into the synaptic cleft by binding to one or more of the transport protein chains with high specificity [27, 28]. The serotypes are different in their protein sequences which accounts for their affinities and antigenicities. Two antigenically different serotypes are available as type A and B; both of these are proved to be generally safe and provide attractive therapeutic options. BoNT-A cleaves synaptosome-associated protein 25, whereas BoNT-B cleaves the vesicle-associated membrane protein, synaptic proteins which are essential for fusion and rupture of the vesicles leading to acetylcholine release [29]. Some studies have shown BoNT-B to have more anticholinergic, unwanted side effects such as dry mouth, dysphagia, and voiding difficulties compared to BoNT-A [30–32].

Three type A and one type B toxins are approved by FDA for the treatment of the patients in the US. The type A toxins are: onabotulinum toxinA (onaA, Botox), incobotulinumtoxinA (incoA, Xeomin), abobotulinumtoxinA (aboA, Dysport), and the type B is rimabotulinumtoxinA (myobloc). Although in research protocols units are sometimes compared with approximation (1unit Botox = 1 unit xeomin = 2.5–3 units Dysport = 40–50 units of Myobloc), in reality the units are not quite comparable and there is considerable individual variability.

The beneficial effects of BoNTs in post-stroke spasticity have been studied through several randomized clinical trials (RCTs). These placebo controlled, double blind studies indicate reduction of muscle tone, improved ambulation, and in some, the quality of life after treatment of spastic limbs with botulinum toxins [33–52] (Tables 2 and 3). Based on these studies, FDA approved the use of BoNT-A for treatment of upper limb spasticity in 2011 and 2013 (extended approval to include additional muscles) and its use for lower limb spasticity in 2015. The Practice Guideline Committee of American Academy of Neurology has recently published an update on the level of evidence for efficacy of BoNTs in adult onset spasticity. For upper spasticity, "aboBoNT-A, incoBoNT-A, and onaBoNT-A are established as effective and should be offered (Level A). RimaBoNT-B is probably effective and should be considered (Level B), for upper limb spasticity. AboBoNT-A and onaBoNT-A are established as effective and should be offered (Level A) for lower-limb spasticity" [53].

Technical Issues

In spasticity, like any other indication for botulinum toxins, treatment success depends to a large extent on where and how the toxin therapy was administered as well as the appropriateness of the treatment dose. Although, over the past 2–3 decades, a fair amount of knowledge has been accumulated on these issues, the thrive for reaching the "optimum" still continues. The optimum site of injection is generally believed to be as close as possible to the muscle end-plates which, for most muscles, is located close to the middle of the muscle. While electromyography and neurostimulation are helpful for localization, ultrasound technique is more precise and better tolerated by the patient (see Alter in Chap. 16).

The optimal dilution of the toxin for treatment of spasticity has been the subject of some controversy. Most neurologists and physiatrists believe that a 50 unit/CC dilution or less (in case of ona-BoNT-A or Inco-BoNT-A) causes a more desirable effect on spasticity. In line with this view is the recent study of Gracies et al. who compared the effects of different dilutions of ona-BoNT-A in 21 patients with spasticity. The best responders were those who received high volume (20 unit/CC) dilution and had the injections delivered close to the end-plates (on the line closer to the middle of the muscle—biceps brachii, rather than into four quadrants of the muscle) [54]. The total dose injected in one session and the maximum dose per muscle is also subject of frequent investigations. While application

Table 2 Randomized blinded studies assessing the efficacy of BoNTs in upper limb stroke-associated spasticity

Author(s)	Number	Limb	Toxin	Dose (U)	Result
Simpson et al. [33]	39	Upper	BOTOX	75, 100, 300	Improved: Ashworth Scale, PGAC, PGIC
					Not improved: hygiene (−)
Hesse et al. [34]	24	Upper	Dysport	1000	Improved: hygiene
					Not improved: MAS and limb position
Bakheit et al. [35]	82	Upper	Dysport	500, 1000	Improved: MAS
					Not improved: Barthel index, hygiene, range of motion
Bhakta et al. [36]	40	Upper	Dysport	1000	Improved: patient disability scale, MAS, care giver burden scale
					Not improved: passive ROM, arm pain
Bakheit et al. [37]	59	Upper	Dysport	1000	Improved: MAS, PGIC, PGIC
					Not improved: ROM, Barthel index, painscore, goal attainment
Brashear et al. [38]	126	Upper	BOTOX	200, 240	Improved: Ashworth disability score, PGIC, CGIC
Childers et al. [39]	92	Upper	BOTOX	90, 180, 320	Improved: MAS
					Not improved: pain, SF36, PGIC, FIM
Brashear et al. [40]	15	Upper	MYOBLOC	10,000	Improved: Ashworth scale
					Not improved: PGIC
Marco et al. [41]	31	Upper	Dysport	500	Improved: VAS
					Not improved: shoulder ROM and MAS
McCrory et al. [42]	96	Upper	Dysport	750, 1000	Improved: MAS, PGIC and patient goal attainment
					Not improved: pain, mood, disability, QOL (−)
Kanovsky et al. [43]	148	Upper	XEOMIN	320	Improved: DAS, global efficacy, Ashworth scale, and care giver burden scale
Kaji et al. [44]	109	Upper	BOTOX	120, 150	Improved: MAS and DAS
					No difference between high- and low-dose groups
Shaw et al. [45]	333	Upper	Dysport	100–200	Improved: Ashworth Scale, pain, arm functional tasks, and action research arm test

(continued)

Table 2 (continued)

Author(s)	Number	Limb	Toxin	Dose (U)	Result
Rosales et al. [46]	163	Upper	Dysport	500	Improved: MAS, global pain scale, and goniometry
					Not improved: functional motor assessment scale
Elovic et al. [47]	347	Upper	XEOMIN	400	Improved: MAS, PGIC and DAS
Gracies et al. [48]	243	Upper	Dysport	500, 1000	Improved in the1000 unit group: MAS, PGA, DAS

MAS modified Ashworth scale, *PGA* physicians global impression, *DAS* disability assessment scale, *BoNT* botulinum neurotoxin

Table 3 Randomized, blinded, clinical trials with botulinum neurotoxins in lower limb spasticity after stroke

Authors	Number	Limb	Toxin	Dose (U)	Result
Pittock et al. [49]	234	Lower	Dysport	500, 1000	Improved: MAS, need for aids, pain
					Not improved: walking, global score, ROM, Rivermead motor assessment
Kaji et al. [50]	120	Lower	BOTOX	300	Improved: MAS, clinical global impression
					Not improved: Gait pattern and gait speed, PGIC
Dunne et al. [51]	85	Lower	BOTOX	300	Improved: Spasm frequency, pain, quality of pain
					Not improved: Ashworth scale
Tao et al. [52]	23	Lower	BOTOX	200	Improved: MAS, gait, muscle tone, FMA, MBI

MAS modified Ashworth scale, *FMA* Fugel-Myer assessment, *MBI* modified Barthel index

of high doses can cause undesirable muscle weakness, suboptimal dosage will deprive the patient from optimal results. In the blinded clinical trials, the maximum dose used for both ona-BoNT-A and inco-BoNT-A was 320 units and for abo-BoNT-A and rima-BoNT-B was 1000 and 10,000 units, respectively (Tables 2 and 3). However, more recent data indicate that considerably higher doses can be used without producing undesirable side effects. For instance, the European Consensus Committee recommended up to 600 units/session for ona and inco-BoNT formulations and 1500 units of abo-BoNT-A for adult spasticity [55]. Others have found doses up to 800 units of ona and inco-BoNT-A more effective for some patients and feasible to use [56, 57].

The number and type of muscles included in the plan of treatment also plays an important role in obtaining satisfactory results. Omission of muscles with important function in a certain indication may result in insufficient or no functional improvement. For instance, lumbrical muscles play an important role in hand spasticity and clinched fist. Many clinical trials of upper limb spasticity did not include these muscles in the plan of injection. Lumbrical muscles flex the metacarpophalangeal joints and enhance wrist flexion. Each of the four lumbricals can be injected at the mid-palm with a 30-gauge needle. We have found injections of these four muscles (15–25 units/muscle) extremely helpful in treatment of clinched fist and severe hand spasticity. The palm of the hand is first treated with Emla cream for an hour before the injection. The palm is then cleaned and injections are performed swiftly after short exposure to additional spray anesthetics.

Side Effects

The RTCs of botulinum toxin treatment of spasticity (Tables 2 and 3) have shown that serious side effects are rare and most side effects are mild and transient. This is supported by a recent study which compared the safety and efficacy of inco-BoNT-A with conventional therapy of spasticity over a period of 1 year through repeated injections [58]. The mean dose of incoA for the first and last injections was 215 and 268 units, respectively. Patients who received inco-BoNT-A showed more improvement in hygiene, dressing, limb position, and pain compared to the conventional therapy; this was statistically significant for improvement of dressing and pain relief in favor of inco-BoNT-A ($P < 0.01$). As to the quality of life, the improvement of both physical and mental scores was statistically more significant in the inco-BoNT group ($P < 0.01$). Adverse effects occurred in 8% of inco-BonT-A and 16% of conventional therapy groups. All adverse effects, but one, were unrelated to treatment. Statistically, there was no difference between the inco-BoNT-A and the conventional therapy group in regard to adverse effects. It has been suggested that early treatment with BoNTs may be more beneficial to the patient with spasticity [59]. Since, in some, contractures may develop as early as 2 weeks after stroke [60]. Kaku and Simpson have recently published an excellent review and update on the role of botulinum neurotoxin therapy in post-stroke spasticity [61].

Comment

Botulinum toxin therapy is now established as a major mode of treatment for adult spasticity. This therapy should be part of a larger treatment plan to include physical therapy and, in many cases, the concomitant use of oral anti-spasticity agents. Further research is needed to optimize the dose and the method of injection. Infrequency of treatment sessions (once every 3–4 months) and low incidence of side effects have made BoNT therapy an attractive choice for patients with post-stroke spasticity.

Post-Stroke Pain

In a recent report on 485 patients, the authors cited a prevalence of 29.5% for post-stroke pain [62]. In 75% of cases, pain occurred in the subacute and chronic phase and was 1.7 times more common among women. The most common varieties of pain consisted of musculoskeletal (most commonly felt in the shoulder ipsilateral to the hemiplegia), pain associated with spasticity, headaches, and central pain.

Several investigators have reported efficacy of botulinum toxin therapy in relieving hemiplegic shoulder pain using different methodologies. In 2003, Yelnik et al. [63] first reported improvement of shoulder pain and range of motion (especially abduction and external rotation) after injection of 250 units of Abo-BoNT-A into the ipsilateral subscapularis muscle of three patients with post-stroke painful shoulder. Four years later, the same authors reported the results of a double blind placebo controlled study in 20 patients with stroke (11 ischemic, 9 hemorrhagic) [64]. Injection of Abo-BoNT-A (500 units) into the ipsilateral subscapularis muscle relieved pain measured by VAS significantly when compared with placebo (At week 4; $P = 0.025$). Furthermore, patients who received Abo-BoNT-A demonstrated significant improvement of lateral rotation ($P = 0.018$). In another randomized double blind study (9 toxin and 9 placebo), Kong et al. [65] failed to show improvement of shoulder pain with the same dose of Abo-BoNT A (500 units) injected into biceps brachii and pectoralis muscles. Marco et al. [41], however, reported that injection of 500 units of Abo-BoNT-A into the pectoralis muscle reduced post-stroke shoulder pain 2.4–3.1-fold compared to the placebo. Their study included 15 stroke and 15 placebo subjects. In another blinded study of patients with post-stroke shoulder pain, the effect of intra-articular injection of 100 units of Ona-BoNT-A was compared with triamcinolone acetate (TA), 40 mg [66]. At week 12, Ona-BoNT-A was found superior to TA in relieving pain measured by VAS score reduction (toxin 4.2 versus placebo 2.4—$P = 0.051$ on a 0–10 scale) and improving the shoulder range of motion (toxin 82.9 versus placebo 51.8° $P = 0.059$). Marciniak et al. [67], in a blinded study, compared the effect of 140–200 units of ona-BoNT-A (10 subjects) with saline (11 subjects) injected into the pectoralis major muscle of the patients with post-stroke shoulder pain. They found no difference between toxin and placebo in term of pain relief (both relieved pain), but subjects who received Ona-BoNT-A demonstrated significant improvement of hygiene on disability assessment scale ($P = 0.05$) and displayed a strong trend for improvement of dressing scale ($P = 0.061$) compared to the placebo. Choi et al. [68] injected 60–80 units (depending on body weight) of onabotulinumtoxinA (botox) into subscapularis muscle of six patients with intractable hemiplegic shoulder pain. Using an 11 point pain scale, the authors found significant improvement of pain in all patients ($p = 0.004$). There was also improvement of shoulder abduction ($p = 0.003$), external rotation ($p = 0.005$), and spasticity of the internal rotator ($p = 0.005$). In another study, the effect of ona-BoNT-A injection into subscapularis muscle (100 units) was compared with injection into pectoralis major (150 units) in 21 patients with post-stroke shoulder pain [69]. Injection into the subscapular was found to be superior to the pectoralis muscle in reducing pain scores (measured by VAS), especially at week 12 after injection (24 versus 7.6 points on 0–100 scale). Castiglione et al. [70] reported significant relief of post-stroke shoulder pain after intra-articular injection of BoNTA in five patients with intractable post-stroke shoulder pain (Fig. 1). Two patients received ona-BoNT-A (100 units), two Inco-BoNT-A (100 units), and one Abo-BoNT-A (500 units). The relief of pain and improvement of arm abduction was significant compared to baseline both at 2 and 8 weeks post-injection ($P = 0.01$).

Comment

Local injection of botulinum toxins can improve post-stroke pain through a variety of mechanisms. These include inhibition of the release of pain modulators (calcitonin gene-related peptide, substance P, glutamate, and others) from both peripheral and central synapses and via retrograde transport reaching the central neurons [71]. One class II and several class IV studies have reported efficacy of Abo-BoNT-A in relieving the intractable shoulder pain in stroke patients. Based on this data, injection of BoNT-A into subscapular muscle is possibly effective (Level C evidence) in ameliorating the post-stroke shoulder pain. The data on the pectoralis muscle injection is contradictory.

One comparator study (class II) and one small Class IV study have also suggested efficacy of intra-articular injection of botulinum toxins in post-stroke shoulder pain. Although these data are encouraging, proof of the efficacy of BoNT injections (intramuscular or intra-articular) in post-stroke shoulder pain requires conduction of RCTs of higher quality.

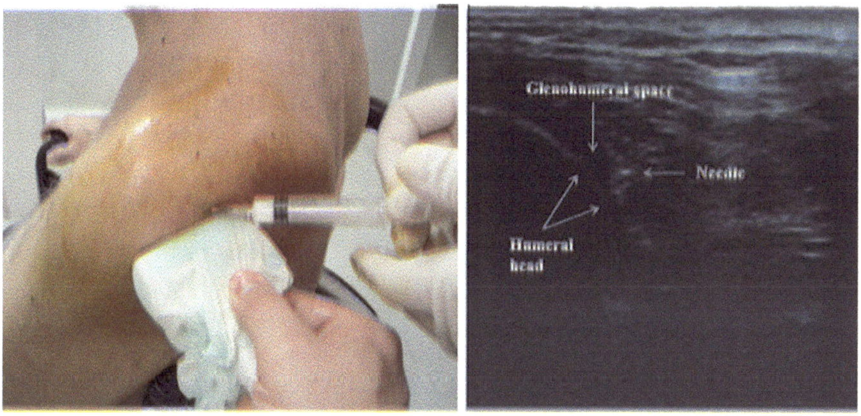

Fig. 1 Glenohumeral injection of botulinum neurotoxinA for a patient with persistent shoulder pain in the hemiplegic side. From Castiglione et al. 2011 with permission from Elsevier Publishing

Focal Muscle Spasms

Focal painful spasms occur in affected muscles after stroke, but the true incidence of such spasms is not known. BoNT-A has been reported to decrease focal muscle spasms in stroke patients when injected under ultrasound guidance [72]. Patients with brain stem infarct sometimes manifest sustained spasms of masseter muscles (trismus), a condition which has been successfully treated with botulinum toxin injection into the masseter muscles [73].

Muscle Pain Associated with Post-Stroke Spasticity

Although most experienced clinicians who inject botulinum toxins for spasticity believe that this treatment relieves spasticity-associated pain in a sizeable number of patients, the data from the blinded clinical trials is scant and disclose mixed results (Table 3). A closer examination of the data shows, however, that failure of BoNT therapy to relieve the spasticity-associated pain has been reported in the studies that either did not mention the applied pain scale or used the pain scales which by today's standards are considered suboptimal. Additional studies using more appropriate pain scales are needed (Table 4).

Post-Stroke Headaches

In a study of 222 patients, Hansen et al. [77] reported the prevalence of chronic post-stroke headaches as 12%. These include tension type headaches (50%), migraine (30.2%), and headaches related to drug overuse (6.25%). It is not clear what percentage of patients with post-stroke migraine fit the category of chronic migraine (>15 headaches/month), which is amenable to botulinum toxin treatment. The role of botulinum toxin therapy in post-stroke chronic migraine is not known due to lack of data.

Involuntary Movements After Stroke

A variety of involuntary movements can develop after cerebral infarcts which further deteriorate the patient's quality of life. The prevalence of hyperkinetic movement disorders after stroke had been reported between 1 and 3.7% from Lausane and Ecuador stroke registries, screening 2900 and 1500 patients, respectively [78, 79] . In the Lausane registry [78], chorea and dystonia were the most common movement disorders; 38 and 17%. Tremor/limb shaking was noted in 13% of the patients. Other movement disorders included myoclonus or myoclonic dystonia

Table 4 Blinded studies of spasticity which reported the effect of BoNT treatment on the spasticity-associated pain

Authors	Number	Limb	BoNT	Dose (units)	Pain scale	Results	Comment
Bakheit et al. [37]	59	upper	aboA	1000	0–3 scale	NI	Suboptimal scale?
Pittock et al. [49]	234	Lower	aboA	500, 1000	Subjective global assessment of arm pain	Improved	
Brashear et al. [40]	15	Upper	rimaB	5000, 10,000	–	NI	Pain scale not mentioned
Childers et al. [39]	91	Upper	onaA	90/180/360	5 point scale	NI	Suboptimal scale? Low level of baseline pain
Suputtitada and Suwanwela [74]	50	Upper	aboA	375, 500, 1000	–	Pain improved	Scale not defined
Shaw et al. [45]	333	Upper	aboA	100, 200	VAS	Wks 4 and 12: NI but at Wk 52 improved ($P = 0.002$)	
Rosales et al. [46]	163	Upper	aboA	500	VAS	Wks 4 and 24: significant pain reduction	
Lam et al. [75]	55	Upper	aboA	1000	Scale 0–5	NI	Suboptimal scale?
Dunne et al. [51]	85	Lower	OnaA	300	VAS	Improved ($P = 0.02$)	
Gracies et al. [76]	24	Upper	rimaB	5000, 1000	Global self-assessment of arm pain	Wk 4: Pain Improved ($P = 0.017$)	

aboA abobotulinumtoxinA (Dysport), *onaA* onabotulinumtoxinA (Botox), *rimaB* rimabotulinum-toxinB (Myobloc), *VAS* visual analogue scale, *NI* not improved

(10%), asterixis (7%), stereotopy (7%), and hemi-akathisia (3%). Post-stroke dystonia is usually in the form of focal limb dystonia. In a study of 32 patients with focal limb dystonia after stroke, 31 had focal limb dystonia and one had cervical dystonia [80]. With the exception of hemi-ballismus and some cases of hemichorea, post-stroke, basal ganglia-generated involuntary movements (dystonia, chorea, tremor) often appear with a delay of weeks to months after the initial insult. Majority of the abnormal movements gradually improve and may not need treatment. In case of persistent movements, administration of oral pharmacologic agents such as anticholinergic drugs or baclofen may help (for dystonia), but the results are usually modest. The responsible lesions for majority of these disorders are located in the basal ganglia [81]. Marsden and his colleagues should be credited for the first detail description of responsible basal ganglia structures in the development of secondary hemidystonia using computed tomography [82]. The lesions were mostly located in the contralateral putamen, with the globus pallidus and thalamus being the next most common sites. This observation was confirmed later by the Magnetic Resonance Imaging (MRI), which identified contralateral post-commisural part of putmen and the lateral and ventral head of the caudate nucleus as the two most common lesion locations for post-stroke hemidystonia [83]. Post-stroke hemichorea and hemi-ballismus (which may precede hemichorea) usually result from lesion(s) of the striatum (caudate and putamen) and subthalamic nucleus (or its vicinity), respectively. Isolated tremor is rare after stroke. The causative lesion for post-stroke tremor is often located in the posterior nucleus of the thalamus.

A favorable response to botulinum toxins has been reported in few patients with post-stroke dystonia caused by deep brain lesions. Walker [84] reported a 56 year old man who suffered from myoclonic dystonia of the right shoulder secondary to an acute infarct in the left posterior thalamus. A modest improvement of dystonia was noted with administration of trihexiphenidyl 5 mg, three times daily. Injection of botulinum toxin (type and dose was not identified) into the right triceps, right trapezius, and cervical muscles resulted in marked improvement of the involuntary movements. Kowacs et al. [85] described a 79 year-old women with a history of left putaminal infarct 9 years prior leading to mild right hemiparesis who developed painful dystonic extensor posturing of the right foot during sleep. A polysomnography revealed that dystonic posturing occurred during REM sleep and coincided with periodic limb movements. Passive extension of the right large toe also produced painful extension dystonia. Injection of 20 units of Abo-BoNT-A into the extensor hallusis longus abolished the dystonic movements. In another study, post-stroke intermittent flexion dystonia of the right knee was treated successfully with 400 units of Ona-BoNT-A injection into the leg muscles (biceps femoris125 units; iliopsoas100 units, semitendineous 75 units; tibialis anterior 60 units) [86]. In a blinded study of 17 patients with secondary dystonias (2 after stroke), authors mentioned satisfaction with botulinum toxin treatment of the affected muscles in 83% of the patients [87].

Cerebellar infarct or intra-cerebellar hemorrhage can also cause a variety of involuntary movements [88]. These movements include intentional tremor, Holms (midbrain) tremor (rest, posture, and intention), palatal tremor, myoclonus, dystonia, stereotypy, and asterixis. A limited literature is available on the use of botulinum toxin for some of these movement disorders including palatal tremor and cerebellar intention tremor.

Palatal tremor (PT) is caused by a lesion which disrupts the dentate-rubro-olivary pathway. The tremor has a frequency ranging between 60 and 180/s. Palatal tremor has an essential and a secondary form. In the secondary PT, the lesion can be either in the cerebellum or brain stem (central tegmental tract). Stroke is one of the common causes of secondary palatal tremor. There is great individual variability in terms of tolerance of PT. Some people are not bothered by it, whereas others poorly tolerate tremoring of soft palate. Secondary PT is also associated with hearing a clicking sound in the ear which adds to the patients' discomfort. Injections are given into the tensor veli palatini. For Ona-BoNT-A, 5–15 units and for Abo-BoNT-A, 30–60 units have been used by different investigators [89].

Recently, Viellote published data from a retrospective observation of 14 patients with cerebellar intention tremor who were treated with intramuscular injection of BoNT-A for cerebellar intentional tremor. BoNT-A was injected into the pronator muscle of the affected arm. Response was measured by assessing the volume of remaining water in a cup after five attempts at drinking from the cup. A significant improvement of nearly 50% was noted in volumetric tests 1 month after botulinum toxin therapy [90].

Sialorrhea

Drooling or excessive salivation is defined as excessive saliva production beyond the margin of the lip and it is a common problem in neurologically impaired adults who have had a stroke [91]. The main functions of saliva include mechanical cleansing of the mouth, contributing to oral homeostasis, and regulation of the oral pH. The parasympathetic nervous system innervates the parotid, submandibular, and sublingual glands with fibers that originate in the pons and medulla, and synapse in the otic and submandibular ganglia. Sympathetic innervation enhances the flow of saliva by promoting the contraction of muscle fibers around the salivary ducts. Typically, drooling results from weak or uncoordinated oropharyngeal muscles and it potentially increases the risk of aspiration. It may also lead to social isolation and depression. These side effects greatly increase the need for nurses—a need that has increased dramatically and increased the burden of care in these patients [92]. Regardless of the cause, treatment of drooling includes anticholinergic medications, radiation of the salivary glands, and various surgical procedures [93]. Botulinum neurotoxins have shown efficacy in reducing saliva in several high-quality studies, although currently there are no clear treatment guidelines regarding the appropriate dose, technique, and selection of salivary glands [94]. Mazlan et al. [95] conducted a blinded study comparing three doses of Abo-BoNT-A (50, 100 and 200 units) in a mixed group of patients suffering from severe sialorrhea. Among 17 subjects who completed the study at 24 weeks, sialorrhea was secondary to stroke in 13 patients. All three doses were more effective than placebo (Fig. 2) with the best results observed in the high-dose group (200 unit dose).

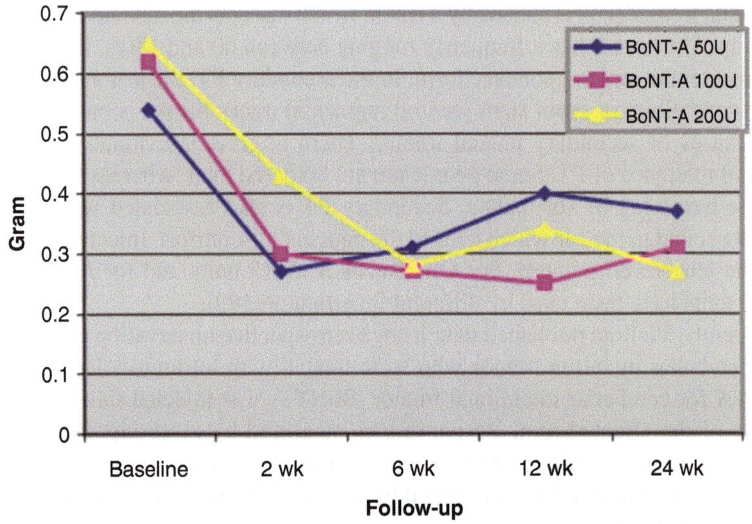

Fig. 2 Mean gauze weight (wet versus dry) after abobotulinumtoxinA injection into parotid and submandibular glands bilaterally—All three doses 50, 100, and 200 reduce saliva effectively, but the effect is more sustained with the higher doses. From Mazlan et al., Toxins 2015

Conclusion

Several sequelae of stroke are amenable to botulinum neurotoxin therapy. Using the guidelines of the American Academy of Neurology [53], there is a level A (effective) evidence (two or more class I studies) of efficacy for post-stroke spasticity. In regard to post-stroke (PS) pain associated with spasticity, available data also support a level A evidence for its utility. Post-stroke shoulder pain could qualify for a level C evidence (possibly effective) based on one class II and several class IV studies. In the area of post-stroke involuntary movements, BoNTs are effective in improving dystonia associated with spasticity. There are case observations that suggest efficacy of BoNTs in intermittent PS-dystonia. Open label studies demonstrate a favorable response to BoNT therapy for PS-palatal tremor. The injections for palatal tremor (PT), in particular, require technical expertise as well as familiarity of the injector with the region's anatomy. Sialorrhea responds well to BoNT therapy [94]. In the specific area of post-stroke sialorrhea, one double blind class II study [95] has demonstrated an excellent response to different doses of abobotulinumtoxinA (Level B- probably effective).

References

1. Barker-Collo S, et al. Sex differences in stroke incidence, prevalence, mortality and disability-adjusted life years: results from the Global Burden of Disease Study 2013. Neuroepidemiology. 2015;45(3):203–14.

2. Kochanek KD, et al. Deaths: final data for 2009. Natl Vital Stat Syst. 2011;60(3):1–116.
3. Ovbiagele B, Nguyen-Huynh MN. Stroke epidemiology: advancing our understanding of disease mechanism and therapy. Neurotherapeutics. 2011;8(3):319.
4. Roger VL, et al. Heart disease and stroke statistics—2011 update. A report from the American Heart Association. Circulation. 2011;123(4):e18–e209.
5. Chong JY, Sacco RL. Risk factors for stroke, assessing risk, and the mass and high-risk approaches for stroke prevention. Continuum: Lifelong Learn Neurol. 2005;11(4):18–34.
6. Go AS, et al. Heart disease and stroke statistics--2014 update: a report from the American Heart Association. Circulation. 2014;129(3):e28–e292.
7. Centers for Disease Control and Prevention (CDC). Prevalence of stroke--United States, 2006-2010. MMWR Morb Mortal Wkly Rep. 2012;61(20):379.
8. Demaerschalk BM, Hwang HM, Leung G. US cost burden of ischemic stroke: a systematic literature review. American J Managed Care. 2010;16(7):525–33.
9. Mozaffarian D, et al. Executive summary: heart disease and stroke statistics-2016 update: a report from the American Heart Association. Circulation. 2016;133(4):447.
10. Brown D, et al. Projected costs of ischemic stroke in the United States. Neurology. 2006;67(8):1390–5.
11. Leal J, et al. Economic burden of cardiovascular diseases in the enlarged European Union. Eur Heart J. 2006;27(13):1610–9.
12. Lance JW. The control of muscle tone, reflexes, and movement Robert Wartenberg lecture. Neurology. 1980;30(12):1303–13.
13. Sommerfeld DK, et al. Spasticity after stroke. Stroke. 2004;35(1):134–9.
14. Watkins C, et al. Prevalence of spasticity post stroke. Clin Rehabil. 2002;16(5):515–22.
15. Leathley MJ, et al. Predicting spasticity after stroke in those surviving to 12 months. Clin Rehabil. 2004;18(4):438–43.
16. Welmer AK, Widén Holmqvist L, Sommerfeld D. Location and severity of spasticity in the first 1–2 weeks and at 3 and 18 months after stroke. Eur J Neurol. 2010;17(5):720–5.
17. Verplancke D, et al. A randomized controlled trial of botulinum toxin on lower limb spasticity following acute acquired severe brain injury. Clin Rehabil. 2005;19(2):117–25.
18. Malhotra S, et al. An investigation into the agreement between clinical, biomechanical and neurophysiological measures of spasticity. Clin Rehabil. 2008;22(12):1105–15.
19. Moeini-Naghani I, Hashemi-Zonouz T, Jabbari B. Botulinum toxin treatment of spasticity in adults and children. Semin Neurol. 2016;36(1):64–72.
20. Sheean G. Botulinum toxin treatment of adult spasticity. Drug Saf. 2006;29(1):31–48.
21. Lindsay C, et al. Pharmacological interventions other than botulinum toxin for spasticity after stroke. Cochrane Database Syst Rev. 2016;10:CD010362.
22. Bogey RA, et al. Stroke and neurodegenerative disorders. 3. Stroke: rehabilitation management. Arch Phys Med Rehabil. 2004;85:15–20.
23. Jang SH, et al. Alcohol neurolysis of tibial nerve motor branches to the gastrocnemius muscle to treat ankle spasticity in patients with hemiplegic stroke. Arch Phys Med Rehabil. 2004;85(3):506–8.
24. Gallichio JE. Pharmacologic management of spasticity following stroke. Phys Ther. 2004;84(10):973.
25. Chou R, Peterson K, Helfand M. Comparative efficacy and safety of skeletal muscle relaxants for spasticity and musculoskeletal conditions: a systematic review. J Pain Symptom Manag. 2004;28(2):140–75.
26. Jankovic J, Brin MF. Botulinum toxin: historical perspective and potential new indications. Muscle Nerve. 1997;20(S6):129–45.
27. Dressler D, Adib Saberi F. Botulinum toxin: mechanisms of action. Eur Neurol. 2005;53(1):3–9.
28. Thakker MM, Rubin PA. Pharmacology and clinical applications of botulinum toxins A and B. Int Ophthalmol Clin. 2004;44(3):147–63.
29. Aoki KR. Pharmacology and immunology of botulinum toxin type A. Clin Dermatol. 2003;21(6):476–80.
30. Comella C, et al. Comparison of botulinum toxin serotypes A and B for the treatment of cervical dystonia. Neurology. 2005;65(9):1423–9.

31. Ozcakir S, Sivrioglu K. Botulinum toxin in poststroke spasticity. Clin Med Res. 2007;5(2):132–8.
32. Tintner R, et al. Autonomic function after botulinum toxin type A or B: a double-blind, randomized trial. Neurology. 2005;65(5):765–7.
33. Simpson D, et al. Botulinum toxin type A in the treatment of upper extremity spasticity: a randomized, double-blind, placebo-controlled trial. Neurology. 1996;46(5):1306–10.
34. Hesse S, et al. Botulinum toxin type A and short-term electrical stimulation in the treatment of upper limb flexor spasticity after stroke: a randomized, double-blind, placebo-controlled trial. Clin Rehabil. 1998;12(5):381–8.
35. Bakheit A, et al. A randomized, double-blind, placebo-controlled, dose-ranging study to compare the efficacy and safety of three doses of botulinum toxin type A (Dysport) with placebo in upper limb spasticity after stroke. Stroke. 2000;31(10):2402–6.
36. Bhakta BB, et al. Impact of botulinum toxin type A on disability and carer burden due to arm spasticity after stroke: a randomised double blind placebo controlled trial. J Neurol Neurosurg Psychiatry. 2000;69(2):217–21.
37. Bakheit A, et al. A randomized, double-blind, placebo-controlled study of the efficacy and safety of botulinum toxin type A in upper limb spasticity in patients with stroke. Eur J Neurol. 2001;8(6):559–65.
38. Brashear A, et al. Intramuscular injection of botulinum toxin for the treatment of wrist and finger spasticity after a stroke. N Engl J Med. 2002;347(6):395–400.
39. Childers MK, et al. Dose-dependent response to intramuscular botulinum toxin type A for upper-limb spasticity in patients after a stroke. Arch Phys Med Rehabil. 2004;85(7):1063–9.
40. Brashear A, et al. Botulinum toxin type B in upper-limb poststroke spasticity: a double-blind, placebo-controlled trial. Arch Phys Med Rehabil. 2004;85(5):705–9.
41. Marco E, et al. Is botulinum toxin type A effective in the treatment of spastic shoulder pain in patients after stroke? A double-blind randomized clinical trial. J Rehabil Med. 2007;39(6):440–7.
42. McCrory P, et al. Botulinum toxin A for treatment of upper limb spasticity following stroke: a multi-centre randomized placebo-controlled study of the effects on quality of life and other person-centred outcomes. J Rehabil Med. 2009;41(7):536–44.
43. Kanovský P, et al. Efficacy and safety of botulinum neurotoxin NT 201 in poststroke upper limb spasticity. Clin Neuropharmacol. 2009;32(5):259–65.
44. Kaji R, et al. Botulinum toxin type A in post-stroke upper limb spasticity. Curr Med Res Opin. 2010;26(8):1983–92.
45. Shaw LC, et al. Botulinum Toxin for the Upper Limb After Stroke (BoTULS) Trial. Stroke. 2011;42(5):1371–9.
46. Rosales RL, et al. Botulinum toxin injection for hypertonicity of the upper extremity within 12 weeks after stroke: a randomized controlled trial. Neurorehabil Neural Repair. 2012;26(7):812–21.
47. Elovic EP, et al. Randomized, placebo-controlled trial of incobotulinumtoxinA for upper-limb post-stroke spasticity. Muscle Nerve. 2015;53(3):415–21.
48. Gracies J-M, et al. Safety and efficacy of abobotulinumtoxinA for hemiparesis in adults with upper limb spasticity after stroke or traumatic brain injury: a double-blind randomised controlled trial. Lancet Neurol. 2015;14(10):992–1001.
49. Pittock SJ, et al. A double-blind randomised placebo-controlled evaluation of three doses of botulinum toxin type A (Dysport®) in the treatment of spastic equinovarus deformity after stroke. Cerebrovasc Dis. 2003;15(4):289–300.
50. Kaji R, et al. Botulinum toxin type A in post-stroke lower limb spasticity: a multicenter, double-blind, placebo-controlled trial. J Neurol. 2010;257(8):1330–7.
51. Dunne JW, et al. A prospective, multicentre, randomized, double-blind, placebo-controlled trial of onabotulinumtoxinA to treat plantarflexor/invertor overactivity after stroke. Clin Rehabil. 2012;26(9):787–97.
52. Tao W, et al. Gait improvement by low-dose botulinum toxin A injection treatment of the lower limbs in subacute stroke patients. J Phys Ther Sci. 2015;27(3):759–62.

53. Simpson DM, et al. Practice guideline update summary: botulinum neurotoxin for the treatment of blepharospasm, cervical dystonia, adult spasticity, and headache: Report of the Guideline Development Subcommittee of the American Academy of Neurology. Neurology. 2016;86(19):1818–26.
54. Gracies J-M, et al. Botulinum toxin dilution and endplate targeting in spasticity: a double-blind controlled study. Arch Phys Med Rehabil. 2009;90(1):9–16. e2
55. Wissel J, et al. European consensus table on the use of botulinum toxin type A in adult spasticity. J Rehabil Med. 2009;41(1):13–25.
56. Baricich A, et al. High doses of onabotulinumtoxinA in post-stroke spasticity: a retrospective analysis. J Neural Transm. 2015;122(9):1283–7.
57. Simpson D, et al. Increasing doses of incobotulinumtoxinA (Xeomin; 400-800 U) improve the functional impact of upper limb spasticity. Toxicon. 2016;123:S78.
58. Dressler D, et al. Long-term efficacy and safety of incobotulinumtoxinA and conventional treatment of poststroke arm spasticity: a prospective, non-interventional, open-label, parallel-group study. BMJ Open. 2015;5(12):e009358.
59. Mohammadi B, et al. Long-term treatment of spasticity with botulinum toxin type A: an analysis of 1221 treatments in 137 patients. Neurol Res. 2010;32(3):309–13.
60. Allison R, et al. Incidence, time course and predictors of impairments relating to caring for the profoundly affected arm after stroke: a systematic review. Physiother Res Int. 2016;21(4):210–27.
61. Kaku M, Simpson DM. Spotlight on botulinum toxin and its potential in the treatment of stroke-related spasticity. Drug Des Devel Ther. 2016;10:1085.
62. Paolucci S, et al. Prevalence and time course of post-stroke pain: a multicenter prospective hospital-based study. Pain Med. 2016;17(5):924–30.
63. Yelnik AP, Colle FM, Bonan IV. Treatment of pain and limited movement of the shoulder in hemiplegic patients with botulinum toxin a in the subscapular muscle. Eur Neurol. 2003;50(2):91–3.
64. Yelnik AP, et al. Treatment of shoulder pain in spastic hemiplegia by reducing spasticity of the subscapular muscle: a randomised, double blind, placebo controlled study of botulinum toxin A. J Neurol Neurosurg Psychiatry. 2007;78(8):845–8.
65. Kong K-H, Neo J-J, Chua KS. A randomized controlled study of botulinum toxin A in the treatment of hemiplegic shoulder pain associated with spasticity. Clin Rehabil. 2007;21(1):28–35.
66. Lim JY, Koh JH, Paik NJ. Intramuscular botulinum toxin-A reduces hemiplegic shoulder pain: a randomized, double-blind, comparative study versus intraarticular triamcinolone acetonide. Stroke. 2008;39(1):126–31.
67. Marciniak CM, et al. Does botulinum toxin type A decrease pain and lessen disability in hemiplegic survivors of stroke with shoulder pain and spasticity?: a randomized, double-blind, placebo-controlled trial. Am J Phys Med Rehabil. 2012;91(12):1007–19.
68. Choi J-G, Shin J-H, Kim B-R. Botulinum toxin A injection into the subscapularis muscle to treat intractable hemiplegic shoulder pain. Ann Rehabil Med. 2016;40(4):592–9.
69. Larrazet S, et al. Hemiplegic shoulder pain: comparison of two sites of intramuscular injections of botulinum toxin type A, "epautox" study. Ann Phys Rehabil Med. 2016;59:e72.
70. Castiglione A, et al. Efficacy of intra-articular injection of botulinum toxin type A in refractory hemiplegic shoulder pain. Arch Phys Med Rehabil. 2011;92(7):1034–7.
71. Mittal SO, Safarpour D, Jabbari B. Botulinum toxin treatment of neuropathic pain. Semin Neurol. 2016;36(1):73–83.
72. Chen H, et al. Ultrasound-guided botulinum toxin injections and EMG biofeedback therapy the lower limb muscle spasm after cerebral infarction. Eur Rev Med Pharmacol Sci. 2014;19(9):1696–9.
73. Fietzek U, et al. Botulinum toxin B increases mouth opening in patients with spastic trismus. Eur J Neurol. 2009;16(12):1299–304.
74. Suputtitada A, Suwanwela N. The lowest effective dose of botulinum A toxin in adult patients with upper limb spasticity. Disabil Rehabil. 2005;27(4):176–84.

75. Lam K, et al. Can botulinum toxin decrease carer burden in long term care residents with upper limb spasticity? A randomized controlled study. J Am Med Dir Assoc. 2012;13(5):477–84.
76. Gracies J-M, et al. Botulinum toxin type B in the spastic arm: a randomized, double-blind, placebo-controlled, preliminary study. Arch Phys Med Rehabil. 2014;95(7):1303–11.
77. Hansen AP, et al. Development of persistent headache following stroke: a 3-year follow-up. Cephalalgia. 2015;35(5):399–409.
78. Ghika-Schmid F, et al. Hyperkinetic movement disorders during and after acute stroke: the Lausanne Stroke Registry. J Neurol Sci. 1997;146(2):109–16.
79. Alarcon F, et al. Post-stroke movement disorders: report of 56 patients. J Neurol Neurosurg Psychiatry. 2004;75(11):1568–74.
80. Strader S, Rodnitzky RL, Gonzalez-Alegre P. Secondary dystonia in a botulinum toxin clinic: clinical characteristics, neuroanatomical substrate and comparison with idiopathic dystonia. Parkinsonism Relat Disord. 2011;17(10):749–52.
81. Park J. Movement disorders following cerebrovascular lesion in the basal ganglia circuit. J Mov Dis. 2016;9(2):71.
82. Marsden C, et al. The anatomical basis of symptomatic hemidystonia. Brain. 1985;108(2):463–83.
83. Chuang C, Fahn S, Frucht S. The natural history and treatment of acquired hemidystonia: report of 33 cases and review of the literature. J Neurol Neurosurg Psychiatry. 2002;72(1):59–67.
84. Walker RH. Jerky dystonic shoulder following infarction of the posterior thalamus. J Clin Mov Dis. 2015;2(1):12.
85. Kowacs PA, et al. Botulinum-A toxin in the treatment of painful post-stroke nocturnal paroxysmal dystonia triggered by periodic limb movements of sleep: case report. Arq Neuropsiquiatr. 2006;64(4):1027–9.
86. Jung TM, et al. Precise muscle selection using dynamic polyelectromyography for treatment of post-stroke dystonia: a case report. Ann Rehabil Med. 2016;40(3):551–5.
87. Yoshimura DM, Aminoff MJ, Olney RK. Botulinum toxin therapy for limb dystonias. Neurology. 1992;42(3):627–30.
88. Choi S-M. Movement disorders following cerebrovascular lesions in cerebellar circuits. J Mov Dis. 2016;9(2):80.
89. Penney SE, Bruce IA, Saeed SR. Botulinum toxin is effective and safe for palatal tremor. J Neurol. 2006;253(7):857–60.
90. Vielotte J. Effectiveness of intramuscular injections of botulinum toxin in the treatment of disabling cerebellar tremor of the hand. Ann Phys Rehabil Med. 2016;59:e142.
91. Stuchell R, Mandel I. Salivary gland dysfunction and swallowing disorders. Otolaryngol Clin North Am. 1988;21(4):649–61.
92. Hockstein NG, et al. Sialorrhea: a management challenge. Am Fam Physician. 2004;69(11)
93. Turk-Gonzales M, Odderson IR. Quantitative reduction of saliva production with botulinum toxin type B injection into the salivary glands. Neurorehabil Neural Repair. 2005;19(1):58–61.
94. Hosp C, Naumann MK, Hamm H. Botulinum toxin treatment of autonomic disorders: focal hyperhidrosis and sialorrhea. Semin Neurol. 2016;36(1):20–8.
95. Mazlan M, et al. A double-blind randomized controlled trial investigating the most efficacious dose of botulinum toxin-A for sialorrhea treatment in Asian adults with neurological diseases. Toxins (Basel). 2015;7(9):3758–70.

Clinical Uses of Botulinum Toxin in the Skin

James Yen Wang

Introduction

Botulinum toxin (BTX) is a potent neurotoxin produced by the bacteria *Clostridium botulinum* and its use has been a staple of both medical and cosmetic treatment in dermatology [1]. In the medical context, BTX can be helpful for decreasing hyperhidrosis, or excessive sweating, in the axilla, palms, and soles. However, the most notable uses within dermatology are the cosmetic applications for dynamic rhytids, or fine lines and wrinkles, that occur upon initiation of facial expressions [2]. Its use for wrinkles was first described in 1989 by plastic surgeon Richard Clark and was approved at that time for strabismus and blepharospasm [3]. Currently, BTX has been FDA-approved to treat hyperfunctional lines resulting from contraction of underlying facial muscles in the glabella (2002) and lateral canthal lines (2013) as well as hyperhidrosis (2012), although off-label uses in other areas of the face have become common practice [4–7].

Clinically, the effects of the toxin are noticed by the patient within 24–72 h after injection, with maximal efficacy attained at 2 weeks [7]. The results generally last 2–4 months, although effects have been reported to last up to 11 months. Currently, there are several types of BTX on the market, including onabotulinum toxin A (Botox by Allergan, Inc.), abobotulinum toxin A (Dysport by Ipsen), incobotulinum toxin A (Xeomin by Merz Pharmaceuticals), and rimabotulinum toxin B (Myobloc by Elan Pharmaceuticals) [8].

J.Y. Wang, M.D., M.B.A. (✉)
Memorial Sloan Kettering Cancer Center, Weill Cornell Medicine,
New York, NY 10065, USA

American Board of Dermatology and Dermatopathology, Newton, MA 02459, USA
e-mail: jameswang.derm@gmail.com

B. Jabbari (ed.), *Botulinum Toxin Treatment in Clinical Medicine*,
DOI 10.1007/978-3-319-56038-0_13

Mechanisms of Action

The biology of BTX is well-known, with many different subtypes including seven toxin serotypes designated A through G (although only types A and B are commercially available as of this writing) [9]. Each serotype acts upon a different player, but all within the same pathway in the motor nerve terminal. BTX binds to various sites within these terminals to prevent the release of acetylcholine neurotransmitters from the motor neurons, leading to flaccid paralysis of the downstream striated muscles responsible for movement [1].

Botulinum toxins consist of a light chain and heavy chain linked by disulfide bonds. Both components are necessary for the uptake of the toxin into the motor neuron (heavy chain) and for the subsequent blockade of neurotransmitter vesicles from fusing with the terminal membrane (light chain) via the soluble N-ethylmaleamide-sensitive factor attachment protein receptor (SNARE). Type A is known to be the most potent serotype and cleaves the synaptosomal-associated protein (SNAP-25) of the SNARE complex [10]. Other subtypes cleave synaptobrevin and syntaxin. Although the paralysis of the muscle is temporary, the blockade of neurotransmitter release is irreversible in the affected nerve terminal, leading to the lasting effect seen clinically. For recovery of movement, the affected nerve must sprout new terminals, which can take from 3 to 5 months [11].

One unit of BTX corresponds to the lethal dose in 50% of the mice tested in preclinical trials (LD50). The different formulations of BTX, however, were tested in different mouse models, leading to non-comparable units among the different manufacturers of BTX. The LD50 in a 70-kg human for Botox Cosmetic (Allergan) is around 2500–3000 units [12, 13].

Contraindications for BTX use include a history of neuromuscular disease such as myasthenia gravis or amyotrophic lateral sclerosis, history of known sensitivity to commercially available BTX or albumin, pregnancy, lactation, and age younger than 12 years [14].

Some individuals can develop neutralizing antibodies to the heavy chain of the BTX molecule, decreasing its efficacy. This is usually seen with doses of more than 300 units at a time. The neutralizing antibodies do not cross-react between the BTX serotypes. Therefore, loss of efficacy in BTX-A could be circumvented clinically by administration of BTX-B. Risk factors for neutralizing antibodies include young age at initiation of injections, larger doses, and shorter injection intervals [15–17].

Side Effects

Side effects are generally mild and include injection site erythema and occasional bruising. The risk of bruising can be minimized by asking the patient to avoid anticoagulants such as aspirin, NSAIDs, and Vitamin E 1–2 weeks prior to BTX injection. During the injection itself, application of ice packs can both lessen patient discomfort and prevent bruising, even when small vessels are penetrated by the needle [18].

The more common serious side effects include ptosis and ectropion when BTX is injected in the upper face. The incidence is believed to be 4% for new injectors and 0.5% with experienced injectors. Lower face injections can cause lip drooping, drooling, and trouble swallowing. Injections for hyperhidrosis or masseter muscle reduction can cause weakness in the injected muscles [19, 20].

There have been rare reported cases of serious side effects when the injected toxin spreads systemically, causing botulism. Hence, there is a black-box warning from the Food and Drug Administration (FDA). BTX remains one of the most lethal toxins known when introduced systemically [21].

Hyperhidrosis

Excessive sweating is caused by hyperactivity of eccrine sweat glands in the dermis. These eccrine sweat glands excrete sweat by contracting sympathetically-innervated smooth muscle around the glands, pushing the fluid through the dermal coils and onto the skin surface. These smooth muscles are innervated by acetylcholine, causing them to be responsive to the effects of BTX [22]. The method of injecting BTX into areas of excessive sweating, most commonly the axilla, hands, and feet, can cause decreased and even complete cessation of sweating in these areas.

Botulinum toxin type A, specifically Botox (Allergan), has been FDA-approved for severe primary axillary hyperhidrosis that has no other known cause and has been recalcitrant to topical antiperspirants such as aluminum chloride. Patients are usually numbed topically prior to injections. Areas of sweating can be identified using the starch-iodine test, where iodine is applied to the axillary area followed by starch. When sweat contacts the iodine, the starch will turn black [22]. This may form the basis for the areas of injection. The standard treatment for axillary hyperhidrosis in clinical practice is 50 units of Botox injected into each axilla in a grid-like pattern with injections performed via a 30-gauge needle and injection sites spaced 1–1.5 cm apart. The level of injection should be in the subcutis and avoiding the underlying musculature. Injection methods vary among providers. Lowe *et al.* performed a study where patients received either 50 or 75 units of Botox, both groups showing significant improvement in sweating compared to placebo (75% vs. 25%, respectively [23]).

For palmar and plantar surfaces, 75–100 units of Botox are used with an average efficacy range of around 5–6 months [24]. The use of BTX for hyperhidrosis in this area is very painful and can require a distal ulnar and/or radial nerve block. Side effects of weakened grip or decreased fine motor skills have been reported in less than 15% of patients. Most of these symptoms resolve within days to weeks. Application of ice as pretreatment can also be helpful. Topical anesthetics have been shown to have minimal efficacy.

Additional uses include inguinal sweating, which starts in affected patients during adolescence and can be very bothersome. The areas affected include the medial thighs, genitals, pubic and suprapubic areas, and inguinal folds. The sweating can be decreased with small aliquots of BTX spaced 1 cm apart. No significant side effects have been reported [25].

Cosmetic Applications

Upper Face

The upper face is the most often-injected area for BTX and the only area where it is FDA-approved to be used. The regions within this area include the glabellar complex, forehead muscles, periocular muscles, and nasalis muscles.

Glabellar Complex Lines ("Elevens" or "Brow Furrow")

The use of BTX to treat rhytids is now an established practice. The first and, until recently, the only FDA-approved indication is for moderate to severe rhytids in the glabellar complex of muscles. These muscles lie centrally and immediately inferior to the forehead, medial to the eyebrows, and superior to the nasal bridge (Fig. 1). The three main muscles that are responsible for the contraction centrally and inferiorly, creating a nasal crease or the "eleven" crease between the eyebrows, are the

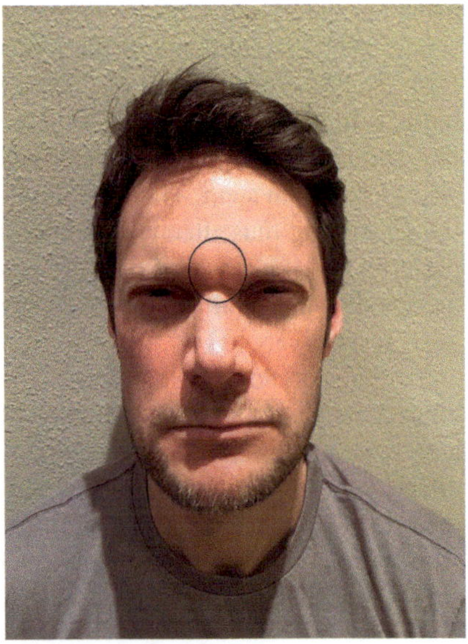

Fig. 1 Illustration of the Glabellar complex of muscles

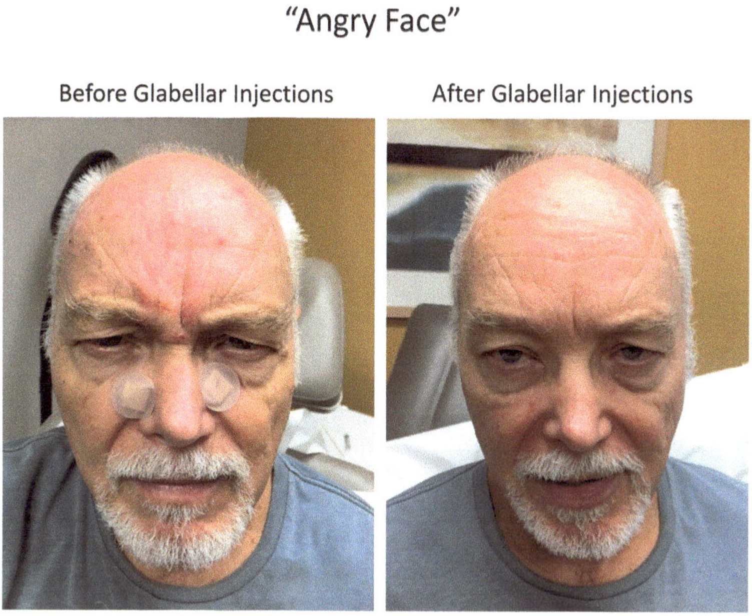

Fig. 2 Botulinum toxin injection into the glabellar complex

procerus, corrugator supercilii, and depressor supercilii. There is also some action of glabellar injections on the medial fibers of the orbicularis oculi muscle [26].

The standard injection technique involves the use of approximately 20 units for the entire glabellar complex with one injection of 4–6 units of Botox midline directly into the belly of the procerus muscle. Mild massage may help with diffusion of BTX laterally to paralyze the depressor supercilii fibers. The effect will be a slight rise of the medial eyebrows and causing a more youthful happier appearance (Fig. 2). The next injection points will be the lower and upper portions of the corrugator muscle on both sides. Having the patient frown will reveal the outline of the muscles. Some patients exhibit more vertically oriented fibers, while others will have a gently sloping corrugator muscle that lies just superior to the eyebrows. Two injections of 4–6 units of Botox along the length of the corrugators are usually sufficient to paralyze them [25].

The main side effect for this area when injected with BTX is medial lid ptosis if the toxin migrates to the levator palpebrae superioris muscle that is responsible for elevating the eyelids. This is especially true if one is "chasing" a low-lying corrugator muscle. As with all BTX injections, additional "reactive" rhytids can form as the balance of muscular strength is shifted. Care should be taken not to inject into the supratrochlear vein or artery, which is located in this area and could theoretically lead to systemic distribution of the neurotoxin [14, 27].

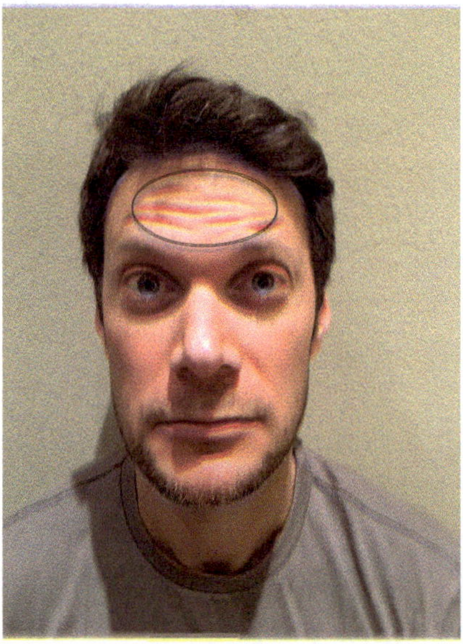

Fig. 3 Illustration of contracted frontalis muscle, producing the transverse forehead wrinkles

Lateral Canthal Lines ("Crow's Feet")

In 2013, onabotulinum toxin received its second FDA-approved injection site for improvement in the appearance of moderate to severe lateral canthal lines, known colloquially as "Crow's Feet." Microaliquots of BTX are injected into the area immediately lateral to the orbital rim, usually 1–3 units of Botox at each site, and targets the orbicularis oculi muscle, which encircles the orbital rim superficially (Fig. 3) [28, 29].

The most common side effect in this area is lateral drooping of the upper eyelid if the diffusion of toxin reaches the levator palpebrae superioris muscle. Injection near the cheek can cause paralysis of the lower eyelid muscles with reported cases of eyelid swelling due to decreased ability of muscles to pump fluid out of the area. A rare but reported side effect is ipsilateral drooping of the mouth. This is due to paralysis of the zygomaticus major or minor muscles, which are responsible for elevating the corner of the mouth.

In some cases, the periocular area can be treated to tailor specific effects to the preferences of the patient. Small aliquots around the maximal arch of the eyebrow can either raise or drop the eyebrow in that location (Fig. 4). In addition, some clinicians inject 1–2 units directly into the belly of the lower eyelid for decreasing the eyelid wrinkles or to widen the appearance of the eyes. These other periocular treatments have a somewhat higher rate of complication, including upper lid ptosis and possible ectropion of the lower eyelid. Edema and an undesirable increase in the "bagginess" of the lower eyelids have been reported [30–32].

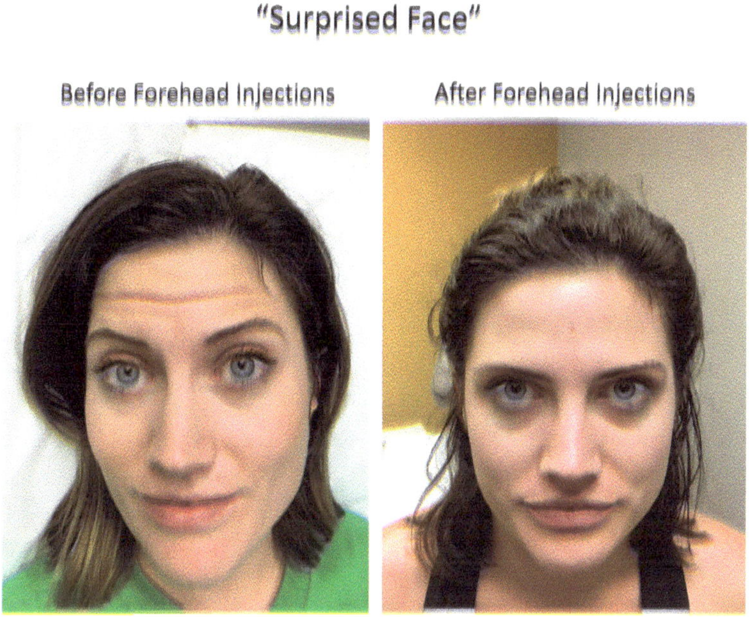

Fig. 4 Botulinum toxin injection into the frontalis muscle

Transverse Forehead Lines

Although one of the most popular treatments for transverse lines across the forehead, injection in this area is not FDA-approved and is considered "off-label." The target being treated is the frontalis muscle, which has a sheet-like architecture over the entire forehead extending from the hairline to the nasal bridge and eyebrows (Fig. 5). Interestingly, this muscle has no bony attachments, but is instead an extension of the galea aponeurotica on the scalp and inserts into the skin under the eyebrows and at the root of the nose. This muscle is important for raising the eyebrows and creating the "surprised" facial expression. There is some phenotypic variation in the structure of the muscle, with some people exhibiting a bifid split toward the upper forehead. These patients do not have transverse forehead lines toward the upper central forehead. Therefore, injection of BTX into this area does result in any noticeable change in the appearance of the skin [33, 34].

The most common way to inject the forehead is to have patients raise their eyebrows to reveal the transverse forehead lines (Fig. 6). Aliquots of BTX, usually 1–2 units, are injected 2 cm apart, allowing for diffusion between injection sites. In general, the mid to upper forehead are safe areas of injection because they will not cause hooding of the upper eyelids from an excessively heavy and unsupported forehead.

The most common side effect is a sensation of heaviness. In severe cases, the upper eyelid hoods, which can obstruct vision. In patients with a short forehead-to-eyebrow distance, BTX injection is not recommended as there is an increased

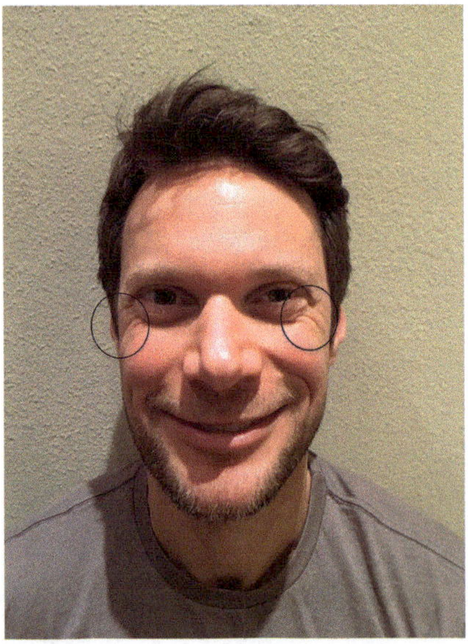

Fig. 5 Illustration of the lateral periocular lines

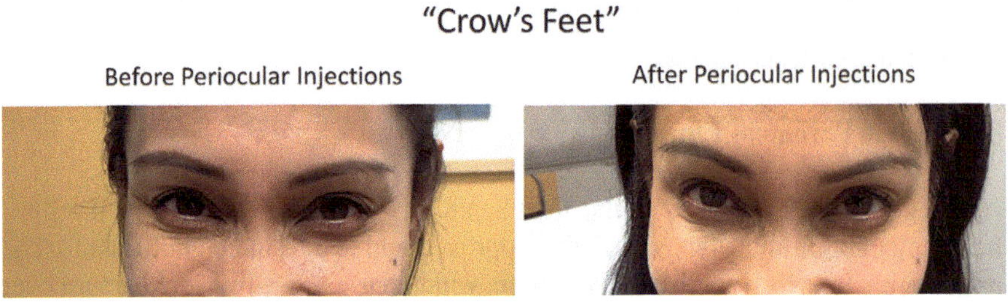

Fig. 6 Botulinum toxin injection in the periocular area

chance for dropping of the eyebrows. Another commonly seen side effect is the "quizzical look" complication of injection. When BTX is injected across the central frontalis muscle with sparing of the lateral portions ("temples"), there is often a noticeable compensatory raising of the lateral eyebrows. In some cases, especially in some female patients, the look is desirable as it increases the appearance of the classically feminine eyebrow arch [31, 32]. It is important to ask the patient his or her preference prior to injection [35, 36].

Brow Shape Correction

While injecting the forehead, the side effect of brow shape alteration can also be a useful and desirable outcome [31, 32]. There are many techniques for this, but for a more classically "feminine" appearing eyebrow with an enhanced arch, injection of the glabellar complex in general will cause a compensatory raising of the lateral

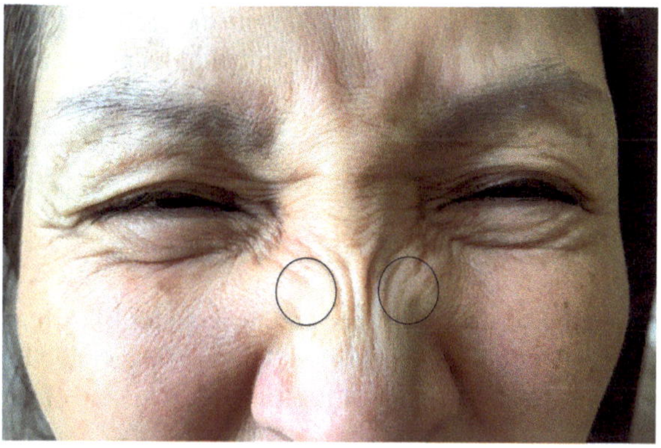

Fig. 7 Illustration of the "bunny lines" caused by contraction of the nasalis muscles

eyebrows. Injection of a small BTX aliquot under the peak of the eyebrow arch paralyzes the lateral depressors of the brow. In fact, Ahn *et al.* have shown that injection at this site, on average, causes a brow elevation of 4.83 mm. However, in some cases, additional muscles can be affected and there can be a paradoxical lowering of the lateral brow. To flatten the eyebrow arch, 2 units of Botox can be injected 1 cm superior to the apex of the arch. This injection relaxes the frontalis muscle there and causes diminution of the arch for a more "masculine" appearance. As always, injection around the eyes can cause unwanted side effects such as ptosis. In those with excessive upper eyelid sagginess, care should be taken as not to cause obstruction of vision [36].

Nasalis Lines ("Bunny Lines")

This is a less common site of injection, but is indicated for dynamic lines along the nasal sidewall when squinting or smiling (Fig. 7). The muscles responsible for the formation of these lines are the anomalous nasalis, levator labii superioris alaeque nasi, and transverse nasalis. Injection requires, on average, 2–3 units of Botox on both side of the superior lateral nasal sidewall. A potential complication is diffusion of BTX to the adjacent levator labii superioris muscle, which is responsible for raising the ipsilateral upper lip. Paralyzing this muscle can cause focal immobility of the upper lip. Care should be taken to avoid the angular artery and vein, which courses lateral to the usual injection site [37].

Nasal Tip Lift

Another off-label use of BTX has been to lift the nasal tip, called nasal tip ptososis. The muscles that affect the nasal tip include the nasalis, depressor septi nasi, levator labii superioris, and alaeque nasi. Injection of 2–4 units of Botox into these muscles, including injection in the base of the columella, has been studied by various groups.

Care should be taken not to elongate the distance significantly between the columella and the upper lip. A dermal filler could be more appropriate for correction depending on the patient [38, 39].

Lower Face

Injection of the lower face and neck is not FDA-approved and tends to be trickier and dependent on injection technique. Care should be taken when injecting in these areas because of underlying structures that can affect movement of the mouth [40].

Drooping Oral Commissure

The sagging corners of the mouth are a common complaint of aging. The effect is a persistent frown and may make a person seem sad or worried (Fig. 8). The best way to address this area with BTX is injection of a small aliquot of 2–4 units of Botox just 1 cm lateral to the marionette line at the level of the mandible, about 1 cm above the jawline. The targeted muscle is the depressor labii oris, which is responsible for pulling down the corners of the mouth. The most common side effect is paralysis of the mental nerve, which can cause ipsilateral lower lip paralysis and asymmetrical lip movement [41].

Melomental Folds ("Marionette Lines")

Melomental folds, also called marionette lines, constitute a common cosmetic complaint among patients. The lines extend from the oral commissure to the jawline, defining the physical chin area. The muscle in the area that pulls down the corners of the mouth is the depressor anguli oris, which acts in opposition to the zygomaticus group of muscles. This area is usually treated with dermal fillers, but some have

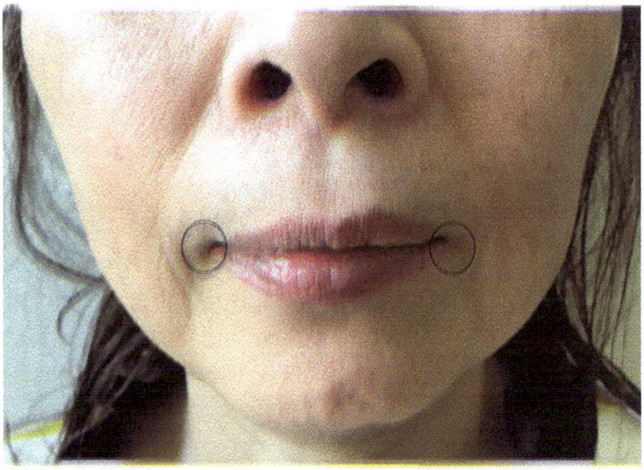

Fig. 8 Illustration of mild drooping of the oral commissures

found that the addition of BTX can also help soften the appearance of the marionette lines. One approach is the injection of 2–4 units of Botox into the depressor anguli oris muscle 1 cm above the mandible. This point is usually located 1 cm lateral to the marionette line as it meets the chin. Some also inject 2 units of Botox 1 cm lateral to the oral commissure. This method is similar to that used for drooping oral commissures because the oral commissure is the superior border of the marionette lines. The most common side effect, as in treatment of oral commissure drooping, is paralysis of the mental nerve, which can cause ipsilateral lower lip paralysis and asymmetrical lip movement [42].

Perioral Lines

Botulinum toxin is effective for the treatment of fine lines and wrinkles around the lips, which are caused by chronic photodamage as well as smoking (Fig. 9). This area is quite sensitive to the effects of BTX, so only small amounts should be used. The standard way to inject is the placement of eight total aliquots of 1 unit of Botox into the orbicularis oris muscle, which is responsible for the pursing of the lips. Two injections should be performed per quadrant of lip, 0.5 cm above the vermillion border, taking care to avoid the central lip. Injection into the midline lip can blunt the desirable Cupid's bow shape of the upper lip. The most common side effect is an inability to drink through a straw or pucker the lips. This is often frustrating to the patient [41, 43].

"Gummy" Smile Correction

Some individuals have an unusually prominent visibility of the upper gingiva when they smile due to overactive upper lip muscles. The main muscle responsible for this action is the levator labii superioris alaeque nasi. It is possible to correct the activity of the muscle by injecting just 1–2 units of Botox into each side of the nasal prominence, at a location called "Yonsei point." A side effect, however, is that relaxation of the muscle causes elongation of the nasal-to-lip distance [44, 45].

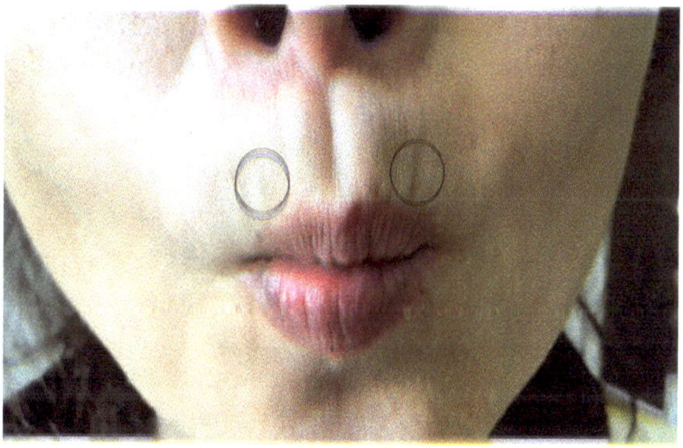

Fig. 9 Illustration of the perioral lines by asking the patient to pucker her mouth

Indistinct Jawline (Nefertiti Lift)

Sometimes used to counter the effects of gravity on early jowl formation, small aliquots of 2–3 units of Botox are injected 1 cm apart just inferior to the jawline. The total amount required is usually 20 units per side. This theoretically decreases the downward pull of the platysma muscle and provides a small lift to the lower face as the balance shifts toward the face elevator muscles. The result is a more defined jawline, hence the nickname "Nefertiti Lift" for an ancient queen known for the perfect jawline. Complications include injecting the marginal mandibular nerve, which can cause an ipsilateral lateral lip droop [46, 47].

Chin Puckering/Mentalis Muscle

Chin puckering is the appearance of small dimples in the skin of the chin with certain facial movements. This is caused by the mentalis muscle, which can become overactive. For correction, a single injection of 4–6 units of Botox can be placed directly into the center of the chin. A side effect is weakness in the lower lip, causing drooling or dribbling of liquid from the corners of the mouth [48].

Enlarged Masseter

A common application of BTX, and the most popular in Asia, is injection into the masseter muscles, which are responsible for chewing and can hypertrophy from overuse or bruxism. This injection is also used medically to treat bruxism or for temporomandibular joint problems. However, cosmetically, BTX injection can cause these muscles to shrink and feminize the face by decreasing the lateral girth of the jaw. The injection technique may vary among providers, but the usual injection point includes three areas in the lower belly of the masseter above the jawline. Some providers will also target the superior portion of the masseter just inferior to temporomandibular joint. The total units used will vary among individuals, but generally, a total of 15–35 units are injected per side [40, 49–51].

Complications are generally limited, with the most common being mild jaw weakness. Injection in the upper portion of the masseter can occasionally cause parotid gland inflammation and possible fistula formation.

Platysmal Bands

Platysmal bands are vertical folds of skin that protrude from the neck when the underlying platysma muscle contracts. This is often distressing to patients who have prominent bands. The standard method of injection is directly into the bands, which are elicited when patients are told to show their lower teeth. The band is grabbed and BTX injections corresponding to 2 units of Botox are spaced 2 cm apart along the length of the band from 1 cm below the jawline to the lower neck, depending on severity. Injection should remain superficial and should never be deep into neck tissue. Deep injections can affect the laryngeal nerves and lead to dysphagia and dysphonia. The amount used will vary depending on the severity of the platysmal bands, but doses larger than 30 units of Botox at a time are not recommended [52–55].

Other Uses

Scrotal Wrinkles ("Scrotox")

This relatively new and controversial application of BTX is now entering clinical practice. The treatment is for scrotal wrinkles that some men find unappealing. Small aliquots of toxin are injected into the muscular layer immediately under the skin, called the dartos muscles. These muscles are responsible for the elevation of the scrotum dependent on temperature changes or other stimuli. The potential complications for this procedure include sterility as the testes may not be appropriately thermoregulated. Unintentional deeper injections can also affect the blood flow and lead to testicular necrosis. As of this writing, there have been no peer-reviewed articles on the practice, but many online sources confirm the presence of such a practice.

Summary

Botulinum toxin is a potent neurotoxin that has been adapted for clinical and cosmetic use in dermatology with great efficacy and safety. As the science and art of facial aesthetics evolve, new methods of injection will be explored.

References

1. Montecucco C, Molgó J. Botulinal neurotoxins: revival of an old killer. Curr Opin Pharmacol. 2005;5(3):274–9.
2. Carruthers A, Carruthers J. Clinical indications and injection technique for the cosmetic use of botulinum A exotoxin. Dermatol Surg. 1998;24:1189–94.
3. Clark RP, Berris CE. Botulinum toxin: a treatment for facial asymmetry caused by facial nerve paralysis. Plast Reconstr Surg. 1989;84(2):353–5.
4. Lew MF. Review of the FDA-approved uses of botulinum toxins, including data suggesting efficacy in pain reduction. Clin J Pain. 2002;18(6):S142–6.
5. Glogau R, et al. Results of a randomized, double-blind, placebo-controlled study to evaluate the efficacy and safety of a botulinum toxin type A topical gel for the treatment of moderate-to-severe lateral canthal lines. J Drugs Dermatol. 2012;11(1):38–45.
6. Ting PT, Freiman A. The story of Clostridium botulinum: from food poisoning to Botox. Clin Med. 2004;4(3):258–61.

7. Small R. Botulinum toxin injection for facial wrinkles. Am Fam Physician. 2014;90(3):168–75.
8. Walker TJ, Dayan SH. Comparison and overview of currently available neurotoxins. J Clin Aesthet Dermatol. 2014;7(2):31–9.
9. American Society of Health-System Pharmacists. Botulinum Toxin Type A. 2011. *drugs.com*.
10. Hill KK, Smith TJ. Genetic diversity within Clostridium botulinum serotypes, botulinum neurotoxin gene clusters and toxin subtypes. In: Rummel A, Binz T, editors. Botulinum neurotoxins. Heidelberg: Springer; 2013.
11. Burgen ASV, Dickens F, Zatman LJ. The action of botulinum toxin on the neuro-muscular junction. J Physiol. 1949;109(1–2):10–24.
12. Wohlfarth K, et al. Botulinum A toxins: units versus units. Naunyn Schmiedeberg's Arch Pharmacol. 1997;355(3):335–40.
13. Sampaio C, et al. DYSBOT: A single-blind, randomized parallel study to determine whether any differences can be detected in the efficacy and tolerability of two formulations of botulinum toxin type A—Dysport and Botox—assuming a ratio of 4: 1. Mov Disord. 1997;12(6):1013–8.
14. Klein AW. Contraindications and complications with the use of botulinum toxin. Clin Dermatol. 2004;22(1):66–75.
15. Göschel H, et al. Botulinum A toxin therapy: neutralizing and nonneutralizing antibodies—therapeutic consequences. Exp Neurol. 1997;147(1):96–102.
16. Stanker LH, et al. Development and partial characterization of high-affinity monoclonal antibodies for botulinum toxin type A and their use in analysis of milk by sandwich ELISA. J Immunol Methods. 2008;336(1):1–8.
17. Siatkowski RM, et al. Serum antibody production to botulinum A toxin. Ophthalmology. 1993;100(12):1861–6.
18. Coté TR, et al. Botulinum toxin type A injections: adverse events reported to the US Food and Drug Administration in therapeutic and cosmetic cases. J Am Acad Dermatol. 2005;53(3):407–15.
19. Glogau RG. Review of the use of botulinum toxin for hyperhidrosis and cosmetic purposes. Clin J Pain. 2002;18(6):S191–7.
20. FDA. FDA Notifies public of adverse reactions linked to Botox use. 2008. *Fda.gov*.
21. Chertow DS, et al. Botulism in 4 adults following cosmetic injections with an unlicensed, highly concentrated botulinum preparation. JAMA. 2006;296(20):2476–9.
22. Heckmann M, et al. Botulinum toxin A for axillary hyperhidrosis (excessive sweating). N Engl J Med. 2001;344:488.
23. Lowe NJ, Glaser DA, Eadie N, et al. Botulinum toxin type A for axillary hyperhidrosis: a 52-week multicenter double-blind, randomized, placebo-controlled study of efficacy and safety. J Am Acad Dermatol. 2007;56:604.
24. Goldman A. Treatment of axillary and palmar hyperhidrosis with botulinum toxin. Aesthet Plast Surg. 2000;24:280.
25. Barankin B, Wasel N. Treatment of inguinal hyperhidrosis with botulinum toxin type A. Int J Dermatol. 2006;45:985.
26. Lorenc ZP, et al. Understanding the functional anatomy of the frontalis and glabellar complex for optimal aesthetic botulinum toxin type A therapy. Aesthet Plast Surg. 2013;37(5):975–83.
27. Carruthers J, Fagien S, Matarasso SL. Consensus recommendations on the use of botulinum toxin type A in facial aesthetics. Plast Reconstr Surg. 2004;114(6):1S–22S.
28. Fagien S. Botox for the treatment of dynamic and hyperkinetic facial lines and furrows: adjunctive use in facial aesthetic surgery. Plast Reconstr Surg. 1999;103(2):701–13.
29. Lowe NJ, et al. Double-blind, randomized, placebo-controlled, dose-response study of the safety and efficacy of botulinum toxin type A in subjects with crow's feet. Dermatol Surg. 2005;31(3):257–62.
30. Ahn MS, Catten M, Maas CS. Temporal brow lift using botulinum toxin A. Plast Reconstr Surg. 2000;105(3):1129–35.
31. Maas CS, Kim EJ. Temporal brow lift using botulinum toxin A: an update. Plast Reconstr Surg. 2003;112(5):109S–12S.

32. Wollina U, Konrad H. Managing adverse events associated with botulinum toxin type a. Am J Clin Dermatol. 2005;6(3):141–50.
33. Koch RJ, Troell RJ, Goode RL. Contemporary management of the aging brow and forehead. Laryngoscope. 1997;107(6):710–5.
34. Matarasso A, Hutchinson OH. Evaluating rejuvenation of the forehead and brow: an algorithm for selecting the appropriate technique. Plast Reconstr Surg. 2000;106(3):687–94.
35. Sarrabayrouse MA. Indications and limitations for the use of botulinum toxin for the treatment of facial wrinkles. Aesthet Plast Surg. 2002;26(4):233–8.
36. Huilgol SC, Carruthers A, Carruthers JD. Raising eyebrows with botulinum toxin. Dermatol Surg. 1999;25(5):373–6.
37. Tamura BM, et al. Treatment of nasal wrinkles with botulinum toxin. Dermatol Surg. 2005;31(3):271–5.
38. Ghavami A, Janis JE, Guyuron B. Regarding the treatment of dynamic nasal tip ptosis with botulinum toxin A. Plast Reconstr Surg. 2006;118(1):263–4.
39. Goldman A, Wollina U. Elevation of the corner of the mouth using botulinum toxin type A. J Cutan Aesthet Surg. 2010;3(3):145.
40. Park MY, Ahn KY, Jung DS. Botulinum toxin type A treatment for contouring of the lower face. Dermatol Surg. 2003;29(5):477–83.
41. Semchyshyn N, Sengelmann RD. Botulinum toxin A treatment of perioral rhytides. Dermatol Surg. 2003;29(5):490–5.
42. Carruthers A, et al. A validated grading scale for marionette lines. Dermatol Surg. 2008;34(Suppl 2):S167–72.
43. Cohen JL, et al. OnabotulinumtoxinA dose-ranging study for hyperdynamic perioral lines. Dermatol Surg. 2012;38(9):1497–505.
44. Polo M. Botulinum toxin type A (Botox) for the neuromuscular correction of excessive gingival display on smiling (gummy smile). Am J Orthod Dentofac Orthop. 2008;133(2):195–203.
45. Hwang W-S, et al. Surface anatomy of the lip elevator muscles for the treatment of gummy smile using botulinum toxin. Angle Orthod. 2009;79(1):70–7.
46. Levy PM. The 'Nefertiti lift': a new technique for specific re-contouring of the jawline. J Cosmet Laser Ther. 2007;9(4):249–52.
47. Petchngaovilai C. Midface lifting with botulinum toxin: intradermal technique. J Cosmet Dermatol. 2009;8(4):312–6.
48. Beer K, Yohn M, Closter J. A double-blinded, placebo-controlled study of Botox for the treatment of subjects with chin rhytids. J Drugs Dermatol. 2004;4(4):417–22.
49. von Lindern JJ, et al. Type A botulinum toxin for the treatment of hypertrophy of the masseter and temporal muscles: an alternative treatment. Plast Reconstr Surg. 2001;107(2):327–32.
50. Castro WH, et al. Botulinum toxin type A in the management of masseter muscle hypertrophy. J Oral Maxillofac Surg. 2005;63(1):20–4.
51. Ahn J, Horn C, Blitzer A. Botulinum toxin for masseter reduction in Asian patients. Arch Facial Plast Surg. 2004;6(3):188–91.
52. Kane MAC. Nonsurgical treatment of platysmal bands with injection of botulinum toxin A. Plast Reconstr Surg. 1999;103(2):656–63.
53. Matarasso A, et al. Botulinum A exotoxin for the management of platysma bands. Plast Reconstr Surg. 1999;103(2):645–52.
54. Brandt FS, Bellman B. Cosmetic use of botulinum A exotoxin for the aging neck. Dermatol Surg. 1998;24(11):1232–4.
55. Matarasso SL. Complications of botulinum A exotoxin for hyperfunctional lines. Dermatol Surg. 1998;24(11):1249–54.

The Role of Botulinum Toxins in Treatment of Cancer-Related Issues: Post-radiation and Post-surgical Pain and Radiation-Induced Damage to the Salivary Glands

Delaram Safarpour and Bahman Jabbari

Introduction

As cancer survival has improved due to earlier detection, improved diagnostic procedures, and advanced surgical and radiotherapeutic treatments, new challenges have surfaced in survivors. After treatment, many cancer survivors return to their baseline functional state, but a sizeable number continue to suffer from the long-term side effects of treatment (s) [1]. Chronic pain, a disabling complaint in cancer patients, has a prevalence of approximately 30% that can increase with increased survival [2]. Severity and persistence of pain exerts a negative effect on overall well-being of patients [3]. While pain can be caused by the primary malignancy, different treatment options have been shown to contribute to its origin and chronicity through a variety of mechanisms.

Advanced cancer and end of life state is associated with moderate to severe pain in 70–80% of patients [4], compared to 41–77% and 34–77% reported for non-malignant, advanced medical disorders such as heart disease and chronic obstructive pulmonary disease, respectively [5, 6]. Palliative treatment of this form of pain is often difficult and side effects of analgesic medications are poorly tolerated by debilitated patients [7].

Damage to salivary glands is common in patients with head and neck cancer after radiotherapy. The submandibular glands are often more severely involved due to the proximity of these glands to jugulo-digastric nodes as well as the recent practice of image-guided radiotherapy, which spares a good part of the parotid glands [8]. Dysfunction of salivary glands after radiotherapy for cancer leads to serious complications

D. Safarpour, M.D.
University of Pennsylvania, Philadelphia, PA, USA
e-mail: Delaram.safarpour@gmail.com

B. Jabbari, M.D., F.A.A.N. (✉)
Neurology—Emeritus, Yale University, New Haven, CT, USA
e-mail: Bahman.jabbari@yale.edu

B. Jabbari (ed.), *Botulinum Toxin Treatment in Clinical Medicine*,
DOI 10.1007/978-3-319-56038-0_14

such as irreversible xerostomia, impaired sense of taste, dysphagia, infectious diseases of the oral and pharyngeal mucosa as well as dental and periodontal diseases [9].

This chapter will start with a discussion of the pathophysiology and therapy of post-radiation and post-surgical pain in cancer patients, followed by descriptions of the available evidence for botulinum neurotoxin (BoNT) effect on preventing and alleviating such pain. Sample case reports relevant to these issues will be provided from the senior author's experience. A brief account on the potential role of botulinum toxins on relieving intractable pain of advance cancer is also provided. The second part of the chapter discusses the available literature on potential benefit of botulinum toxin therapy in preventing damage to the salivary glands following radiation to the face and neck.

Focal Pain After Head and Face Radiation in Cancer Patients

The pathophysiology of radiation-induced pain is not well-understood. However, radiation-induced fibrosis leading to nerve compression along with direct axonal damage and demyelination along with blood vessels ischemia following capillary network failure have been suggested to be the main culprits for such pain [10–12]. List and Bilir [13] have attributed the post-radiation pain observed in 15–30% of patients with head and neck cancer to the development of fibrosis, scar, and keloid. Severe local pain after radiation may require potent systemic analgesic medications such as opioids which, although effective, often cause undesirable side effects. Among the multitude of side effects with these agents are nausea, somnolence, and constipation, each noted in more than 20% of the patients [14]. Topical application of trolamine, hyaluronic acid, and lidocaine patch may provide transient relief [15–17], but sustained relief is uncommon and was noted in only 25% of patients who applied lidocaine patch to the allodynic region [18].

Focal Pain After Surgery

Etiology of pain related to surgery is multifactorial and in most cases depends on the site and type of procedure. For example, the subpectoral tissue expansion phase of breast reconstruction surgery that uses an expander to provide a precise pocket over several months to contain the permanent implant can be associated with severe discomfort and pain. The pain can start immediately after the procedure and continue throughout this phase [18]. In other surgical procedures, damage to sensory nerves can cause persistent neuropathic pain, while in others, focal pain in the area of surgery may be related to the development of muscle spasms and increased tone.

Among all cancer types, prevalence of moderate to severe pain is highest in head/neck cancer patients (70%; 95% CI 51–88%) [19]. A review of literature shows that 48% of patients undergoing surgery for malignant head and neck disease reported a pain intensity greater than four (out of ten) at visual analogue scale (VAS) [20].

The current practice in management of pain after surgery is based on surgical complexity and includes: (1) for minor surgeries: NSAIDS (ketoprofen of ketorolac), paracetamol, or tramadol. (2) for medium or major surgeries: opioids (morphine), NSAIDs in elastomeric pump (i.e., ketoprofen)± paracetamol [21]. However, as mentioned earlier, most of these medications have sedative side effects and, in most cases, lead to suboptimal pain management.

Botulinum Neurotoxin Therapy for Post-radiation/Post-surgical Pain in Cancer Patients

The literature on this subject includes one double blind study and eight open label case series (Table 1) as well as a few case reports. Among eight open label studies, five were prospective and three were retrospective. The data collectively indicate that local injection of BoNTs into areas of pain (muscle or skin) significantly alleviates this form of pain in cancer patients.

Table 1 Open studies of BoNTs in post-radiation/post-surgical pain of cancer patients

Study	Pts	Toxin type	Dose	Treatment	Location	PO	Results
Van Daele et al. [28]	6 R	BoNT-A	20–25	Rad/chemo	Head and neck	Pain	Complete pain relief in four out of six patients
Wittekindt et al. [23]	23 P	BoNT-A	60–120 160–240	Rad/surg	Head and neck	VAS at day 28	Only low dose was effective ($P < 0.05$)
Hartel et al. [24]	19 P	onA/aboA	50/250	Chemo/rad	Head/neck	VAS and function, 4 weeks	VAS ($P = 0.02$), Function ($P = 0.04$)
Stubblefield et al. [29]	23 R	onaA	25–200	Rad/surg	Head/neck	Pain	Improved in 87%
Vuong et al. [25]	15 P	onaA	100	Rad/surg	Prostate	VAS	Improved ($P < 0.05$)
Mittal et al. [30]	7 R	onaA	100	Rad/surg	Head/neck and breast	VAS, PGIC at week 4	VAS ($P < 0.05$) PGIC: satisfactory
Bach et al. [27]	9 P	aboA	100–400(SCM) 125–200 (PF)	Rad/surg	Head and neck	FDSNP at week 4	FDSNP ($P = 0.01$) Pain ($P = 0.01$)
Rostami et al. [26]	12 P	incoA	100	Rad/surg	Head and neck VAS	VAS and PGIC	VAS, PGIC (P < 0.05)

BoNT botulinum neurotoxin, *P* prospective, *R* retrospective, *DB* double blind, *VAS* visual analogue scale, *PGIP* patient global impression of pain, *FDSNP* functional disability scale for neck pain, *SCM* sternocleidomastoid, *PF* pectoralis flap

Randomized, Double Blind, Placebo-Controlled Study (1)

Gabriel et al. [22] investigated the effect of the injection of onabotulinum toxinA into pectoralis muscle in 30 patients (15 toxin, 15 saline) who had undergone mastectomy with immediate expander or acellular dermal matrix reconstruction. A total of 40 units of onabotulinum toxin A was injected into each pectoralis muscle. The saline group received a comparable volume. Patients in the toxin group demonstrated significant improvement of VAS score for pain and were able to tolerate more volume of expansion per visit ($p < 0.05$). The toxin group also showed a significant decrease in the use of narcotics from the post-injection day 7–45 ($p < 0.05$).

Prospective Studies (5)

Wittekindt et al. [23] examined the efficacy of BoNT-A (type not specified) in 23 patients who reported neuropathic pain in the neck and shoulder following neck dissection for squamous cell carcinoma of upper "aero-digestive tract." Patients were divided into low-dose (80–120 units) and high-dose (160–240 units) groups. Patients and physicians were blinded to the dose of injections. Injections were performed in 8–12 locations subcutaneously into targeted neck and shoulder regions. Patients' response to BoNT injection was measured by visual analog scale (VAS) at baseline prior to injections and at day 28 after injections. The mean baseline pain was 4.3 on VAS (0–10) scale. The quality of life was evaluated by a questionnaire from the European Organization for Research and Treatment of Cancer (EORTC), specifically prepared for head and neck cancers, at the same time frames. At day 28, mean VAS score for the low-dose group changed from 4.3 to 3.6 ($P < 0.05$), but the change for the high-dose group was not statistically significant. Furthermore, the low-dose group also showed a trend for improvement of quality of life.

In another prospective study [24], the efficacy of onabotulinum toxinA (OnaA) and abobotulinum toxinA (AboA) was assessed in 19 patients with nasopharyngeal and oropharyngeal cancer who developed severe spasm of masseter muscles and trismus, on the average, 5.6 years after radiotherapy for cancer. Eleven patients had received chemotherapy in addition to radiation. The location of cancers was in the nasopharynx ($n = 3$), oropharynx ($n = 9$), oral cavity ($n = 2$), oral cavity and nasopharynx ($n = 1$), larynx ($n = 3$), and parotid gland ($n = 1$). Each masseter muscle was injected at two points, with the total dose of 50 units (onaA) or 250 units (aboA). At 4 weeks post-injection, pain, spasms, and functional score (measured in a 20 subset questionnaire) all improved significantly compared to baseline ($P = 0.002$, $P = 0.004$, $P = 0.04$, respectively). No difference was noted between onaA and AboA.

Voung et al. [25] studied the effect of BoNT injection into the rectal wall immediately after high dose-rate-endorectal brachytherapy (HDREBT) in 15 patients with prostatic cancer and used non-injected patients as controls. The patients who received 100 units of onaA into the rectal wall had a lower incidence of acute radiation prostatitis with significant reduction of bowel frequency and urgency ($P < 0.05$) and lesser degrees of pain ($P = 0.07$).

More recently, the Yale group published their experience with patients who had head, neck, and breast cancer and suffered from moderate to severe pain (VAS 5 or more) at the site of cancer resection or radiation [26]. Patients were prospectively enrolled in an open label study. A total of up to 80–100 units of incobotulinum toxin A, diluted in 1 cc of saline, was injected into the area of local pain indicated by the patient. The injections were subcutaneous or intramuscular depending on the type of pain, neuropathic (subcutaneous), or focal muscle spasm (intramuscular). The efficacy of treatment was assessed via VAS, Patient Global Impression of Change (PGIC), and American Chronic Pain Association questionnaire (Quality of Life Scale for pain), at 4, 6, 8, 10, 12 weeks post-injection. The primary outcome was two grades or more improvement in VAS score plus subject satisfaction expressed in the PGIC at 6 weeks. The secondary outcome was improvement of quality of life at 6 weeks. Twenty-five patients were screened and 12 were enrolled in the study. Two patients died during the study from complications of cancer and two were too sick to attend the follow-up sessions. Eight subjects, 31–70 years of age—four female four males—completed the study. Their baseline mean pain score in VAS was 7.4 (range 5–10). Four had breast cancer, two tonsillar, one base of the tongue, and one dermal squamous cell carcinoma of the neck.

At 4 weeks, all eight subjects reported significant pain relief with the mean baseline VAS of 7.4 dropping to 3.8 ($P < 0.05$). Five of eight patients maintained the same degree of pain relief at 12 weeks. Seven of eight patients reported their pain as much improved or very much improved on the PGIC assessment. Three of eight patients reported significant improvement of the quality of life at 6 weeks.

Bach et al. [27] prospectively followed nine patients with post-surgical contracture of sternocleidomastoid or pectoralis major muscle related to head and neck cancer. AbobotulinumtoxinA was injected into the sternocleidomastoid (100–400 units) and into the pectoralis major flap (125–200 units). All patients expressed pain relief. The cervical disability score fell from 33 to 23 ($P < 0.01$). There were no side effects.

Retrospective Studies (3)

In the study of Van Daele et al. [28], injection of onabotulinum toxin A into the tight and painful sternocleidomastoid muscle relieved the pain and tightness in four of six patients. All patients had received radiotherapy for head and neck cancer. The injected dose was 20–25 units administered at one or two points into the sternocleidomastoid muscle.

Stubblefield et al. [29] also found BoNT-A injection helpful in relieving focal pain caused by radiation fibrosis. In this retrospective study of 23 patients, 30% had painful trismus and 43% had trigeminal and cervical plexus neuralgia.

Mittal et al. [30] reviewed the results of onabotulinum toxinA treatment in eight patients with head and neck and breast cancer. Injection of 80–100 units of onA into the painful region alleviated muscle spasms and neuropathic pain in these patients. Five of eight patients reported treatment as “very satisfactory” in the Patient Global Impression of Change (PGIC).

The following case reports describe two patients who have participated in the Yale protocol assessing the effect of BoNT therapy on cancer-related pain.

Case 1—Carcinoma of the Base of the Tongue Associated with Painful Upper Neck Spasms and Burning Pain Interfering with Speaking and Swallowing A 47 year old, right-handed gentleman was referred to the Yale Neurotoxin Treatment Clinic for evaluation of right upper neck pain, difficulty in swallowing, and speaking of 5 years duration. Six years ago, he was found to have a tumor at the base of the tongue and cervical lymphadenopathy on the right side. He underwent resection of the tumor with removal of lymph nodes and neck muscles on the right side. The tumor was a squamous cell carcinoma. Shortly after resection, he received radiotherapy to the base of the tongue and right side of the neck. A few months later, he experienced tingling and pulling of the base of the tongue which gradually evolved into painful spasms and burning sensation below the angle of the right jaw interfering with speaking and eating. Treatment with a variety of analgesic drugs was only minimally helpful.

General medical and neurological examinations were normal except for loss of muscles on the right side of the neck and mild weakness of the tongue. A vertical surgical scar was visible on the right side of the neck extending from lower neck to the lower edge of the mandible. Several areas of induration and keloid formation were present, the hardest and most painful being located anterior to and slightly below the angle of the right jaw.

Twenty units of Onabotulinum toxin A was injected into each of the three areas of indurated, scar tissue on the right side of the neck (Fig. 1). The dilution was 100 units/cc. A ¾ inch long, 27.5 gauge needle was used for injections. After a week, patient reported total cessation of muscle spasms and burning pain as well as marked improvement of his swallowing and speech. He reported no side effects. The pain and discomfort returned after 6 months. Patient reported the same favorable results over 8 years of follow-up with slightly higher doses of onaA (30, 30, and 20 units) applied in the last 3 years.

Case 2—Intense Left Cervical Pain Following Laryngectomy and Neck Dissections for Squamous Cell Carcinoma of the Piriform Sinus A 48-year-old man underwent laser supraglottic laryngectomy with bilateral neck dissections for squamous cell carcinoma of the left piriform sinus. This was followed by courses of chemotherapy and radiation. Two years later, patient developed intense left cervical pain and left shoulder pain beginning with spasms of the left sternocleidomastoid (SCM) muscle. The pain was described as deep and aching, but at times sharp and jabbing. A variety of medications including fentanyl 25 μg/h. patch and hydromorphone 2 mg tablets, given as needed, provided no significant pain relief. He was then injected with a total dose of 200 units of Onabotulinum toxin A into the left cervical and shoulder muscles: left SCM, left trapezius, left splenius, and left levator scapulae muscles at several points, 15–20 units per site (Fig. 2). After a week, he reported marked reduction of pain (from VAS 8 to 1); on PGIC, he expressed the outcome as "very satisfactory." The response continued over a period of 3 years with repeat injections performed every 4 months. The patient did not report any side effects.

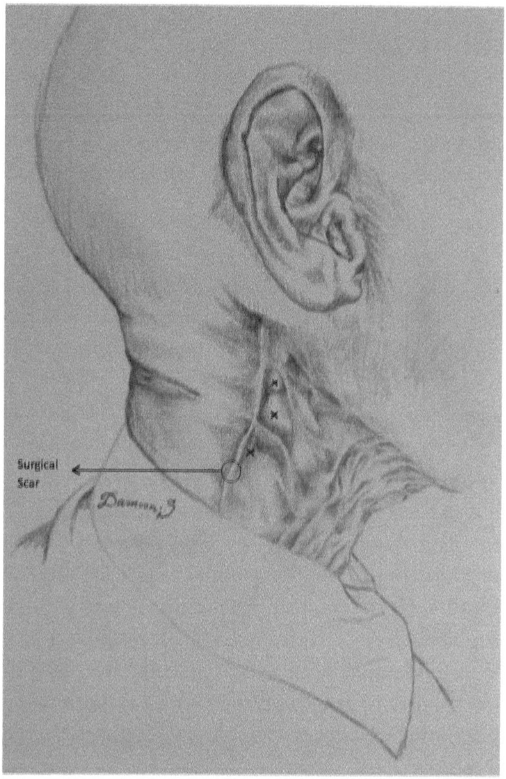

Fig. 1 Onabotulinum toxin A injection sites in the right side of the neck into areas of keloid, induration, and fibrosis

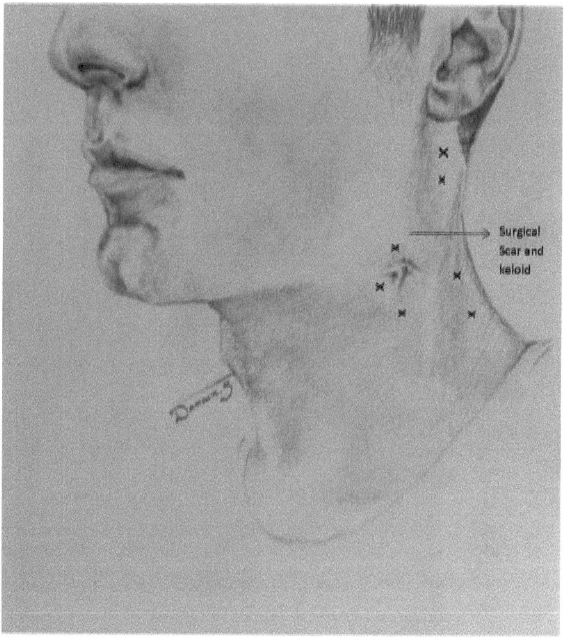

Fig. 2 Injection sites in the left side of the neck and shoulder into the sternocleidomastoid, levator scapulae, splenius, and trapezius muscles

Palliative Effects of Botulinum Toxins in Patients with Terminal Cancer and Recalcitrant Pain

Pain can be a major issue in cancer patients close to end of life. Such fragile patients often poorly tolerate potent analgesics. Anectodal observations attest to the analgesic and palliative action of BoNTs in the end of the life pain [31]. The patient reported below was treated by the senior author of this chapter for pain relief.

Case 1: Severe Jaw Pain and Trismus Due to the Direct Invasion of Masseter Muscle and Jaw Bone by a Non-small Cell Cancer of the Lung A 69-year-old female with non-small cell carcinoma of the lungs (stage IV) and metastasis to the bones (femur, petrous) and brain underwent multiple courses of radiation and chemotherapy. Three months after the completion of radiotherapy, she complained of jaw stiffness, inability to open the mouth fully, and right masseter pain when attempting to open the mouth. Over the next few weeks, the pain reached a point that she refrained from eating. Administration of oxycodone (10 mg, twice daily) and fentanyl (25 μg patch every 72 h) provided partial pain relief, but did not alleviate the trismus. An MRI showed enlargement of right masseter due to neoplastic involvement (Fig. 3).

Injection of onabotulinum toxinA (50 units) into the right masseter and 20 units into the right temporalis decreased the right masseter pain and improved jaw opening for 6 weeks. Subsequent injections of a larger dose of onaA into the right masseter (70 units) with additional injection into the left masseter (30 units) improved her quality of life (pain relief, less eating difficulty) over the next 18 months before her demise from complications of cancer.

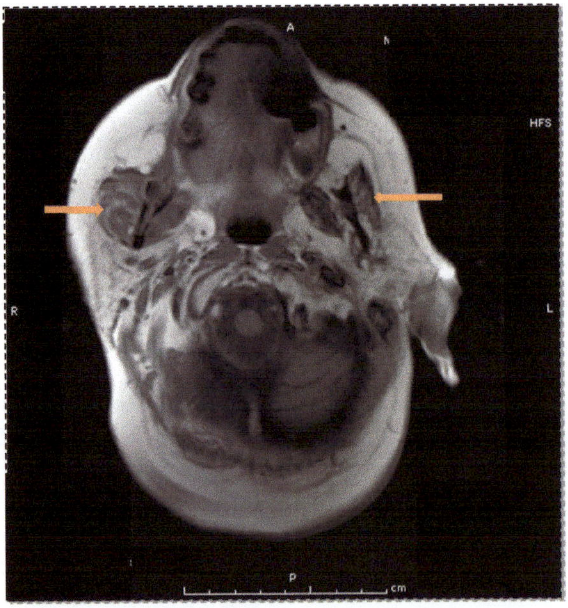

Fig. 3 Magnetic resonance imaging (MRI) with special base view showing the right masseter enlargement presumably from cancerous involvement

Comment

Botulinum neurotoxins can influence and reduce pain via a variety of mechanisms [32–34]. These include inhibition of pain mediator (CGRP, SP, glutamate) release from nerve endings, dorsal root ganglia, and spinal neurons as well as reduction of local inflammation. Further mechanisms involve inhibition of sodium and purinergic channels (ATP), decreased discharge of sympathetic neurons, and muscle spindles [32–34]. These effects collectively subdue peripheral and ultimately central sensitization, the principal factors of pain chronicity. Intra-lesional injection of botuliumtoxinA into keloids formed at the site of surgery or radiation softens and reduces the volume of keloids in a manner similar to steroid injection and is superior to steroids in regard to symptom relief (including pain) [35].

Cancer-related pain is hard to treat and introduction of a novel therapeutic modality with a safe and low side effect profile is welcome, given the fragility of the patients and their higher propensity for developing side effects. Although current literature in this area does not include high-quality clinical trials, the available data collectively support a place for all three types of BoNTs (onaA, incoA, and AboA) in the treatment of cancer-related pain.

The Role of BoNTs in Prevention of Post-radiation Damage to the Salivary Glands

As was mentioned in the introduction, radiation to the face and neck damages the salivary glands and leads to a variety of unpleasant symptoms caused by salivary glands dysfunction [9]. The submandibular gland is often more damaged as it is less protected than parotid gland by the modern radiotherapeutic techniques [8]. Submandibular glands provide 60–67% of the unstimulated and 50% of stimulated saliva. There is evidence in animals and human that injection of BoNTs into the salivary gland prior to radiotherapy reduces the damage to these glands substantially.

Teymoortash et al. [36] showed that injection of BoNT-A or B into submandibular glands of the rat before irradiation of the gland prevented the marked radiation-induced parenchymal loss and acinar fibrosis compared to the saline-injected rats. The weight of submandibular gland after radiation was also markedly reduced in the saline-injected rats, but not in the BoNT-injected rats ($P = 0.008$).

In another study of irradiated salivary glands, at third day post-irradiation, mice pre-injected with BoNT-A demonstrated 25% reduction in the flow of saliva compared to 50% reduction in the BoNT-untreated mice ($P < 0.05$). Local neutrophil infiltration, detected by myeloperoxidase staining, was threefold lower for the BoNT-treated mice. At 4 weeks post-irradiation, the saline (control) group showed a 40% reduction in basal SMG weight, compared with 20% in weight reduction in the BoNT group. Histologically, BoNT-pretreated glands showed relative preservation of acinar structures after radiation [37].

In a recent prospective, randomized, placebo-controlled, double-blinded study conducted in human subjects affected by head and neck cancer, investigators assessed safety of BoNT A and B injection into the submandibular gland prior to radiotherapy. Subjects were divided into four groups, each consisting of three subjects. The injected doses were 20 units for type A and 750 units for the type B toxin. Injections were safe, but authors found no difference between BoNTs (A or B) and placebo regarding the gland's uptake of technetium pertechnetate or regarding the salivary excretion fraction. The authors concluded that due to the small number of patients, further investigation of various doses and timing of BoNT injection is required for a more precise analysis of toxin's efficacy in humans [38].

Chapter Conclusion

Several studies in human indicate that local injection of BoNTs into the scar and keloid tissue and into adjacent muscles substantially reduces the post-surgical pain in cancer patients after surgery and radiation. Case observations strongly suggest that local injection of BoNTs can ease the pain in some terminal cancer patients with recalcitrant local pain. Data in animals indicate that injection of BoNTs into the submandibular gland prior to irradiation of the gland prevents paranchymal damage, gland atrophy, and reduction of salivation. In human, additional studies are needed for assessing the efficacy of BoNTs in this setting.

References

1. Stein KD, Syrjala KL, Andrykowski MA. Physical and psychological long-term and late effects of cancer. Cancer. 2008;112:2577–92. doi:10.1002/cncr.23448.
2. Brown MR, Ramirez JD, Farquhar-Smith P. Pain in cancer survivors. Br J Pain. 2014;8:139–53. doi:10.1177/2049463714542605.
3. Elliott J, Fallows A, Staetsky L, Smith PW, Foster CL, Maher EJ, Corner J. The health and well-being of cancer survivors in the UK: findings from a population-based survey. Br J Cancer. 2011;105(Suppl 1):S11–20. doi:10.1038/bjc.2011.418.
4. Caraceni A, Hanks G, Kaasa S, Bennett MI, Brunelli C, Cherny N, Dale O, De Conno F, Fallon M, Hanna M, Haugen DF, Juhl G, King S, Klepstad P, Laugsand EA, Maltoni M, Mercadante S, Nabal M, Pigni A, Radbruch L, Reid C, Sjogren P, Stone PC, Tassinari D, Zeppetella G. Use of opioid analgesics in the treatment of cancer pain: evidence-based recommendations from the EAPC. Lancet Oncol. 2012;13:e58–68. doi:10.1016/s1470-2045(12)70040-2.
5. Harris DG. Management of pain in advanced disease. Br Med Bull. 2014;110:117–28. doi:10.1093/bmb/ldu010.
6. Solano JP, Gomes B, Higginson IJ. A comparison of symptom prevalence in far advanced cancer, AIDS, heart disease, chronic obstructive pulmonary disease and renal disease. J Pain Symptom Manag. 2006;31:58–69. doi:10.1016/j.jpainsymman.2005.06.007.
7. Borsook D. Neurological diseases and pain. Brain J Neurol. 2012;135:320–44. doi:10.1093/brain/awr271.

8. Cannon DM, Lee NY. Recurrence in region of spared parotid gland after definitive intensity-modulated radiotherapy for head and neck cancer. Int J Radiat Oncol Biol Phys. 2008;70:660–5.
9. Bansal M, Mohanti BK, Shah N, et al. Radiation related morbidities and their impact on quality of life in head and neck cancer patients receiving radical radiotherapy. Qual Life Res. 2004;13:481–8.
10. Kehlet H, Jensen TS, Woolf CJ. Persistent postsurgical pain: risk factors and prevention. Lancet. 2006;367:1618–25. doi:10.1016/s0140-6736(06)68700-x.
11. Kanner RM, Foley KM. Patterns of narcotic drug use in a cancer pain clinic. Ann N Y Acad Sci. 1981;362:161–72.
12. Delanian S, Lefaix JL, Pradat PF. Radiation-induced neuropathy in cancer survivors. Radiother Oncol. 2012;105:273–82. doi:10.1016/j.radonc.2012.10.012.
13. List MA, Bilir SP. Functional outcomes in head and neck cancer. Semin Radiat Oncol. 2004;14:178–89. doi:10.1053/j.semradonc.2003.12.008.
14. Straube C, Derry S, Jackson KC, Wiffen PJ, Bell RF, Strassels S, Straube S. Codeine, alone and with paracetamol (acetaminophen), for cancer pain. Cochrane Database Syst Rev. 2014;Cd006601. doi:10.1002/14651858.CD006601.pub4.
15. Fisher J, Scott C, Stevens R, Marconi B, Champion L, Freedman GM, Asrari F, Pilepich MV, Gagnon JD, Wong G. Randomized phase III study comparing best supportive care to Biafine as a prophylactic agent for radiation-induced skin toxicity for women undergoing breast irradiation: Radiation Therapy Oncology Group (RTOG) 97-13. Int J Radiat Oncol Biol Phys. 2000;48:1307–1310.
16. Chargari C, Fromantin I, Kirova YM. Importance of local skin treatments during radiotherapy for prevention and treatment of radio-induced epithelitis. Cancer Radiother. 2009;13:259–66. doi:10.1016/j.canrad.2009.04.003.
17. Kirova YM, Fromantin I, De Rycke Y, Fourquet A, Morvan E, Padiglione S, Falcou MC, Campana F, Bollet MA. Can we decrease the skin reaction in breast cancer patients using hyaluronic acid during radiation therapy? Results of phase III randomised trial. Radiother Oncol. 2011;100:205–9. doi:10.1016/j.radonc.2011.05.014.
18. Fleming JA, O'Connor BD. Use of lidocaine patches for neuropathic pain in a comprehensive cancer centre. Pain Res Manag. 2009;14:381–8.
19. van den Beuken-van Everdingen MH, de Rijke JM, Kessels AG, Schouten HC, van Kleef M, Patijn J. Prevalence of pain in patients with cancer: a systematic review of the past 40 years. Ann Oncol. 2007;18:1437–49. doi:10.1093/annonc/mdm056.
20. Sommer M, Geurts JW, Stessel B, Kessels AG, Peters ML, Patijn J, van Kleef M, Kremer B, Marcus MA. Prevalence and predictors of postoperative pain after ear, nose, and throat surgery. Arch Otolaryngol Head Neck Surg. 2009;135:124–30. doi:10.1001/archoto.2009.3.
21. Bianchini C, Malago M, Crema L, Aimoni C, Matarazzo T, Bortolazzi S, Ciorba A, Pelucchi S, Pastore A. Post-operative pain management in head and neck cancer patients: predictive factors and efficacy of therapy. Acta Otorhinolaryngol Ital. 2016;36:91–6. doi:10.14639/0392-100x-499.
22. Gabriel A, Champaneria MC, Maxwell GP. The efficacy of botulinum toxin A in post-mastectomy breast reconstruction: a pilot study. Aesthet Surg J. 2015;35:402–9. doi:10.1093/asj/sjv040.
23. Wittekindt C, Liu WC, Preuss SF, Guntinas-Lichius O. Botulinum toxin A for neuropathic pain after neck dissection: a dose-finding study. Laryngoscope. 2006;116:1168–71. doi:10.1097/01.mlg.0000217797.05523.75.
24. Hartl DM, Cohen M, Julieron M, Marandas P, Janot F, Bourhis J. Botulinum toxin for radiation-induced facial pain and trismus. Otolaryngol Head Neck Surg. 2008;138:459–63. doi:10.1016/j.otohns.2007.12.021.
25. Vuong T, Waschke K, Niazi T, Richard C, Parent J, Liberman S, Mayrand S, Loungnarath R, Stein B, Devic S. The value of Botox-A in acute radiation proctitis: results from a phase I/II study using a three-dimensional scoring system. Int J Radiat Oncol Biol Phys. 2011;80(5):1505–11.

26. Rostami R, Mittal SO, Radmand R, Jabbari B. Incobotulinum toxin-A improves post-surgical and post-radiation pain in cancer patients. Toxins. 2016;8(1):22. doi:10.3390/toxins8010022.
27. Bach CA, Wagner I, Lachiver X, Baujat B, Chabolle F. Botulinum toxin in the treatment of post-radiosurgical neck contracture in head and neck cancer: a novel approach. Eur Ann Otorhinolaryngol Head Neck Dis. 2012;129:6–10. doi:10.1016/j.anorl.2011.07.002.
28. Van Daele DJ, Finnegan EM, Rodnitzky RL, Zhen W, McCulloch TM, Hoffman HT. Head and neck muscle spasm after radiotherapy: management with botulinum toxin A injection. Arch Otolaryngol Head Neck Surg. 2002;128:956–9.
29. Stubblefield MD, Levine A, Custodio CM, Fitzpatrick T. The role of botulinum toxin type A in the radiation fibrosis syndrome: a preliminary report. Arch Phys Med Rehabil. 2008;89:417–21. doi:10.1016/j.apmr.2007.11.022.
30. Mittal S, Machado DG, Jabbari B. Onabotulinum toxin A for treatment of focal cancer pain after surgery and/or radiation. Pain Med. 2012;13:1029–33. doi:10.1111/j.1526-4637.2012.01437.x.
31. Fu J, Ngo A, Shin K, et al. Botulinum toxin injection and phenol nerve block for reduction of end-of-life pain. J Palliat Med. 2013;16:1637–40.
32. Aoki RK, Francis J. Update on the nociceptive mechanism hypothesiss and related disorders. Parkinsonism Relat Disord. 2011;17:S28–33.
33. Brown EA, Schutz SG, Simpson DM. Botulinum toxin for neuropathic pain and spasticity: an overview. Pain Manag. 2014;4:129–51.
34. Mittal SO, Safarpour D, Jabbari B. Botulinum toxin treatment of neuropathic pain. Semin Neurol. 2016;36:73–83.
35. Shaarawy E, Hegazy RA, Abdel Hay RM. Intralesional botulinum toxin type A equally effective and better tolerated than intralesional steroid in the treatment of keloids: a randomized controlled trial. J Cosmet Dermatol. 2015;14:161–6.
36. Teymoortash A, Müller F, Juricko J, Bieker M, Mandic R, Librizzi D, Höffken H, Pfestroff A, Werner JA. Botulinum toxin prevents radiotherapy-induced salivary gland damage. Oral Oncol. 2009;45:737–9.
37. Zeidan YH, Xiao N, Cao H, Kong C, Le QT, Sirjani D. Botulinum toxin confers radioprotection in murine salivary glands. Int J Radiat Oncol Biol Phys. 2016;94:1190–7.
38. Teymoortash A, Pfestroff A, Wittig A, Franke N, Hoch S, Harnisch S, Schade-Brittinger C, Hoeffken H, Engenhart-Cabillic R, Brugger M, Strauch K. Safety and efficacy of botulinum toxin to preserve gland function after radiotherapy in patients with head and neck cancer: a prospective, randomized, placebo-controlled, double-blinded phase I clinical trial. PLoS One. 2016;11(3):e0151316. doi: 10.1371/journal.pone.0151316. eCollection 2016.

Ultrasound, Electromyography, Electrical Stimulation; Techniques Aiding More Effective Botulinum Toxin Therapy

Katharine E. Alter and Barbara I. Karp

Introduction

Over the past two decades, the clinical applications of botulinum (BoNT) have expanded from the initial use and approval in ophthalmology to include many other conditions which depend upon neurotransmitter release and the SNARE protein complex. Current approvals and proposed applications of BoNTs include conditions ranging from its widely accepted use for muscle overactivity (spasticity, dystonia, tremor, and rigidity) to include neurosecretory, urological, gastrointestinal, and other disorders including pain for which the mechanism of action of BoNTs is incompletely understood.

As the clinical use and regulatory agency approvals of BoNTs have expanded, extensive experience and published studies support that these agents are effective and safe when administered by experienced practitioners. However, there is little data and continued debate on the safest, most accurate, or most effective method to deliver BoNTs to the intended target. This chapter will review the most common guidance techniques for BoNT therapy including anatomic or manual guidance and instrumented guidance techniques including electromyography (EMG), electrical stimulation (E-Stim), ultrasound (US), and fluoroscopy (Flouro), including discussion of the current level of evidence for the advantages and limitations of each of these techniques.

K.E. Alter, M.D. (✉) • B.I. Karp, M.D.
National Institute of Health, Bethesda, MD, USA
e-mail: kalter@mail.nih.gov; karpb@ninds.nih.gov

B. Jabbari (ed.), *Botulinum Toxin Treatment in Clinical Medicine*,
DOI 10.1007/978-3-319-56038-0_15

Guidance Techniques

Anatomic or Manual Guidance

Anatomic (manual) guidance relies on visual identification of surface anatomy, palpation of anatomic landmarks, and/or passive or active range of motion (PROM, AROM) to estimate a muscle position and depth. Once the clinician identifies the muscle, a skin site for needle entry is selected that provides the most direct approach to the intended target and avoids blood vessels and other critical structures. The skin at the site for needle insertion is disinfected and the needle is inserted through the skin and advanced blindly to the estimated muscle position and depth. With manual guidance, standard hypodermic needles are used for injection, typically 25–30 gauge and 0.5–2 1/2 in. in length depending on the estimated depth of the target. The anatomic/manual technique was especially common in the early days of BoNT therapy when many clinicians relied solely on their knowledge of gross and surface anatomy, cross-sectional, or functional anatomy to identify the site for needle insertion and BoNT injection. While a detailed knowledge of anatomy is critical for all injections including chemodenervation procedures, most physicians no longer recommend relying solely on this technique for the majority of BoNT procedures [1] as it has been shown to be inaccurate (see below) [2–4]. However, regardless of what supplementary guidance technique is used, all physicians must rely first and foremost on their knowledge of surface, cross-sectional, and functional anatomy when performing chemodenervation procedures.

Advantages

1. All physicians receive education and training in gross and functional anatomy during medical school and perhaps again during residency training.
2. Anatomic guidance requires no specialized equipment and minimal resources, usually only anatomic reference guides. There are many useful print and online resources which can serve as a starting point for estimating the site of needle insertion and target injection [5–8].
3. Some muscles are easily palpated and/or localized by their anatomic landmarks and position on the limb, trunk, or neck. Examples of easily identified and palpated muscles include the biceps brachii and tibialis anterior.

Limitations: While knowledge of surface and functional anatomy is required for all chemodenervation procedures, relying solely on this technique without supplemental guidance has many limitations [9, 42].

1. *Inadequate familiarity with anatomy*: Many clinicians who perform chemodenervation procedures had their last exposure to gross anatomy in medical school, often in the distant past, leaving them with only remote memories of the course material. It is difficult for practicing physicians to arrange time and get access to gross anatomy training courses.

2. *Individual anatomic variations in location and size*: There is substantial individual variation in muscle anatomy, including shape or form, relative size, location or depth, as well as the absence or presence of certain muscles. It is difficult or impossible to determine by inspection or palpation alone whether such an anatomic variation exists in a patient. For example, the palmaris longus (PL), reportedly the most variable muscle in humans, is absent in 4–26% of individuals. Even when present, the PL varies in size; can have one or more bellies and can be either tendinous or muscular at either the proximal or distal end [10, 11]. In some individuals, the PL is unusually large, thereby potentially having a greater contribution to wrist flexion force than expected (Fig. 1a, b). When treating a patient with wrist flexor spasticity, this anatomic variation alone may impact the outcome of BoNT injections. The PL is often left untreated as it is thought to contribute little to wrist flexion. If, however, a large PL is present, failure to target this muscle may contribute to treatment failure and a false conclusion of insufficient dosing in other wrist flexor muscles rather than recognizing the need to inject the PL.
3. *Disease processes can also distort anatomy*: Spastic muscles may be shortened and shifted in position. Dystonic muscles may hypertrophy from repeated over-contraction.
4. *Complex overlapping anatomy and muscle depth*: There are approximately 20 muscles in the forearm alone, with so many deep and overlapping that it may be difficult or impossible to estimate the position of these muscles by palpation or inspection. The same is true for estimating the position and depth of muscles in other areas, such as the neck or lower limb where the muscles are deep to overlying adipose tissue.
5. *Interposed critical structures*: As well as hitting the intended target, proper injection must avoid hitting nerves, blood vessels, and other critical structures. By visual inspection, it is impossible to project the site of vessels, nerves, or other structures that are in the path to the target muscle and that should be avoided.
6. *Patient positioning*: When estimating a muscle's location, most physicians rely on one or more of the available anatomic reference guides [5–7]. The majority of these guides were developed for use in diagnostic electromyography, not for botulinum toxin or other chemodenervation procedures. These guides require that the patient's limb be placed in a specific position, often the standard anatomic position. When treating patients with movement disorders or spasticity, it is often difficult or impossible to position patients as described in the book, limiting the accuracy of the guides' recommended position for needle insertion.

Caveats: A thorough knowledge of anatomy is mandatory for all physicians who perform BoNT injections or other chemodenervation regardless of what supplemental technique may be used, as anatomy serves as the basis for utilizing other targeting techniques. Most physicians and all of the toxin manufacturers recommend supplemental guidance along with anatomic assessment when guiding most BoNT procedures. Neurolytic chemodenervation procedures with phenol or denatured ethyl alcohol should not be performed without guidance with E-Stim or E-Stim + US.

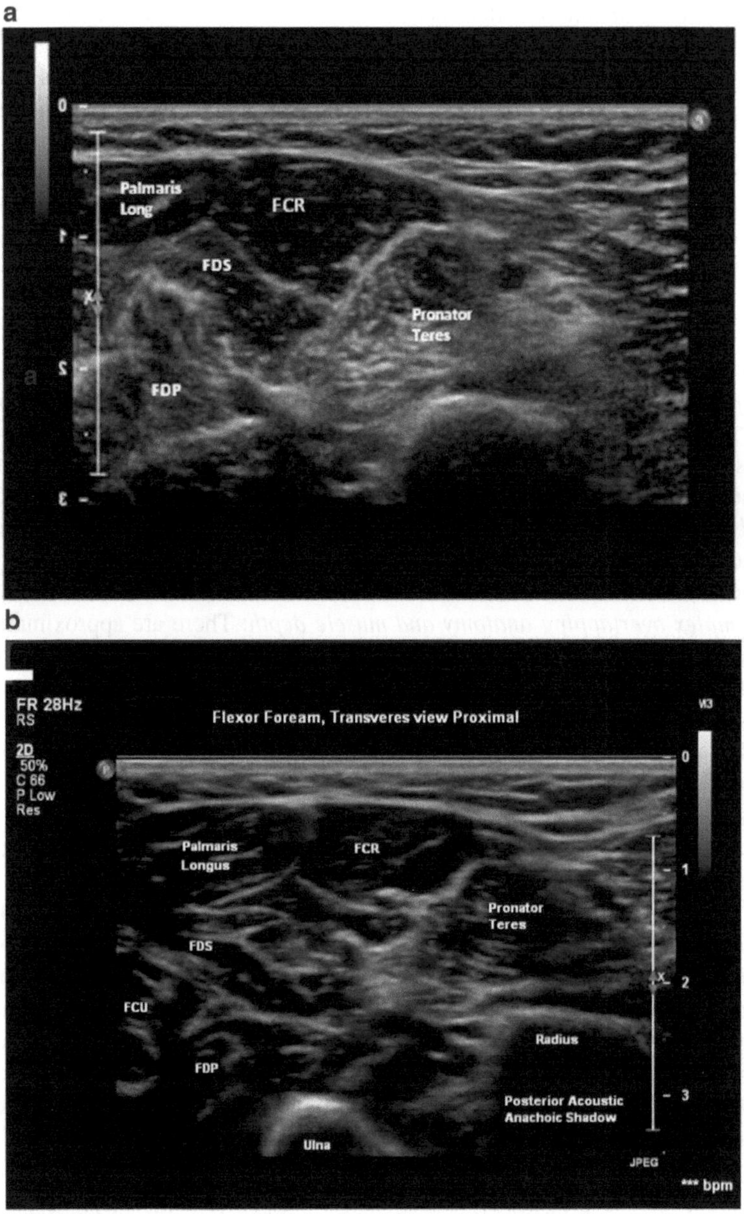

Fig. 1 (**a**) Palmaris longus anatomical size variant, typical size. (**b**) Palmaris longus anatomical size variant large muscle size

Electromyography/EMG Guidance

EMG is the most commonly reported or recommended localization techniques for BoNT injections involving muscle targets [2, 12–16]. EMG guidance requires equipment either a standard electrodiagnostic machine, EMG amplifier, or combined EMG amplifier-E-Stim unit as well as insulated (usually Teflon-coated) injecting needle electrodes of the appropriate length to reach the intended target muscle or muscles and ground and reference electrodes (Fig. 2a–c).

When using EMG to guide BoNT injections, the patient should be situated comfortably both to provide easy access to the muscles and facilitate a relaxation in the target muscle groups. The steps in identifying the optimal site for the needle electrode insertion using anatomic localization include inspection, measurement, and palpation with or without performing PROM or AROM of the muscle. The area of the body to be injected is exposed to reveal the region of interest and the patient positioned to allow access to this region. Proper positioning typically requires the assistance of other staff especially for patients who have significant spasticity, involuntary movements, or ROM limitations, as well as for those who have difficulty cooperating or following directions. If many muscles are to be injected, the patient should be carefully repositioned to optimize each injection site. Once the patient is positioned, the reference and ground electrodes are placed; the insulated injection needle serves as the active electrode.

The skin over the selected site is then disinfected and the needle electrode is inserted through the skin and advanced to the target while listening for audible EMG activity. Insertional activity will be heard when the needle enters the muscle. Insertional activity is then followed by a tonal change from a low, dull pitch to the crisp high frequency of motor unit action potentials (MUAPs), which confirms that the electrode is in an actively contracting muscle. If the tone remains dull (i.e., low frequency), the needle position should be adjusted, advanced, or redirected until a high frequency "crisp" tone is obtained.

If possible, the patient should be instructed to relax completely, then to voluntarily contract the target muscle. This facilitates muscle localization as the injector can hear the muscle interference pattern with voluntary activation of the target muscle, but there should be no sound (or only the sound of distant motor units) with activation of surrounding muscles.

EMG alone can be effective in localizing muscles for BoNT procedures if the patient is able to simultaneously contract the target muscle and relax adjacent muscles, even those with a similar action and/or antagonist muscles. This approach, however, may be difficult or impossible for many patients with spasticity or secondary dystonia due to impaired selective motor control and/or co-contraction or mass synergies [17]. For example, when targeting the flexor carpi radialis (FCR) for BoNT in a patient with post-stroke spasticity (PSS), co-contraction may be present in other forearm muscles making it impossible to determine in which of the simultaneously firing muscles (flexor digitorum superficialis (FDS), pronator teres (PT), or flexor digitorum profundus (FDP)) the needle electrode is located. In this

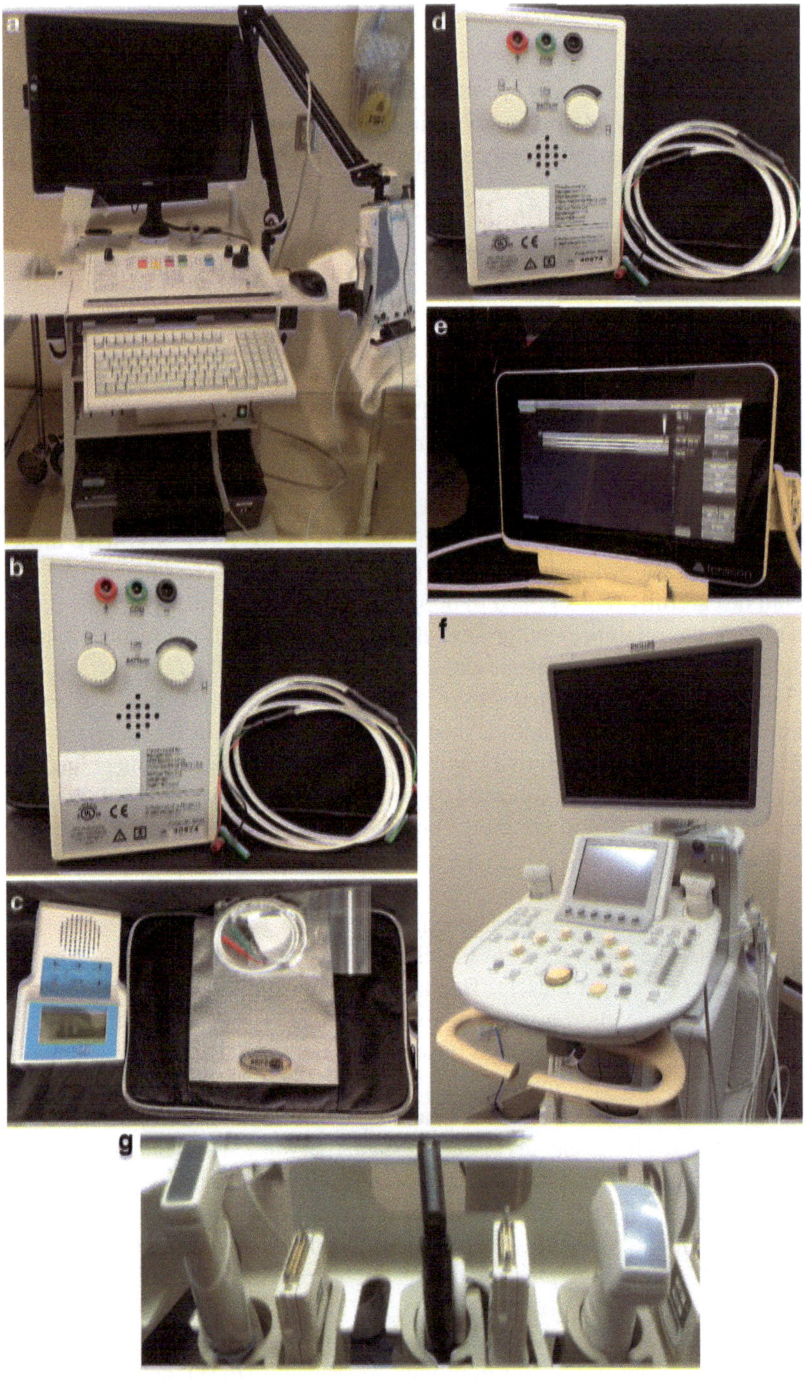

Fig. 2 Equipment for instrumented guidance. (**a**) Electrodiagnostic machine, (**b**) EMG audio amplifier, (**c**) electrical stimulation unit, (**d**) combined electrical stimulation/EMG unit, (**e**) portable ultrasound machine, (**f**) cart-based ultrasound machine, (**g**) ultrasound transducers

situation, it may be possible to ascertain the position of the needle by PROM of the target muscle, as stretching the muscle may elicit increased firing. Similarly, careful inspection of the patient's abnormal posture may also help determine which muscle the needle is in. However, many physicians faced with this situation would choose E-Stim (E-Stim) to guide the BoNT procedure rather than EMG [15, 18].

Advantages and Limitations of EMG for BoNT Procedures

1. *Identification of over-contracting muscles*: The primary advantage of EMG is that it provides feedback (auditory or visual, depending on the equipment used) indicating the level of activity or overactivity in a muscle. It is particularly useful in patients with complex patterns of cervical dystonia (CD) or limb dystonia where EMG can demonstrate whether a muscle is actively firing when it should be at rest and thereby contributing to the abnormal head, neck, or limb posture [19, 20].
2. *Fine or discrete localization*: In focal hand dystonia, there is often dystonic contraction of just part of a larger muscle. Such patients may have, for example, flexion in a single finger, indicating dystonic involvement of just one fascicle of the FDS or FDP. Thus, in limb dystonia, EMG is useful when it is important to isolate individual muscle fascicles for injection.

Limitations

1. *Inadequate familiarity with EMG procedures and EMG equipment*: The use of EMG requires training for safety and proper use of the equipment. The need for training can be minimized by using commercially available audio EMG units without stimulation capability. Inexpensive units are widely available, so that cost is not a major limiting factor.
2. *Factors limiting accuracy*: The accuracy of muscle localization by EMG is limited by;
   (a) Co-contraction and muscle synergies
   (b) Loss of reciprocal inhibition, leading to diffuse activation of multiple muscles including co-contraction of agonists and antagonists.
   (c) Loss of EMG signal when patients are sedated for BoNT injections, particularly if general anesthesia is used.
3. *Not always needed*: EMG is not generally used for chemodenervation of orbicularis oculi in patients with blepharospasm or many of the thin, superficial muscles of facial expression.
4. *Non-muscle targets*: EMG is not helpful for localizing non-muscle targets such as glands for sialorrhea or hyper-secretory disorders.
5. *Blind insertion*: EMG uses blind insertion of the needle that may penetrate vessels, nerves, organs, or other structures in the path to the target muscle.
6. *Pain/discomfort*: Patients often report more pain with the insertion of insulated needle electrodes than with standard hypodermic needles.
7. *Cost*: Insulated needle electrodes are more costly than hypodermic needles.

Caveats: When considering BoNT treatment for muscle overactivity, EMG can provide useful information related to the level of activity in a muscle. EMG is likely more useful in patients with focal dystonia than in those with spasticity. Some of the limitations of EMG guidance can be resolved by carefully selecting the patient in whom EMG will be used and combining EMG with other guidance, such as E-stim or US. US has the advantage of reducing the risks of blind needle insertion and can be combined with EMG-guided procedures.

Electrical Stimulation (E-Stim)

E-Stim is an EMG technique whereby the muscle with the needle in place is stimulated through the injection EMG needle. It is used or recommended by many clinicians who perform chemodenervation procedures including BoNT injections and neurolytic procedures (such as phenol or ethyl alcohol nerve/motor point blocks). We consider E-Stim to be required for all neurolytic procedures or diagnostic nerve blocks. E-Stim is only useful for BoNT injections of muscle targets and is not informative when injecting glands or non-muscle targets. Similar to EMG, E-Stim may not be required or useful when treating the orbicularis oculi in blepharospasm or other superficial muscles of face. When performing neurolytic chemodenervation procedures (with phenol or denatured ethyl alcohol), the physician has several options including performing a motor nerve or nerve trunk block, motor nerve branch block, or motor points/motor endplate blocks (MoEPs) [15, 21]. When the motor nerve trunk or motor nerve is targeted for neurolysis, all of the muscles innervated by that nerve trunk or nerve will be affected by the block. Motor branch blocks are more selective than nerve trunk blocks and can allow targeting of specific muscles and/or fascicles with MoEP targeting being the most selective E-Stim localization technique. E-Stim localization can help guide the injector to the selected level of neurolysis, from broad nerve trunk blocks of multiple muscles to MoEP blocks resulting in focal treatment of a muscle or muscle fascicle. E-Stim is similarly helpful when performing BoNT chemoneurolysis in muscle targets.

E-Stim guidance for neurolysis or BoNT chemodenervation procedures requires either a small hand-held stimulator (Fig. 2c, d) or an electrodiagnostic instrument (Fig. 2a), ground and reference electrodes, and insulated injecting needle electrodes of a length appropriate for the estimated muscle or nerve depth and the trajectory of the needle insertion.

When using E-Stim) guidance to determine the best site for needle insertion, physicians typically use published information for muscle anatomy from reference guides, nerves from anatomy texts or atlases, and MoEPs from published studies/information (see section in this chapter on MoEP targeting) [5, 6, 8]. The area of the body to be injected is then exposed to reveal the region of interest and the patient positioned to allow access to this region.

Proper positioning typically requires the assistance of other staff, especially in patients who have significant spasticity, involuntary movements, or ROM limitations as well as in those who have difficulty cooperating or following directions. If many muscles are to be injected, the patient should be carefully repositioned to optimize each injection site. Once the patient is positioned, the reference and ground electrodes are placed; the injection needle serves as the active electrode. With the site for needle insertion identified, the skin is cleaned or disinfected using the physician or institution's standard protocol and the needle is inserted through the skin and advanced toward the target. US guidance can be used in combination with E-stim to allow continuous visualization and to avoid blind insertion. When the physician estimates (or visualizes with US) that the needle is near the nerve or within the muscle target, the stimulator is turned on starting at a low intensity. The intensity of stimulation for intramuscular injection is gradually increased until there is a visible muscle twitch or joint movement, typically at an intensity of 1–3 mA. The needle can be maneuvered so that successive reductions in stimulation intensity continue to produce a maximum twitch in the desired muscle. Once the needle is in the proper position, the injection then proceeds. If the needle is not at the desired target, it is then advanced, redirected, or repositioned and stimulation repeated until positioning is correct. When performing motor point blocks, the stimulation intensity required has been reported to be at 0.25–0.5 mA [15]. If upon stimulation, contraction occurs in several muscles or a muscle other than the target, the clinician should reposition the needle to isolate the target muscle. Care must be taken to avoid overstimulation which may lead to volume conduction and false localization.

Advantages

1. E-Stim produces a direct visual feedback via muscle twitch and/or joint movement confirming that the needle is likely to be within the target muscle.
    - E-Stim provides more reliable information about the location of the needle than voluntary contraction, especially in patients where co-contraction, mass synergy, or impaired motor control) limit their ability to isolate a muscle for contraction, thereby limiting the utility of EMG.
    - E-Stim can be used when patients are sedated, whereas the EMG is attenuated or absent with sedation.
2. E-Stim can be used to isolate thin muscles (e.g., rectal sphincter) which may be difficult to isolate with EMG.
3. E-Stim may be helpful in isolating deep or overlapping muscles where it is difficult to palpate the muscle or estimate its precise location or depth.
4. Studies have shown that E-Stim is more accurate than manual needle placement [22, 23].

Disadvantages

1. *Inadequate familiarity with E-Stim procedures and E-Stim/EMG equipment*: The use of E-stim requires training for safety and proper use of the equipment. Inexpensive units are widely available, so that cost is not a major limiting factor. Performing E-Stim correctly also requires a certain amount of skill to avoid localization errors. Localization errors with E-stim may occur through;

(a) *Volume conduction*: When excessive current is used by turning the stimulator intensity up too high, the area or zone of depolarization is enlarged. This may lead to stimulation of and twitch in a muscle distant from the stimulating needle electrode. In this situation, the physician may falsely conclude that the needle electrode is in the target muscle when it is located outside of the muscle or in another muscle. Such false localization may lead to an unwarranted conclusion of treatment failure or the need to increase toxin dose, weakness in an untargeted muscle, and/or other adverse events.
(b) *Placement by a nerve*: When the stimulating needle electrode is outside the target muscle but adjacent to the motor nerve branch innervating the muscle, stimulation will lead to a visible twitch even though the needle tip is outside of the intended muscle target for injection.

2. *Pain and prolonged procedure*: The current from electrical stimulation can be quite painful. Pain is minimized by using the lowest stimulation intensity required to produce a twitch in the muscle, typically not exceeding 3mAmp [15, 24]. The use of E-stim can prolong procedure time compared to manual placement or EMG ([18, 19, 23, 25]; Alter et al. 2010).
3. *Possible need for sedation*: Most, if not all children, will require sedation which increases the;

   (a) Risk of the procedure especially in medically fragile patients.
   (b) Time and cost of the chemodenervation or neurolysis procedure.
   (c) Time away from school or work for the patient and/or family members/caregivers

Caveats: The current level of evidence suggests that E-Stim is more accurate than EMG, particularly when treating patients with spasticity or generalized dystonia. E-Stim is required for all nerve blocks and neurolytic procedures and can be combined with US to further increase the accuracy of muscle or nerve targeting.

Motor End Plate Targeting or Localization Technique

BoNTs exert their action in muscle at the neuromuscular junction, found at the motor end plate (MoEP). Therefore, physicians and researchers have questioned, suggested, and investigated whether MoEP targeting can increase toxin uptake into the target muscle and hence the clinical efficacy or, by being provided at the site of action, reduce the required effective dose of BoNT [26–29]. The location of MoEP or end plate zones in animal models and in humans has been studied both by histochemical staining and electrophysiological methods [28, 30–32]. Coers described three arrangements of MoEP in human muscles: (1) a single innervation band, (2) multiple innervation bands, and (3) innervation bands scattered throughout the muscle [31]. Christensson reported that the MoEP in stillborn infants were arranged as a single transverse band at the midpoint of unipennate muscles and in a concave band in bipennate muscles such as the gastrocnemius [30].

More recent anatomical studies detail the location of MoEP in various lower and upper limb muscles [21, 29, 33–35]. In particular:

- *Posterior calf muscles*: In the medial and lateral gastrocnemius and soleus muscles, Kim et al. reported that the MoEPs are arranged along the length of the muscle with the most;
  - Proximal MoEPs in the medial gastrocnemius, lateral gastrocnemius, and soleus at 9.6% (+/– 3.5%), 12.0% (+/– 3.4%), and 20.5% (+/– 3.9%) of calf/leg length, respectively [34].
  - Distal MoEP were reportedly located at 37.5% (+/– 5.5%), 37.9% (+/–2.3%), and 46.7% (+/– 3.6%) of lower limb length, respectively [34].
- *Biceps brachii*: MoEP are arranged in the muscle in an inverted V [33] with the MoEP zone location in cm and as a ratio of olecranon-acromion length as follows;
  - 1 cm in width
  - 7 cm proximal to the olecranon, laterally with a MoEP zone ratio of 0.25
  - 11 cm proximal to the olecranon, midline with a MoEP zone ratio of 0.39
  - 8 cm proximal to the olecranon, medially with a MoEP zone ration of 0.28
- *Psoas Muscle*: In a 2010 cadaver study, Van Campenhaut et al. published information on the number, location, and distribution of MoEP in the psoas muscle of adult cadavers.
  - The psoas muscle was made up of converging muscle fibers of variable lengths
  - An average of 3.7 (range 2–7) nerve branches from the lumbar plexus innervated the psoas muscle along its length.
  - That the majority of MoEPs were located proximal to the sacral promontory and were distributed between 30.83%–70.25% of the distance from T12 to the inguinal ligament [35].

MoEP targeting procedure for BoNT injections: MoEP targeting techniques generally require EMG, E-Stim, or US guidance methods and include;

- The use of published reference data on motor point location and/or distribution combined with anatomic, EMG, E-Stim, or US guidance for BoNT injections.
- With EMG, the location of the needle at the MoEP is identified by hearing the distinctive sound referred to as endplate noise and injecting toxin in this zone/location [26].
- If using a diagnostic EMG unit with a visual display, MoEPs can be targeted by adjusting the needle position within the muscle until the initial deflection of all the motor unit action potentials recorded by the needle electrode is negative [36].
- If using E-Stim, MoEP are targeted by repositioning the needle and reducing the stimulation intensity until the maximal visible muscle twitch is present with minimal intensity [21].
- While the resolution of current US transducers does not allow direct visualization of MoEPs, US can be used to place the needle accurately in the zone of the published location of MoEPs in the target muscle [37].

Advantages of MoEP Targeting

1. *Ease of use*: MoEP targeting is easily incorporated into BoNT procedures regardless of what other guidance technique used in addition to anatomic localization.
2. *Ease of localization*: The published information on the location and distribution of MoEPs in many commonly targeted muscles are easily accessed.
3. *Potential increased benefit*: Studies suggest that utilizing MoEP targeting may reduce the required effective dose and/or improve outcome following BoNT injections [21, 29].

Limitations of MoEP Targeting

1. Lack of data on MoEPs: Maps of the location and distribution of MoEP are not available for all muscles
2. Longer procedure: Utilizing electrophysiological means of MoEP targeting (EMG, E-Stim) may increase the time required to perform the BoNT injection procedure.
3. Lack of applicability for all BoNT uses: MoEP targeting cannot be used for non-muscle targets.

Caveats: MoEP targeting may be a useful addition to traditional guidance techniques, resulting in improved outcomes and reducing the required effective dose. Many clinicians advocate for or recommend using MoEP targeting for BoNT injections [21, 26, 27, 38], but the data comparing other targeting techniques with and without the use of MoEP is limited.

Imaging-Based Guidance

Fluoroscopy and Computerized axial tomography (CT): While fluoroscopy and CT have occasionally been reported as an option to guide chemodenervation procedures [39–45], the use of these techniques is limited by;

- *Inconvenience*: Inconvenient access to and cost of the radiographic imaging equipment may take these procedures out of the office, making them unfeasible for most BoNT injections.
- *Cost and time*: These procedures add substantial cost and time to chemodenervation procedure
- *Repeated exposure to ionizing radiation*: Given that chemodenervation sessions are frequently repeated at 3–4 month intervals over years, the risks associated with repeated exposure to ionizing radiation are significant, especially in children.

Ultrasound (US): US is the most common imaging-based guidance technique for chemodenervation procedures including BoNT. Its increasing use is related to a number of factors including;

- *Convenience*: The portability, accessibility, and relatively low cost of US equipment, making office US feasible
- *Safety*: US does not expose patients to ionizing radiation. There are no identified safety concerns with frequent or repeated exposure to muscle or other US for chemodenervation.
- *Cost*: US entails lower cost when compared with fluoroscopy or CT guidance
- *Patient comfort*: US entails minimal patient discomfort. Patients quickly become familiar with US and readily accept its use.

Ultrasound Guidance for Chemodenervation Procedures

In the last decade, the development of small portable US machines, high frequency linear transducers, physician familiarity/training, and the recognized utility of US for procedural guidance has increased the use of US guidance for invasive interventions including chemodenervation procedures [19, 39, 40, 42, 46–56]. US has an advantage over electrodiagnostic techniques (EMG/E-stim) as it is useful not only for identifying muscle targets, but it can also be used for injections of BoNT into non-muscle targets such as salivary glands or prostate as well as for diagnostic or neurolytic nerve blocks [57, 48].

US guidance for chemodenervation procedures requires an ultrasound instrument (Fig. 2e, f), linear, curvilinear and/or specialty transducers (for prostate injections) of various frequencies (typically 3–17 MHz) (Fig. 2g), gel, transducer covers (if desired), hypodermic needles of various lengths (1–2.5 in., 30–25 g) as well as injection, equipment cleaning, and maintenance supplies. If combining US guidance with EMG or E-Stim, a portable EMG amplifier or combined portable EMG-E-Stim unit, insulated injecting needle electrodes of various lengths, and associated supplies are also required. Additional information on US equipment can be found below.

Basic physics for US Scanning: The following section provides a brief review of US physics and imaging. For additional information, readers are referred to several book chapters or articles which review these topics in more detail [39–42, 49, 58].

Piezoelectric Crystals

The high-resolution images obtained with US scanning are made possible by piezoelectric crystals, devices which are responsible for converting electrical pulses into mechanical vibrations and vice-versa. Piezoelectric crystals are placed into arrays within a transducer, the device used for US scanning. When the transducer is placed in contact with the patient, some of the mechanical vibrations or sound waves generated by the piezoelectric crystals are transmitted through the patient's skin. These sound waves are then transmitted through superficial tissues and on to deeper structures within the body where they are either scattered, refracted, or reflected at tissue interfaces. Those mechanical sound waves reflected back to the transducer are then converted back to electrical pulses by the piezoelectric crystals, transmitted to the US machine, and processed into real-time grey scale images visualized on the display screen using a time-distance co-efficient [58].

Transducer/Ultrasound Frequency

The frequency of the sound waves generated by the piezoelectric crystals within the transducer determines image resolution and the depth of penetration of the generated US waves. The frequency of the sound waves emitted by a given transducer thus determines the structures that can be visualized when scanning. High-frequency sound waves (12–18 MHz) have a higher sampling rate permitting improved lateral resolution and thus better discrimination of adjacent structures. However, while higher US frequency provides better resolution, this is at the expense of reduced depth of penetration of the US waveforms. Soft tissues (muscles, adipose tissue, glands, etc.) absorb the high-frequency US waves, leaving fewer waveforms available to travel onto deeper structures compromising imaging of these deep structures. Lower frequency (3–5 mHz) US waves travel through soft tissues, allowing them to penetrate to deeper structures, but the images created will have a lower resolution and appear grainer due to reduced lateral resolution. To at least partially mitigate these limitations, commercial US transducers all emit a mix of sound wave frequencies (15-4, 5-3 MHz etc.), which allows imaging of tissues at various depths [41, 58]. However, it remains important that the sonographer chose a transducer with the frequencies providing adequate visualization of the target and nearby structures in the region of interest.

Sonoacoustic Properties of Tissues

The impedance of and speed of sound waves in tissues determines their sonoacoustic appearance, i.e., echogenicity or US appearance (Figs. 1a, b, 3a, 4a–c, 5a, b, 6a, b, and 7). When sound waves travel through the body and encounter tissue interfaces of differing acoustic impedances, sound waves are reflected, refracted, or scattered off these interfaces [58, 59]. If only a few sound waves are reflected back to the transducer, then the image on the screen will be dark or hypoechoic (Figs. 1a, b and 3a). If a tissue interface is highly reflective of US, then most of the waveforms are reflected back to the transducer and the image will appear bright or hyperechoic (Figs. 1a, b and 3a). Tissues with higher water content are relatively hypoechoic. Those with low water content and those with a higher content of fibro-connective tissue or calcium (bone cortex) will appear hyperechoic [59] (Figs. 1a, b and 3a). Sound wave cannot penetrate all tissue types, for example bone, and therefore structures deep to these tissues cannot be visualized with US. This is one of several

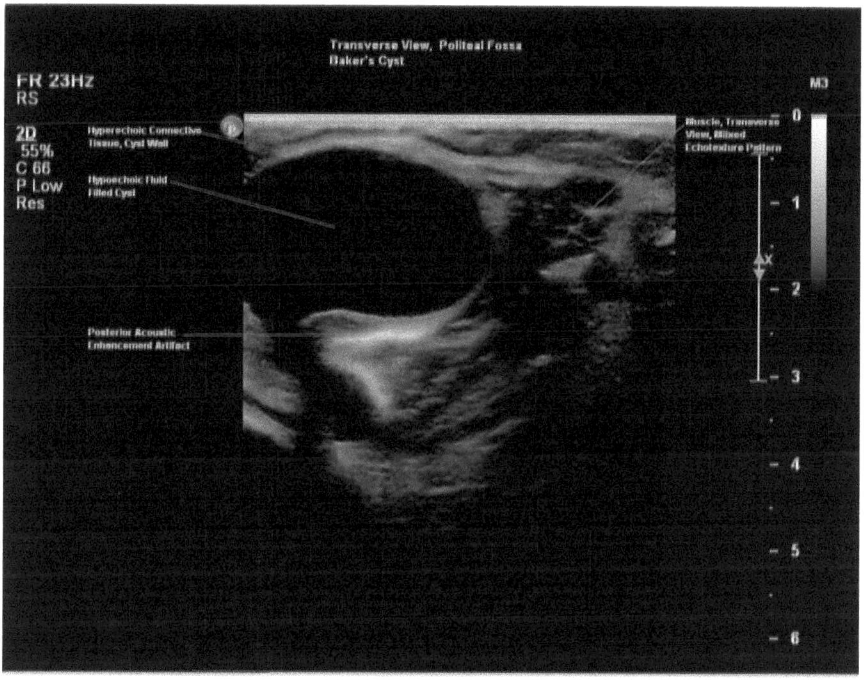

Fig. 3 Transverse ultrasound image popliteal fossa, Baker's cyst with posterior acoustic enhancement

important imaging issues or artifacts that are encountered with US imaging which include;

- *Posterior acoustic shadow*; as noted above, this artifact occurs when US waves encounter a tissue that reflects all of the sound waves (bone, metal) preventing the US from travelling through this tissue and onto tissues below the structure. The reflection of all the sound waves by these US mirror like structures leads to an anechoic area or shadow deep to these tissues [41, 58, 59] (Fig. 1b).
- *Posterior acoustic enhancement*; this artifact is encountered when imaging a tissue that is located deep to a fluid-filled structure, such as a cyst or full urinary bladder. In this circumstance, the majority of the sound waves encounter minimal or no resistance and travel through the fluid-filled structure and then onto the deeper tissues. As a result, more of the sound waves reach the deeper structures, making the deeper tissues underlying fluid-filled structures appear artifactually bright or hyperechoic [41, 58, 59] (Fig. 3b). When performing fetal US, obstetricians take advantage of this fluid artifact and scan the fetus through a full bladder which enhances visualization of the fetus
- *Anisotropy*; is a characteristic of some types of tissue (including tendons and nerves) whereby the appearance of the tissue on US is affected by the incidence angle of sound waves relative to the tissue [58]. When US waves are perpendicular to a tendon, the tendon fibers will appear highly echogenic or hyperechoic.

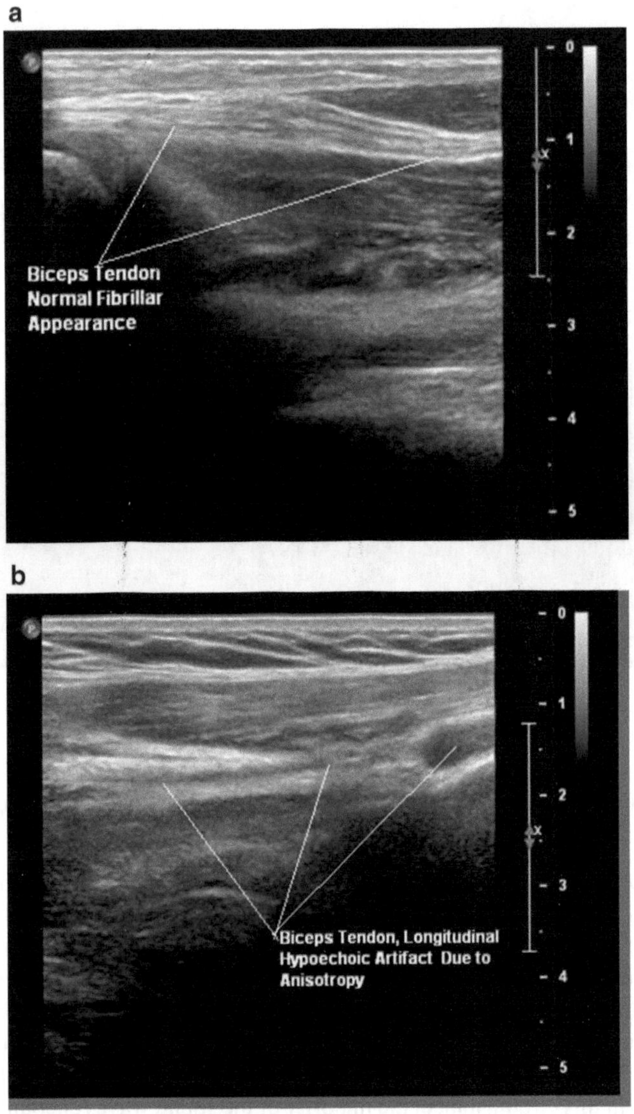

Fig. 4 Longitudinal view, biceps tendon. (**a**) Normal tendon appearance, (**b**) artifactually hypoechoic appearance of tendon due to anisotropy

If the same structure is imaged with the transducer positioned where the incidence angle of the sound waves is at less than 90°, the structure will appear artifactually hypoechoic (Figs. 4a and 5b). This artifact is important when performing diagnostic US because an inexperienced clinician may conclude that a hypoechoic tendon represents a partial or full thickness tear of a tendon when in reality the structure is intact and only appeared hypoechoic because it was not

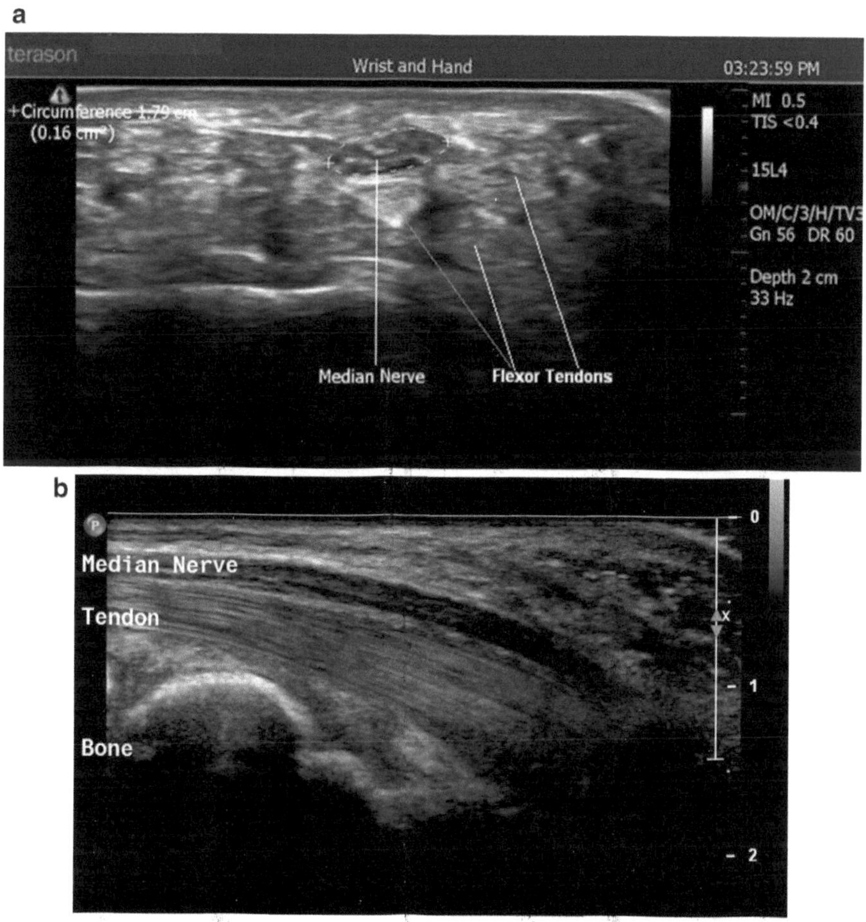

Fig. 5 Distinguishing nerve from tendon using anisotropy. (**a**) Transverse view, (**b**) longitudinal view

imaged at 90°. Anisotropy is useful, however, as it can be used to help distinguish various tissues from one another. For example, nerves which are less anisotropic can be differentiated from tendons which are highly anisotropic (Fig. 5a, b).

As noted above, tissues are described by their sonoacoustic properties including their internal echo-texture and relative echogenicity. Most organs and structures in the human body are comprised of several tissue types, for example, a muscle is comprised of the surrounding fascia (highly echogenic/hyperechoic), contractile elements/fascicles (hypoechoic), and intramuscular connective tissue/tendons (hyperechoic) (Figs. 1a and 6a, b). In contrast to muscle, glandular tissues such as salivary gland or thyroid are homogenous in composition, with a resulting uniform grey-scale echotexture sonoacoustic appearance with US imaging [58, 59] (Fig. 7).

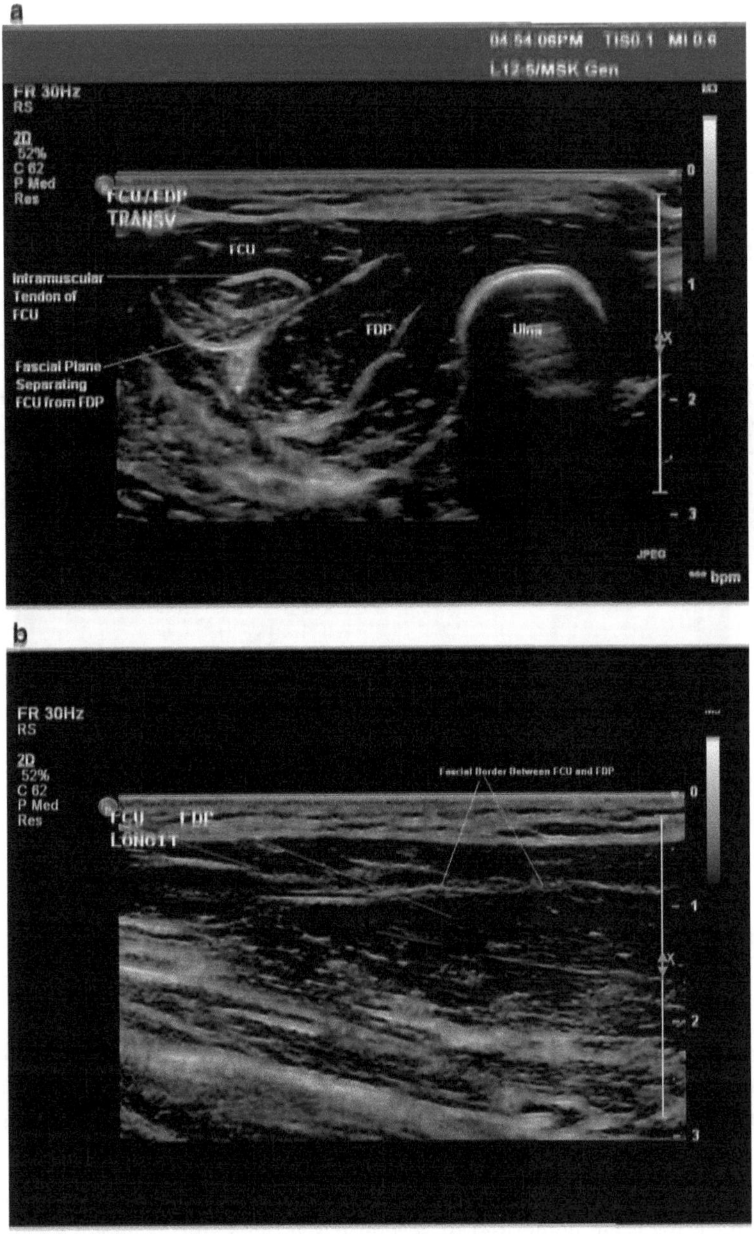

Fig. 6 Sonoacoustic appearance of muscle. (**a**) Transverse view, (**b**) longitudinal view

The appearance of some tissues, like muscle or nerve, will vary with the scanning plane, i.e., in whether the transducer is placed longitudinally vs. transversely on the skin over the structure. For example, when scanned with the transducer placed parallel to the longitudinal plane of the muscle, muscle has the appearance of long, thin, hypoechoic bands (contractile fascicles) that are surrounded by or

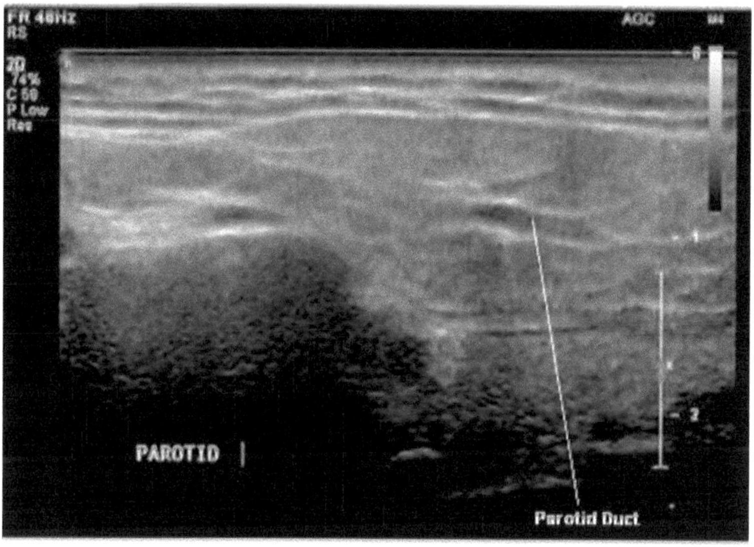

Fig. 7 Sonoacoustic property of parotid gland

interspersed with linear hyperechoic bands (non-contractile fibro-connective tissue/intramuscular tendons) (Fig. 6b). In contrast, in a transverse view, muscles have a speckled appearance, representing the internal mix of hypoechoic contractile fascicles and hyperechoic and hyperechoic intramuscular connective tissue (Figs. 1a, b and 6a). On B-mode scans, blood vessels will appear hypoechoic, tendons are highly echogenic/hyperechoic and fibrillar, whereas nerves have a more mixed hyperechoic, hypoechoic appearance [59] (Figs. 5a, b and 6b).

US Procedural Guidance Techniques for BoNT Injections: As with other instrumented guidance techniques, an US-guided BoNT procedure begins with a physical examination, including evaluation of muscle tone and a functional assessment, external inspection of the body part to be treated (including skin integrity), palpation, PROM and AROM to identify which are the optimal targets for injection. The area of the body to be scanned/injected is then exposed to reveal the region of interest and the patient positioned to allow access to this region. Proper positioning typically requires the assistance of other staff, especially for patients who have significant spasticity, involuntary movements, or ROM limitations as well as for those who have difficulty cooperating or following directions. The patient and the examination or treatment room should be set up in a manner that permits the injector to access both the patient and US machine controls and transducers, with an unobstructed view of the US screen. The room may need to be darkened so that the screen images can be seen more easily.

Once the US machine is turned on, the patient data is entered (this is required on most machines in order for still or video cine-loops to be saved). Most machines have preset parameters for imaging different tissues or body territories. Before staring the US examination, the injector should assure that the correct machine preset is selected, such as that for musculoskeletal, gland, or nerve. This is accompanied by selection of the most appropriate transducer for scanning the region of interest (which should be the transducer of the highest frequency which provides an adequate field of view/depth). The sonographer must adjust various machine settings to optimize imaging including [49] adjustment of the

- Scanning Mode: B or Brightness Mode, Color Doppler, Power Doppler.
- Depth.
- Number of and position of focal zones.
- Overall gain.

B-mode and Color Doppler are the most commonly used scanning modes for US-guided chemodenervation procedures. B-mode scanning provides real-time grey scale images of structures and continuous visualization of the

- Target.
- Structures to be avoided.
- Needle.
- Toxin or other injectate as it is injected.

Color Doppler is useful in identifying blood vessels in the field of view, differentiating arteries from veins and in discriminating vessels from large nerve trunks so as to avoid these non-targets when inserting the needle and directing it into the muscle (Fig. 8a, b).

After cleaning the transducer, gel is applied to the transducer to reduce impedance to sound waves at the air/skin interface, thereby enhancing sound transmission through the skin. The transducer, with an adequate layer of gel, is placed in contact with the patient's skin and the sonographer scans the region of interest in transverse and longitudinal imaging planes (Fig. 9a, b) to determine the depth, location, and safest path to the target. The US beam emitted from the transducer is only 1–2 mm wide, approximately the width of a credit card and therefore only a small slice of the region of interest is visualized if the transducer remains in a static position [41, 58]. To scan the entire region of interest (including the target, structures to be avoided, and path to the target) the entire region must be scanned thoroughly by dynamic imaging. This is accomplished by using different scanning planes/transducer orientations and by moving the transducer in various directions over the region of interest.

Muscles are identified based on their position in the body (based on an understanding of anatomy), and based on their unique pattern, i.e., recognition of each muscle's characteristic shape, contour lines and relationship to identifiable nearby structures such as bones, nerves, vessels, or other muscles (Figs. 1a, b and 6a, b). Identification of muscles on US can often also be verified by observing muscle contraction on US with voluntary contraction by the patient, for those who are able to selectively activate muscles.

Once the muscle's or target's position and depth have been identified, the physician chooses the most appropriate needle and injection technique. There are two techniques for needle insertion when utilizing US guidance; in-plane (Fig. 10a) or

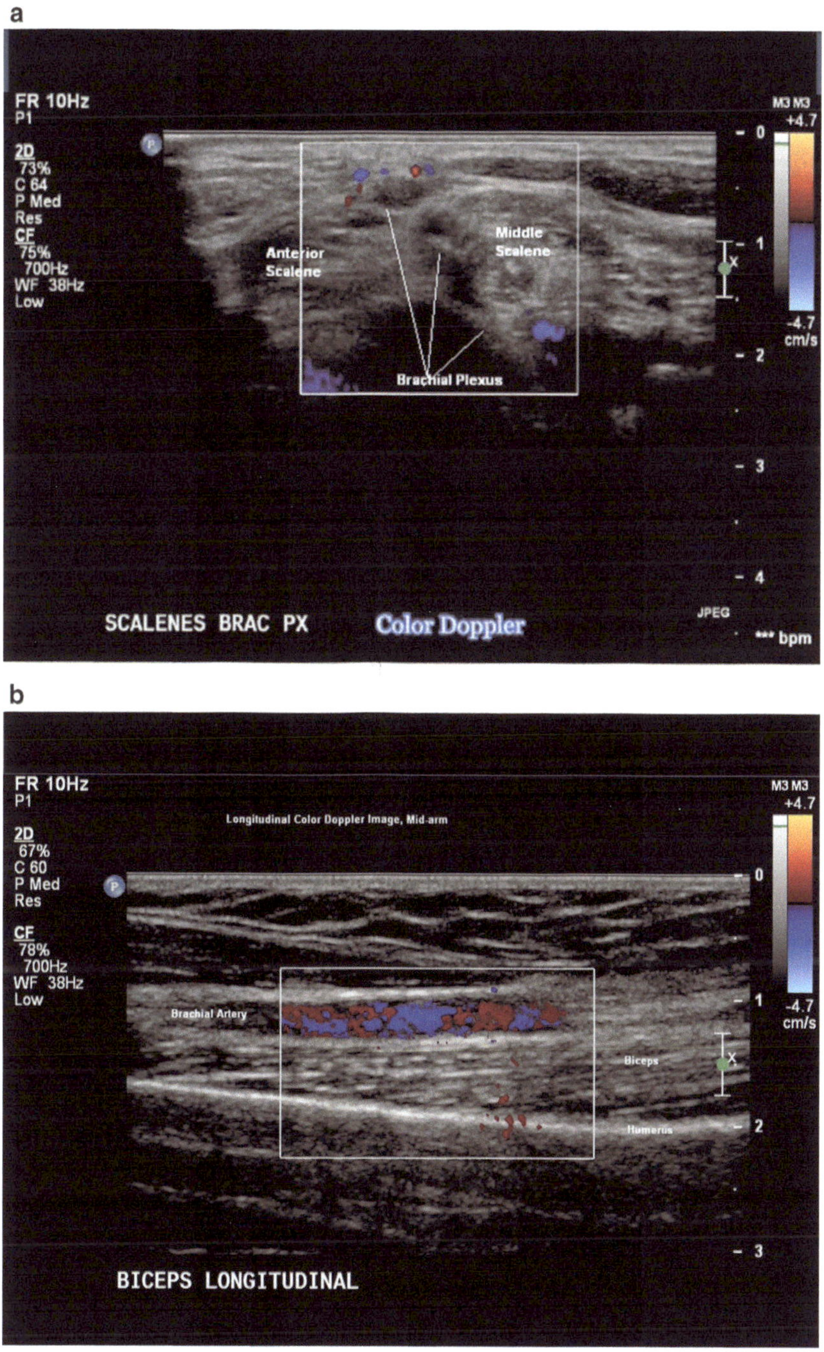

Fig. 8 (**a**) Transverse Color Doppler images inter-scalene triangle, (**b**) longitudinal Color Doppler image, mid-arm, brachial artery, biceps muscle

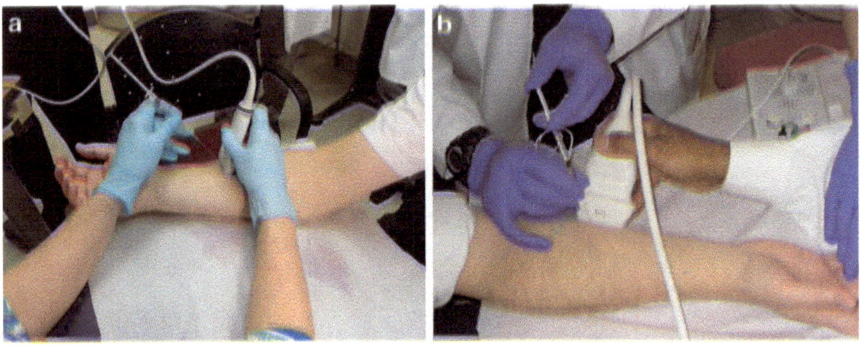

Fig. 9 (**a**) Transverse view, forearm, in plane needle view, (**b**) longitudinal limb view, out of plane needle view

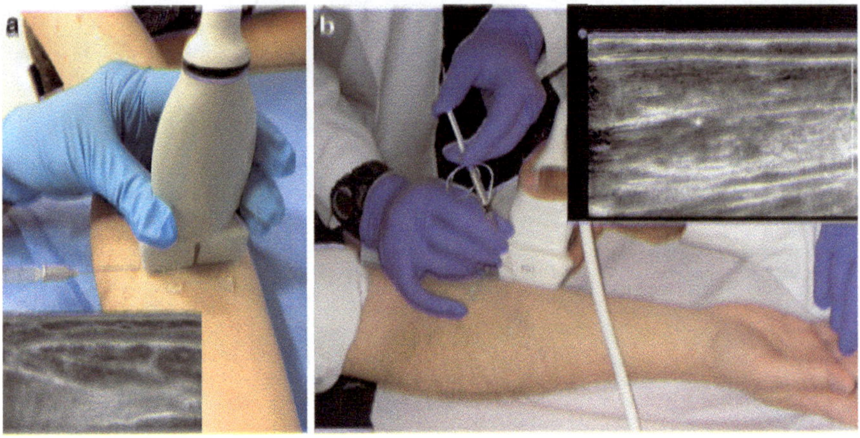

Fig. 10 (**a**) Transverse US view, flexor forarm. In plane view of needle. (**b**) Longitudinal view, flexor digitorum superficialis. Out of plane view of needle

out-of-plane (Fig. 10b) [60]. For the in-plane technique, the needle is inserted down the length of the transducer and the entire needle, including the needle tip, is visualized (Fig. 10a). In contrast, when using an out-of-plane technique, the needle is inserted across the short axis of the transducer and the needle is scanned in cross-section and therefore is visualized as a hyperechoic dot (Fig. 10b). Since the entire needle is scanned in cross section, it appears on the screen as a hyperechoic dot along its entire length, including the tip. Because the entire needle cannot be visualized when using an out-of-plane technique, physicians must use a "walk-down" technique to track the needle to the target [37, 41, 42, 60]. This is accomplished by inserting the needle through the skin, then advancing the needle in very small, brief rapid increments, similar to the technique used when listening for insertional activity during a diagnostic EMG. When using the walk-down technique, the physician should closely observe the movement of the needle through the tissues as it passes from superficial to deep. Once the target muscle or structure is reached, the toxin is injected. To distribute the toxin throughout the muscles or targets, the needle may be repositioned under US guidance to allow for multiple injection sites.

Equipment: Performing US-guided BoNT injections requires an US machine. Machines are available with a range of features, resolution, and portability (Fig. 2e, f). A portable US machine is sufficient for most office-based chemodenervation procedures. If possible, a variety of linear or curvilinear transducers should be available to accommodate imaging the few range of muscles and structures that may require injection. Linear or curvilinear 5-3 MHz transducers are used for the most deeply situated muscles, transducers with a frequency range of 12-5 MHz are used for less deeply seated muscles, and 18-7 MHz transducers are utilized for the most superficial muscles or structures, as well as when scanning small, thin children. A hockey stick linear transducer with a small footprint is frequently best for imaging irregular surfaces such as the hand, in small patients, and for salivary gland injections.

Other supplies for scanning include ultrasound gel (sterile, non-sterile), sterile transducer covers if needed, a manufacturer's approved transducer cleaner, and tissues or towels to remove the gel after the procedure is completed. The use of sterile transducer covers is typically reserved for sterile procedures such as joint injections (including BoNTs) and for joint aspirations. There is no standard recommendation for the use of a non-sterile transducer cover when performing chemodenervation procedures. While some physicians use non-sterile transducer covers for all injections, others rarely or never use these covers when performing chemodenervation procedures [17, 40].

Supplies for injection included syringes, hypodermic needles of narrow gauge, and various lengths. If performing simultaneous US and EMG or E-Stim, then monopolar-insulated injection electrodes, surface needles, surface electrodes, and an EMG machine, EMG amplifier, or E-Stim unit are also required. It is important to note that alcohol-based products must be avoided when cleaning US transducers as these products will damage the transducer membrane and void the product warranty [37, 49].

Advantages and Limitations of US to Guide BoNT Injections

There are a number of advantages and disadvantages or limitations to the use of US guidance for chemodenervation procedures including BoNT injections [17, 37, 39, 41, 42].

Advantages

- US provides a detailed view of the location and depth of the target, structures to be avoided, and the safest path to injection target to avoid penetration or injection of un-intended targets.
- It also allows the needle to be tracked to the target and visual confirmation of the location of the injectate.

- During the procedure, the volume of injectate can be visualized and needle position adjusted to prevent excessive volume administration at any one site.
- When performed by an experienced clinician, US may speed localization of the target.
- US scanning is painless and requires no ionizing radiation.
- Standard hypodermic needles may be used for US-guided procedures, which may be less painful than insulated monopolar-injecting electrodes.
- Watching the US screen provides a helpful distraction during the procedure for some patients.
- Pediatric patients may require no sedation for US-guided BoNT procedures.

Disadvantages of US Guidance for BoNT Injections

- US machines may be costly, which may be a barrier to acquire this equipment.
- The hands-on training required to become proficient in US-guided chemodenervation procedures may be inaccessible, expensive, or require time away from one's medical practice.
- There may be a steep learning curve when learning US guidance skills and pattern recognition of the relevant structures.
- Until one becomes proficient, the use of US may increase the time required for these procedures.
- While US provides very accurate information about the location of the target and position of the needle, it generally does not provide information on the activity level of a muscle target and therefore whether it is contributing to the patient's disability and requires injection. US may need to be combined with EMG to provide the information related to muscle activity.
- US guidance alone is not adequate for nerve or motor point blocks. US used with E-Stim is recommended for these procedures [48].

Caveats: Of the available guidance techniques for chemodenervation procedures, US guidance provides the most anatomically correct information about the location, depth of the target, structures to be avoided, and the safest path to the target.

Guidance Techniques for BoNT Procedures, What Is the Evidence?

Studies Comparing Guidance Techniques

There are a limited number of large and well-controlled trials comparing head-to-head the accuracy or efficacy of all of the available guidance techniques. However, there is an increasing body of literature from high-quality controlled and blinded trials comparing the accuracy and/or efficacy of two or three of the available techniques. All studies, to date, which compared the accuracy of needle placement or outcomes of chemodenervation procedures concluded that procedures guided solely by anatomic means are less accurate and/or less effective than when instrumented guidance techniques of EMG, E-Stim, or US are utilized. The following is a selective review of the available studies:

- *Anatomic guidance vs. EMG for Limb Muscles*: A 2013 randomized controlled trial (RCT) of 27 adult patients with spasticity from an upper motor neuron syndrome (brain injury or spinal cord injury) compared the efficacy of BoNT injections in upper and lower limb muscles guided by anatomic landmarks to injections with EMG guidance [20]. Outcome measures included spasticity rated using the Modified Ashworth Scale (MAS) and a functional outcome assessment using the Modified Barthel Index. Although spasticity and function were improved in all subjects, the degree of improvement in both outcome measures was lower in the group where the injections were based on only anatomic guidance. The authors concluded that EMG guidance was superior to anatomic guidance for BoNT procedures in limb muscles. A 2002 study of adults with focal hand dystonia study compared the accuracy of needle placement by either EMG or anatomic techniques. The authors concluded that EMG was superior to anatomic methods in assuring injection into selected muscles [2].
- *Anatomic Guidance vs. EMG for Cervical Dystonia*: A 2016 RCT compared the outcome of injections using EMG guidance to injections based on palpation for adult patients with cervical dystonia (CD) [61]. The patients in the group receiving injections guided by EMG had a greater improvement in the primary endpoint, Tsui score for CD, at 16 weeks. No between-group differences were noted in their secondary endpoints of pain on a visual analog scale (VAS) or on other secondary endpoints including the Hospital Anxiety and Depression Scale (HADS) and the Clinical and Patient Global Impression of Change (CGIC and PGIC). When comparing adverse events, the group injected with EMG guidance had significantly more injection site pain, but, importantly, significantly lower incidence of dysphagia than the palpation guidance group.
- *Anatomic guidance vs. E-Stim*: A 2009 study in children with hemiplegic or diplegic CP compared the efficacy of BoNT injections guided either by palpation or E-Stim. At 3 months, patients who had injections guided by E-Stim had a statistically greater reduction in MAS scores and Composite Spasticity Scale scores and greater improvement in PROM and Gross Motor Function Measure (GMFM) than patients injected using manual guidance alone [62]. A 2005 study of 226 children with CP investigated the accuracy of manual needle for BoNT injections for 1376 needle insertions in upper and lower limb muscles [22]. Surface anatomy, depth estimated by limb size, and PROM were used for manual placement of the needle. Following manual placement, the position was evaluated using E-Stim with the inserted needle to see whether the muscle that twitched was the target or another muscle. The accuracy of manual placement was as follows: gastrocnemius-soleus 78%, hip adductors 67%, medial hamstrings 46%, tibialis posterior 11%, biceps brachii 62%, pronator teres 22%, flexor carpi radialis (FCR) 13%, flexor carpi ulnaris (FCU) 16%, and adductor pollicis 35%. Thus, the authors concluded that manual placement was adequately

accurate only in the gastrocnemius. They postulated that inaccurate muscle targeting could be responsible, at least in part, for a lack of insufficient clinical response following BoNT injections in children with CP.

- *Anatomic placement checked by ultrasound in limb muscles*: All of the studies, to date, comparing the accuracy and/or efficacy of manual needle placement to US guidance have concluded that US guidance is more accurate in limb muscles [54, 56]. The reported accuracy of manual placement in children with CP ranged from 46–64% in the lateral and 87–93% in the medial gastrocnemius [56], leading authors of the latter study to conclude that supplementary localization techniques should be considered for the medial gastrocnemius muscle in younger patients and for the lateral gastrocnemius for all patients. In another 2009 study of 54 children with CP, the authors evaluated the effect of a number of variables on the efficacy of lower limb BoNT procedures. The authors reported a greater efficacy of injections guided by US when patients were younger than 6 years of age or older than 12 years of age and when the hamstrings or gastrocnemii were targeted. The authors concluded that their study confirmed the usefulness of US guidance for BoNT injections in lower limb muscles [54].
- *Manual placement, E-Stim, and Ultrasound*: A 2012 RCT evaluated the efficacy of a fixed dose and dilution of onabotulinum toxinA in the gastrocnemius muscle of 49 adult patients with PSS comparing three localization techniques, manual/anatomic placement, E-Stim, and US [19]. At 4 weeks after injection, the US guidance group had a greater reduction in MAS scale score than the manual guidance group. The US group also had a greater increase in PROM when compared with the E-Stim and manual injection groups. There was no significant difference in the Tardieu Scale score between the three groups. The authors concluded that, for PSS in the gastrocnemius muscles, US guidance for BoNT provided both a greater reduction in spasticity and greater clinical benefit than injections guided with manual needle placement or E-Stim.
- *Identifying Muscle Fascicle Location by Anatomic Reference Guides compared to US Localization*: A 2010 study of patients with forearm flexor muscle spasticity assessed the location of forearm muscles and of individual muscle fascicles. The authors used published anatomic reference guides to estimate the location of the muscle or muscle fascicles and then identified the actual muscle or fascicle position using US. There were significant differences between the estimated position of the muscle or muscle fascicles when compared to position visible on US for the flexor carpi radialis (FCR), flexor pollicis longus (FPL), and for fascicles of the flexor digitorum superficialis (FDS) [52].
- *EMG vs. Ultrasound for Cervical Dystonia*: In a 2012 study, Hong et al. assessed the incidence of dysphagia following BoNT injections guided by EMG compared to those guided by US. The incidence of dysphagia was 34.7% in patients where the procedure was guided by EMG and 0% in the same patients when the procedure was guided by US [53].

Cadaver studies assessing the accuracy of anatomic guidance for injections or manual needle or wire placement using EMG surface anatomy reference guides

- *Anatomic guidance checked by dissection*: A 2012 study assessed the accuracy of palpation and surface landmarks to guide injections into the gastrocnemius muscles of 30 cadavers. Injections of ink, performed by 121 physicians, were followed by dissection [63]. The authors reported that 43% of the injections were within the target muscles and 57% of the injections were outside of the gastrocnemius, either in the soft tissue superficial to the muscle (19.8%) or in the soleus muscle deep to the target (37.2%).
- A 2011 masked study compared "blind" (anatomic) versus US placement of a wire into 14 lower limb muscles in fresh cadavers. Two clinicians (a resident with 6 months of EMG training and an attending physician with more than 10 years of EMG experience) performed the needle insertions. The accuracy was then verified by CT and assessed by a third clinician [64]. The overall accuracy with anatomic guidance was 39% (range 0–100%), while the accuracy for US guidance was 96% (range 50–100%). When using anatomic guidance, the only muscles where wire placement was 100% accurate were the tibialis anterior and short head of the biceps femoris. Using US guidance, the only muscle targeted with less than 100% accuracy of wire placement was the semitendinosus muscle. Unexpectedly, the accuracy of blind anatomic wire placement was 0% for needle insertions into semitendinosus, rectus femoris, and extensor hallicus longus. Interestingly, there was no significant difference in the accuracy of needle placement between the less experienced and more experienced clinician. The only significant difference between the two clinicians was that the trajectory of the wire path towards the target was more accurate in the experienced clinician.
- A 2003 study assessed the accuracy of wire placement during 263 insertions into 36 lower limb muscles using placement landmarks cited in three standard EMG anatomic reference books; those of Gieringer, Perotto, and Delagi. The wire insertions were performed by three physicians with varying degrees of EMG experience. The location was checked by anatomical dissection by an anatomist. The authors reported that 57% of wire insertions penetrated the target muscle, but that the tip of the wire was located in the target muscle in only 45% of attempts. There was significant variability in the accuracy of targeting for different muscles, ranging from 100% accuracy for vastus medialis to 0% for 12 attempts to place a wire in the hip flexors. The authors also studied the proximity of the wire to undesirable structures, with 17% of insertions either penetrating or passing within 5 mm of a nerve, tendon, artery, vein, or joint. The authors concluded that the accuracy of blind wire placement using EMG reference guides was quite variable and recommended that safer strategies be developed [51].

Systematic Reviews of Guidance Techniques for BoNT Injections

In recent years, several systematic reviews articles on chemodenervation specifically focused on guidance techniques or at least included information on them.

A 2016 systematic review of clinical trials reported on guidance techniques (anatomic, EMG, E-Stim, US techniques, motor end-plate targeting techinques), and toxin dilution [65] for limb spasticity injections. The authors identified 9 of 347 reported trials which met their inclusion criteria (all were RCTs comparing two or more BoNT injection techniques with use of similar doses of BoNT between groups; studies with adult participants (⩾16 years old) with upper and/or lower limb spasticity from various causes; studies with unrestricted methods of injection techniques which could include methods to localize, injection sites, use of different injectate volumes, selection of where to inject within muscles; English language studies). Injection methodology issues reviewed included injection localization technique, injection site selection, and injectate volume. The authors found level 1 evidence that US, EMG, and E-Stim are superior to manual needle placement (greater decrease in Modified Ashworth Scale (MAS), improvement in Tardieu Scale (TS), increase in passive range of motion). They also concluded that endplate targeting improved outcomes (MAS, TS, active elbow range of motion) compared to multisite quadrant injections in the biceps brachii and that injections using motor point localization in the gastrocnemius were equivalent in efficacy (MAS, TS, clonus scale, ambulation measure) to injections distal to the motor endplate. In their review of the effects of dilution, the authors reported that using a high volume was not more effective than delivering the same dose in a smaller volume in flexor forearm muscles.

Another study evaluating the effect of volume on the outcomes (mean rectified voltage, MAS, TS, Active ROM) of injections in the biceps brachii found no effect of volume when the site of the injections was non-selective. A third study of BoNT-A injections in the biceps brachii reported that high volume injections that were distant from the motor endplates were more effective (mean rectified voltage, MAS, TS, Active ROM) than low volumes closer to the endplates. When comparing adverse events with the various guidance techniques, eight of the nine studies reviewed reported no adverse events. One of the cited studies [20] reported transient post-injection pain in two subjects, one subject each in the EMG and manual placement groups [65].

In 2015, Grigoui conducted a systematic review of the impact of guidance techniques (anatomic, EMG, E-Stim, and US) on the effectiveness of BoNT injection for spasticity and dystonia [66]. Seven of their ten reviewed studies were RCTs. The authors concluded that there was;

1. Level 1 evidence that instrumented guidance (EMG, E-Stim, US) was more effective than anatomic/manual needle placement for the treatment of cervical dystonia, upper limb spasticity, and spastic equinus in adults with post-stroke spasticity (PSS) and in children with cerebral palsy (CP).
2. Level 1 evidence from three studies showing similar effectiveness of E-Stim compared to US for upper and lower limb PSS and spastic equinus due to CP.
3. Level 2 evidence in focal hand dystonia (writer's cramp): that while injections under E-Stim guidance were more effective than those using EMG, EMG-guided injections were associated with fewer complaints of weakness in adjacent muscles.
4. Evidence from two studies supported that US-guided injections were more effective than those using E-Stim on two components of the Physician Rating Scale

(PRS) including gait pattern at 1 and 3 months post-treatment and hind-foot position at maximum foot or floor contact during stance at 3 months post-treatment in children with CP and on ankle PROM in adults with PSS.
5. In patients with PSS and children with equinus that there was poor evidence or no available evidence on injections with EMG or other instrumented techniques.

Based on their systematic review, the authors concluded that instrumented guidance for BoNT injections using E-Stim or US is strongly recommended for the treatment of spasticity in adults and children and additionally EMG for focal/cervical dystonia. US appears to be more effective than E-Stim for spastic equinus in adults with PSS.

In another 2015 article, (Walker et al. in 2015) the authors reviewed the available evidence for the impact of guidance techniques for BoNT injections including landmark-based anatomic guidance, EMG, E-Stim, and US. Based on their systematic review, the authors concluded that;

1. Anatomic guidance in children and adults was the least accurate method of guidance.
2. The available studies suggested that supplemental guidance with EMG, E-Stim, or US was all more accurate than anatomic guidance alone.

The authors also concluded that additional studies are required to determine which, if any, of the reviewed supplemental guidance techniques are the most accurate and/or lead to better clinical outcomes.

Consensus Statements and Practice Guidelines

In the 2016 American Academy of Neurology (AAN) Practice Guideline, Simpson et al. [70] reviewed the use of BoNT for various causes of muscle overactivity including blepharospasm, cervical dystonia, spasticity, and for headache. With regard to spasticity, the authors also reviewed reports of methods that aimed to optimize the response to BoNT, including dilution and guidance techniques. Based on their evidence-based systematic review of the data, the authors concluded that for upper limb spasticity, high volume/low potency injections and motor point guidance techniques were "probably effective" at enhancing tone reduction. When comparing E-Stim, EMG, and US, the authors found insufficient data to determine whether one technique was superior to another.

Wissel et al., in 2009, published the European consensus table for BoNT-A treatment of adult spasticity. The authors recommended that when the location of motor points is known, such as in the biceps brachii, this information should be used to target the injections into that muscle. The authors also concluded that when the sites of the motor points are not known or are known to be diffusely spread through the muscle, multiple injection sites should be considered. They noted that additional studies were required to determine the optimal localization method for BoNT chemodenervation procedures [67].

Heinen et al., in 2006, published the European consensus table for BoNT-A for pediatric patients. The authors recommended that injections in children should be performed using accurate localization techniques and that, in addition to the traditional methods of EMG and E-Stim, US could fine-tune localization of targets and would be painless [68].

Summary

Clinicians have a number of guidance techniques from which to choose when performing chemodenervation procedures including BoNT injections. Because of the limitations of and inaccuracy of relying solely on anatomic guidance for BoNT procedures, the majority of physicians now combine initial anatomic guidance with one of the available supplemental localization techniques, EMG, E-STIM, or US. The data from presently published studies indicates that US and E-Stim are superior to manual guidance in terms of accuracy and often in terms of outcome efficacy and also better than EMG for patients with upper motor neuron-related spasticity. The recognized advantages of US guidance over other instrumented techniques are that it provides direct visualization of the location and depth of the target, structures to be avoided, and infusion spread of the injectate. While US guidance provides the most anatomically accurate guidance method, additional studies comparing US to other instrumented techniques needed to determine or confirm whether its use provides additional advantages on, for example, improving efficacy or minimizing adverse effects.

References

1. Schwabe AL. Botulinum toxin in the treatment of pediatric upper limb spasticity. Semin Plast Surg. 2016;30(1):24–8.
2. Malloy FM, Shill HA, Kaelin-Lang A, Karp BI. Accuracy of muscle localization without EMG: implications for treatment of limb dystonia. Neurology. 2002;58(5):805–7.
3. Speelman JD, Brans JWM. Cervical dystonia and botulinum treatment: is electromyographic guidance necessary? Mov Disord. 1995;10:802.
4. Van Gerpen JA, Matsumoto JY, Ahlskog JE, Maraganore DM, McManis PG. Utility of an EMG mapping study in treating cervical dystonia. Muscle Nerve. 2000;23(11):1752–6.
5. Chu-Andrews J, Johnson RJ. Electrodiagnosis: a clinical and anatomic approach. Baltimore: J.B. Lippincott; 1986.
6. Delagi EF, Perotto AO, Daniel M. Anatomical guide for the electromyographer: the limbs and trunk. 5th ed. Springfield: Charles C Thomas; 2011.
7. Jost W, Klaus-Peter V. Pictorial atlas of botulinum toxin injection: dosage, localization, application. 1st ed. Hanover Park: Quintessence Publishing; 2009.
8. Lee J, DeLisa JA. Manual of nerve conduction study and surface anatomy for needle electromyography. Philadelphia: Lippincott Williams & Wilkins; 2004.
9. Walker HW, Lee MY, Bahroo LB, Hedera P, Charles D. Botulinum toxin injection techniques for the management of adult spasticity. PM R. 2015;7(4):417–27.

10. Sebastin SJ, Lim AY, Bee WH, Wong TC, Methil BV. Does the absence of the palmaris longus affect grip and pinch strength? J Hand Surg Br. 2005;30(4):406–8.
11. Thejodhar P, Potu BK, Vasavi RG. Unusual palmaris longus muscle. Indian J Plast Surg. 2008;41(1):95–6.
12. BOTOX® Prescribing Information Allergan. www.allergan.com/assets/pdf/botox_pi.pdf.
13. Dysport PI. [Package insert/prescribing information]. Basking Ridge: Ipsen Biopharmaceuticals, Inc. http://pi.medicis.us/printer_friendly/dysport.pdf.
14. Myobloc. [Package insert/prescribing information]. Louisville: Solstice Neurosciences (US WorldMeds). http://www.myobloc.com/hp_about/PI_5-19-10.pdf.
15. O'Brien CF. Injection techniques for botulinum toxin using electromyography and electrical stimulation. Muscle Nerve. 1997;S6:S176–80.
16. Xeomin PI. [Package insert/prescribing information]. Greensboro: Merz Pharmaceuticals. http://www.xeomin.com/files/Xeomin_PI.pdf.
17. Alter KE, Munin MC. Comparing guidance techniques for chemodenervation procedures. In: Alter KE, Wilson N, editors. Botulinum neurotoxin injection manual. New York: Demos Medical Publishing; 2014. p. 126–9.
18. Lim EC, Quek AM, Seet RC. Accurate targeting of botulinum toxin injections: how to and why. Parkinsonism Relat Disord. 2011;11(S1):S34–9.
19. Picelli A, Tamburin S, Bonetti P, Fontana C, Barausse M, Dambruoso F, Gajofatto F, Santilli V, Smania N. Botulinum toxin type a injection into the gastrocnemius muscle for spastic equinus in adults with stroke: a randomized controlled trial comparing manual needle placement, electrical stimulation and ultrasonography-guided injection techniques. Am J Phys Med Rehabil, 2012;91(11), 957–64.
20. Ploumis A, Varvarousis D, Konitsiotis S, Beris A. Effectiveness of botulinum toxin injection with and without needle electromyographic guidance for the treatment of spasticity in hemiplegic patients: a randomized controlled trial. Disabil Rehabil. 2014;36(4):313–8.
21. Gracies JM, Lugassy M, Weisz DJ, Vecchio M, Flanagan S, Simpson DM. Botulinum toxin dilution and endplate targeting in spasticity: a double-blind controlled study. Arch Phys Med Rehabil. 2009;90(1):9–16.
22. Chin TY, Nattrass GR, Selber P, Graham HK. Accuracy of intramuscular injection of botulinum toxin a in juvenile cerebral palsy: a comparison between manual needle placement and placement guided by electrical stimulation. J Pediatr Orthop. 2005;25(3):286–91.
23. Kwon JY, Hwang JH, Kim JS. Botulinum toxin a injection into calf muscles for treatment of spastic equinus in cerebral palsy: a controlled trial comparing sonography and electric stimulation-guided injection techniques: a preliminary report. Am J Phys Med Rehabil. 2010;89(4):279–86.
24. Gooch JL, Patton CP. Combining botulinum toxin and phenol to manage spasticity in children. Arch Phys Med Rehabil. 2004;85(7):1121–4.
25. Fehlings D, Narayanan U, Andersen J, Beauchamp R, Gorter JW, Kawamura A, Kiefer G, Mason M, McCormick A, Mesterman R, Switzer L, Watt J. Botulinum toxin-a use in paediatric hypertonia: Canadian practice patterns. Can J Neurol Sci. 2012;39(4):508–15.
26. Childers MK. Targeting the neuromuscular junction in skeletal muscles. Am J Phys Med Rehabil. 2004;83(10):S38–44.
27. Childers MK. The importance of electromyographic guidance and electrical stimulation for injection of botulinum toxin. Phys Med Rehabil Clin N Am. 2003;14(4):781–92.
28. Parratte B, Tatu L, Vuillier F, et al. Intramuscular distribution of nerves in the human triceps surae muscle: anatomical bases for treatment of spastic drop foot with botulinum toxin. Surg Radiol Anat. 2002;24(2):91–6.
29. Van Campenhout A, Molenaers G. Localization of the motor endplate zone in human skeletal muscles of the lower limb: anatomical guidelines for injection with botulinum toxin. Dev Med Child Neurol. 2011;53(2):108–19.
30. Christensson E. Topography of terminal motor innervation in striated muscles from stillborn infants. Am J Phys Med. 1959;38:65–78.

31. Coers C. Structural organization of the motor nerve endings in mammalian muscle spindles and other striated muscle fibers. Am J Phys Med Rehabil. 1958;38:166–75.
32. Saitou K, Masuda T, Michikami D, Michikami D, Kojima R, Okada M. Innervation zones of the upper and lower limb muscles estimated by using multichannel surface EMG. J Hum Ergol (Tokyo). 2000;29(1–2):35–52.
33. Amirali A, Mu L, Gracies JM, Simpson DM. Anatomical localization of motor endplate bands in the human biceps brachii. J Clin Neuromuscul Dis. 2007;9(2):306–12.
34. Kim MW, Kim JH, Yang YJ, Ko YJ. Anatomic localization of motor points in gastrocnemius and soleus muscles. Am J Phys Med Rehabil. 2005;84(9):680–3.
35. Van Campenhout A, Hubens G, Fagard K, Molenaers G. Localization of motor nerve branches of the human psoas muscle. Muscle Nerve. 2010;42(2):202–7.
36. Hallett M. Explanation of timing of botulinum neurotoxin effects, onset and duration, and clinical ways of influencing them. Toxicon. 2015;107(Pt A):64–7.
37. Alter KE, Murphy KP. Guidance techniques for Botulinum toxins and other injections. In: Alexander MA, Matthew DJ, editors. Pediatric rehabilitation, principles and practice. 5th ed. New York: Demos Medical Publishing; 2016. p. 153–69.
38. Shaari CM, Sanders I. Quantifying how location and dose of botulinum toxin injections affect muscle paralysis. Muscle Nerve. 1993;16(9):964–9.
39. Alter KE, Munin MC. Comparing guidance techniques for chemodenervation procedures. In: Alter KE, Hallett M, Karp B, Lungu C, editors. Ultrasound-guided chemodenervation procedures: Text and atlas. New York: Demos Medical Publishing; 2012. p. 138–54.
40. Alter KE, Munin MC. US-guided neuortoxin (BoNT) injections: clinical applications. In: Ultrasound-guided chemodenervation procedures: Text and atlas. New York: Demos Medical Publishing; 2012. p. 54–169.
41. Alter KE. High-frequency ultrasound guidance for neurotoxin injections. Phys Med Rehabil Clin N Am. 2010;21(3):607–30.
42. Elovic EP, Esquenazi A, Alter KE, Lin JL, Alfaro A, Kaelin DL. Chemodenervation and nerve blocks in the diagnosis and management of spasticity and muscle overactivity. PM R. 2009;1(9):842–51.
43. Glass GA, Ku S, Ostrem JL, Heath S, Larson PS. Fluoroscopic, EMG-guided injection of botulinum toxin into the longus colli for the treatment of anterocollis. Parkinsonism Relat Disord. 2009;15(8):610–3.
44. Jordan SE, Ahn SS, Gelabert HA. Combining ultrasonography and electromyography for botulinum chemodenervation treatment of thoracic outlet syndrome: comparison with fluoroscopy and electromyography guidance. Pain Physician. 2007;10(4):541–6.
45. Lee IH, Yoon YC, Sung DH, Kwon JW, Jung JY. Initial experience with imaging-guided intramuscular botulinum toxin injection in patients with idiopathic cervical dystonia. AJR Am J Roentgenol. 2009;192(4):996–1001.
46. Alter KE. Ultrasound guidance for botulinum toxin therapy: cervical dystonia. In: Troung D, Hallett M, Zachary C, Dressler D, editors. Manual of botulinum toxin therapy. 2nd ed. New York: Cambridge University Press; 2014. p. 46–59.
47. Alter KE. Ultrasound guidance for botulinum toxin therapy: thoracic outlet syndrome. In: Eds Troung D, Hallett M, Zachary C, Dressler D, editors. Manual of botulinum toxin therapy. 2nd ed. New York: Cambridge University Press; 2014. p. 269–27.
48. Alter KE, Lin J. Ultrasound guidance for nerve and motor point blocks. In: Alter KE, Hallett M, Karp BI, Lungu C, editors. Ultrasound guided chemodenervation procedures, Text and atlas. New York: Demos Medical Publishing; 2012. p. 170–84.
49. Alter KE, Skurow S. Instrumentation and knobology. In: Alter KE, Hallett M, Karp BI, Lungu C, editors. Ultrasound guided chemodenervation procedures; Text and atlas. New York: Demos Medical Publishing; 2012. p. 84–107.
50. Berweck S, Schroeder AS, Fietzek UM, Heinen F. Sonography-guided injection of botulinum toxin in children with cerebral palsy. Lancet. 2004;363(9404):249–50.
51. Haig AJ, Goodmurphy CW, Harris AR, Ruiz AP, Etemad J. The accuracy of needle placement in lower-limb muscles: a blinded study. Arch Phys Med Rehabil. 2003;84(6):877–82.

52. Henzel MK, Munin MC, Niyonkuru C, Skidmore ER, Weber DJ, Zafonte RD. Comparison of surface and ultrasound localization to identify forearm flexor muscles for botulinum toxin injections. PM R. 2010;2(7):642–6.
53. Hong JS, Sathe GG, Niyonkuru C, Munin MC. Elimination of dysphagia using ultrasound guidance for botulinum toxin injections in cervical dystonia. Muscle Nerve. 2012;46(4):535–9.
54. Py AG, Zein Addeen G, Perrier Y, Carlier RY, Picard A. Evaluation of the effectiveness of botulinum toxin injections in the lower limb muscles of children with cerebral palsy. Preliminary prospective study of the advantages of ultrasound guidance. Ann Phys Rehabil Med. 2009;52(3):215–23.
55. Schnabel A, Meyer-Frießem CH, Zahn PK, Pogatzki-Zahn EM. Ultrasound compared with nerve stimulation guidance for peripheral nerve catheter placement: a meta-analysis of randomized controlled trials. Br J Anaesth. 2013;111(4):564–72.
56. Yang EJ, Rha DW, Yoo JK, Park ES. Accuracy of manual needle placement for gastrocnemius muscle in children with cerebral palsy checked against ultrasonography. Arch Phys Med Rehabil. 2009;90(5):741–4.
57. Marina MB, Sani A, Hamzaini AH, Hamidon BB. Ultrasound-guided botulinum toxin A injection: an alternative treatment for dribbling. J Laryngol Otol. 2008;122(6):609–14.
58. Sikdar S. Ultrasound physics. In: Alter KE, Hallett M, Karp BI, Lungu C, editors. Ultrasound guided chemodenervation procedures; Text and atlas. New York: Demos Medical Publishing; 2012. p. 56–83.
59. Alter KE, Skurow S. Chemodenervation: ultrasound characteristics of relevant tissues. In: Alter KE, Hallett M, Karp BI, Lungu C, editors. Ultrasound guided chemodenervation procedures; text and atlas. New York: Demos Medical Publishing; 2012. p. 124–37.
60. Smith J, Finnoff JT. Diagnostic and interventional musculoskeletal ultrasound: part 1. Fundamentals. PM R. 2009;1(1):64–75.
61. Wu C, Xue F, Chang W, Lian Y, Zheng Y, Xie N, Zhang L, Chen C. Botulinum toxin type a with or without needle electromyographic guidance in patients with cervical dystonia. Springerplus. 2016;5(1):1292.
62. Xu K, Yan T, Mai J. A randomized controlled trial to compare two botulinum toxin injection techniques on the functional improvement of the leg of children with cerebral palsy. Clin Rehabil. 2009;23(9):800–11.
63. Schnitzler A, Roche N, Denormandie P, Lautridou C, Parratte B, Genet F. Manual needle placement: accuracy of botulinum toxin A injections. Muscle Nerve. 2012;46(4):531–4.
64. Boon AJ, Oney-Marlow TM, Murthy NS, et al. Accuracy of electromyography needle placement in cadavers: non-guided vs. ultrasound guided. Muscle Nerve. 2011;44(1):45–9.
65. Chan AK, Finlayson H, Mills PB. Does the method of botulinum neurotoxin injection for limb spasticity affect outcomes? A systematic review. Clin Rehabil. 2017;31(6):713–21.
66. Grigoriu AI, Dinomais M, Rémy-Néris O, Brochard S. Impact of injection-guiding techniques on the effectiveness of botulinum toxin for the treatment of focal spasticity and dystonia: a systematic review. Arch Phys Med Rehabil. 2015;96(11):2067–78.
67. Wissel J, Ward TB, Erztgaard P, Bensmail D, Hecht, MJ, Lejeune TM, Schnider P, European consensus table on the use of botulinum toxin type a in adult spasticity. J Rehabil Med. 2009;41:13–25.
68. Heinen F, Molenaers G, Fairhurst C, Carr LC, Desloovere K, Valayer CE, Morel E, Papavassiliou AS, Tedroff K, Pascual-Pascual SI, Bernert G, Berweck S, Di Rosa, Kolanowski E, Brageloh-Mann I. European consensus table 2006 on botulinum toxin for children with cerebral palsy. Eur J Paediatr Neurol. 2006;10:215–225.
69. Geiringer SR. Anatomic localization for needle EMG. 2nd ed. New York: Elsevier Medical Publishers; 1999.
70. Simpson DM, Hallett M, Ashman EJ, Comella CL, Green MW, Gronseth GS, Armstrong MJ, Gloss D, Potrebic S, Jankovic J, Karp BP, Naumann M, So YT, Yablon SA. Practice guideline update summary: botulinum neurotoxin for the treatment of blepharospasm, cervical dystonia, adult spasticity, and headache: report of the guideline Development Subcommittee of the American Academy of Neurology. Neurology. 2016;86(19):1818–26.

Botulinum Toxin Therapy: Future Perspectives

Bahman Jabbari

The preceding chapters have discussed clinical conditions in which high-quality studies have demonstrated the efficacy of BoNTs in alleviating symptoms of various disorders. There are also other important clinical conditions in which the preliminary results of BoNT therapy are promising, though the proof of efficacy still awaits results of high-quality clinical trials. These potential indications, however, pertain to some very common and hard to treat medical disorders; hence, the promising information about them should be of interest to the challenged clinicians.

I have selected four such medical conditions for discussion in this chapter in which human clinical trials have been available.

Orthopedic Disorders

Intra-Articular Use of Botulinum Neurotoxins for Treatment of Arthritic Pain

Pain of chronic arthritis is a hard symptom to treat. Intra-articular injection of steroids (triamcinolone) and hyaluronate, as well as treatment with tropisetron and tanezumab, provides only partial pain relief [1]. Therefore, newer therapeutic agents, for management of arthritic pain, are desirable.

Mahowald et al. [2] first reported positive results with intra-articular injection of onabotulinum toxinA for pain relief in arthritis (nine, shoulder; three, knee; three, ankle). All patients had failed previous intra-articular injection of steroids and/or viscosupplement agents. Onabotulinum toxinA (ona-BoNT-A) (Botox-Allergan) was injected into shoulder (100 units) and limb joints (25–50 units). Following

B. Jabbari, M.D. (✉)
Yale University School of Medicine, New Haven, CT, USA
e-mail: Bahman.jabbari@yale.edu

B. Jabbari (ed.), *Botulinum Toxin Treatment in Clinical Medicine*,
DOI 10.1007/978-3-319-56038-0_16

injection of ona-BoNT-A, the mean maximum reduction in limb joint pain was 55% ($P = 0.02$) and 38% ($P = 0.044$) at 4 and 10 weeks, respectively. For shoulder pain, there was even a higher magnitude of pain reduction (72%, $P = 0.001$). The subjects also demonstrated improved range of motion in the shoulder and limb joints. No significant side effects were reported.

Sing et al. [3] in a double blind placebo-controlled study compared the results of intra-articular injection of ona-BoNT-A (100 units) and lidocaine with lidocaine and saline in 43 patients with chronic shoulder pain (21 onaA, 22 placebo). At 1 month, the mean decrease in visual analogue score was 2.4 for Ona-BoNT-A group and 0.8 for the saline group ($P = 0.014$). Five subscales of SF-36 were also improved significantly in the onaA group ($P = 0.035$) as well as a trend for improvement noted in the Disability Index ($P = 0.083$). A year later, same group of authors reported, in a double blind study of 54 patients, significant relief of pain after knee arthroplasty with intra-articular injection of 100 units of ona-BoNT-A. There was also a statistically significant improvement in Physician Global Impression of Change and in SKF36 pain subscale score [4].

In a prospective, open label study of five patients with post-hemiplegic shoulder pain, Castiglione et al. [5] injected BoNT-A (ona A, two patients; incoA(Xeomin), two patients; aboA(Dysport), one patient) into painful glenohumeral joint. The dose was 100 units for ona-BoNT-A and inco-BoNT-A, but 500 units for abo-BoNT-A. Patients' level of pain was assessed by VAS at rest and during the passive arm abduction at 2 and 8 weeks. At both 2 and 8 weeks, all patients showed marked improvement of shoulder pain measured both at rest and at arm abduction ($P = 0.001$, $P < 0.001$). There was no difference in the level of pain relief at 2 and 8 weeks.

Comparator Studies

Boon et al. [6] compared the efficacy of low dose (100 units) and high dose (200 units) of onabotulinum toxinA injection with 40 units of methylprednisolone acetate in 60 subjects with pain (minimum level six at VAS) and functional impairment due to osteoarthritis of the knee. The primary outcome was defined as reduction of pain in VAS at 8 weeks. All three approaches were effective in reducing pain, but the reduction reached significance only for the low-dose onA group at 8 weeks ($P = 0.01$).

Sun et al. [7] conducted a single blind (assessor), prospective study comparing the efficacy and safety of onaA with hyaluronate plus rehabilitation in 75 patients with symptomatic ankle osteoarthritis. Thirty-eight patients received a single injection of 100 units of onaA into the ankle joint, while 37 received a single injection of hyaluronate plus 12 sessions of physical therapy. The primary outcome was measured on the Ankle Osteoarthritis Scale (AOS), which includes both pain and disability scale; each measures the intensity on a scale of 0–10. Pain-related outcomes were assessed at baseline (before injection) and at 2 weeks, 1, 3, and 6 months. The authors considered 30% or more decline in the pain score as significant. After treatment, subjects in both groups (onaA and hyaluronate) experienced marked reduction of pain measuring 50% or more in the pain subset of AOS and in VAS score. There was no difference between the toxin of hyaluronate injections. Both groups also showed substantial improvement in the disability scores. The injections did not induce any significant side effects in either of the two groups.

Comment

A recent meta-analysis of six clinical trials (placebo-controlled and comparator) [8] assessing the utility of botulinum toxins for pain relief in osteoarthritis concluded that, compared with conventional therapy, intra-articular injection of BoNTs in patients with refractory joint pain has beneficial effects. It improved pain score and Western Ontario McMaster Arthritis Index (WOMAC) score in adult patients. The incidence of side effects in BoNT-injected patients was not more than those who received placebo or other modalities of treatment. Proof of efficacy of BoNT therapy against pain of osteoarthritis awaits the results of future multi-center, placebo-controlled clinical trials.

Psychiatry—Depression

Major depressive disorder (MDD) is a common mental disorder with a life-time prevalence of 5–10% among men and 10–25% among women [9]. The affected patients suffer from lack of interest, low mood, and a variety of vegetative and cognitive problems leading to functional disability. Five clinical trials, [10–14] three randomized and blinded and two open label, suggest that injection of BoNTs into the glabellar muscles alleviates depression (Table 1). The three blinded studies are reviewed in some detail below.

Wollmer et al. [11] have compared the effect of onabotulinum toxinA injection into the glabellar region with placebo injection in 30 patients (15 in each group) with major depression. Six weeks after a single treatment, the scores of 17-item Hamilton Depression Rating Scale (primary outcome measure) were reduced by an average of 41.7% in the toxin group vs. 9.2% in the placebo group ($P < 0.001$). The effect size was even larger at the end of the study (16 weeks). Subjects also demonstrated improvement of Beck depression inventory and clinical global impression scale.

Finizi and Rosenthal [12] assessed the efficacy of onabotulinum toxinA injection into the glabellar muscles (29 units in females and 40 units in males) in a double blind placebo-controlled study. The primary outcome was 50% or more reduction of Montgomery-Asberg Depression Rating Scale (MADRS) at 6 weeks. There was 52% reduction of depression in MADRS for OnaA group compared to 15% for the placebo group ($P < 0.001$). The remission rate (MADRS score of 10 or less), the secondary outcome for the study, was also reduced by an average of 47% in the onaA group, while the placebo group showed only a 21% improvement ($P < 0.03$).

In another placebo-controlled, crossover study [14], the effect of two injections of onaA (weeks 0 and 12) was compared with placebo. The primary outcome was >50% reduction in the scores of Hamilton Depression Rating Scale-21 (HDRS-21). The toxin group demonstrated substantial improvement of depression with the HDRS-21 response rates being 55, 24, and 0% for the first and second onA injection groups and the placebo, respectively.

How injection of onabotulinum toxinA into glabellar muscles (procerus and Corrugator) leads to improvement of major depression is difficult to explain. Finzi and Rosenthal [15] propose that glabellar muscles (procerus and corregator) provide emotional proprioception and communicate with certain brain regions such as amygdala and prefrontal cortex (PFC). In depressed patients, similar to looking at a negative, unpleasant picture, the enhanced tone in glabellar muscles is associated with overactivity of amygdala and decreased activity of PFC. It has been shown by functional magnetic resonance imaging (fMRI) that injection of BoNT-A into contracted glabellar muscles (when subject looks at an unpleasant picture), similar to treatment with Paroxetine and behavioral therapy, decreases the overactivity of amygdala and increases PFC activity [16–19]. Onabotulinum toxinA injection into glabellar region may improve depression by influencing the function of amygdala or PFC via the trigeminal system.

A recent meta-analysis of the literature on the effect of BoNT on depression identified five studies, three of them being of high quality (Table 1) [20]. The analysis concluded that botulinum toxinA can produce significant improvement in depressive symptoms and is a safe adjunctive treatment for patients receiving pharmacotherapy for depression. Future trials are needed to evaluate the antidepressant effect per se of botulinum toxin A and to further elucidate the underlying antidepressant mechanism of botulinum toxin A in patients suffering from depression.

Comment

Each of the three published blinded BoNT studies in depression (Table 1) qualify as a class II [18] study providing an evidence-based efficacy level of B (probably effective) [20] according to the criteria of Assessment Subcommittee of the American Academy of Neurology [21]. Although the results are encouraging, the effect on men has not been assessed yet, since over 90% of the studies, cohorts were women. Furthermore, all randomized clinical trials so far have investigated the effect of onabotulinum toxinA on depression; hence, studies with other type A and type B toxin are also needed. Establishment of an A level of efficacy (definitely effective) for BoNT therapy in depression requires conduction of Class I clinical trials (preferably multi-center RCTs).

Table 1 Clinical trials assessing efficacy of BoNTs in depression

Study	Design	N	F/M	Toxin dose	Primary	Response and remission rates
Finzi and Waserman [10]	Open label	10	10/0	OnaA 29 U	Beck depression inventory (BDI)	Depressive symptoms improved (less than 20 score in BDI) in 8 of 10 patients
Wolmer et al. [11]	Double blind parallel	30	28/2	onaA F: 29 U	Hamilton depression rating scale-21 (HDRS-21) at week 6	Response rate: onaA 60% vs. placebo 13% ($P = 0.02$)
			23/7	M: 39 U		Remission rate: onaA 33% vs. placebo 13% (ns)
Hexsel et al. [12]	Open label	25	?	OnaA 20 U	Beck depression inventory at 8 weeks	54% decrease in BDI scores
Finzi and Rosenthal [13]	Double blind, parallel	74	69/5	Ona-A F: 29 U M: 40 U	50% reduction of Montgomery-Asberg Depression Scale (MASDS) at 6 weeks	Response rate: onaA 61% vs. placebo 12% ($P < 0.001$)
						Remission rate: onaA 48% vs. placebo 12% ($P < 0.001$)
Magid et al. [14]	Double blind, crossover	30	28/2	Toxin injections at weeks 0 and 12–29 U	50% or more reduction in HDRS-21 score at week 6	HDRS-21 Response rate: onaA 55 and 24% vs. placebo 5% ($P = 0.001$)
						Remission rate: onaA 33% vs. placebo 5% (ns)

OnaA onabotulinum toxinA(Botox), *F* female, *M* Male

Cardiology

Atrial Fibrillation (AF)

Atrial ganglionic plexi (GP) are located inside the epicardial fat pads and constitute the intrinsic cardiac autonomic nervous system. Five GP locations have been identified; superior surface of the right atrium, superior surface of the left atrium, posterior surface of the right atrium, posterior medial surface of the left atrium, and inferior and lateral aspects of the posterior left atrium [23]. Inside atrial GPs, there are abundant postganglionic parasympathetic neurons, while sympathetic neurons constitute a small sub-population. Cardiac GP modulate sinus rate, atrioventricular conduction, atrial electrophysiolgical properties, and atrial fibrillation inducibility.

Atrial fibrillation is a major health problem which affects 2.5% of the general population (9% or higher after age 75) [24, 25]. Atrial fibrillation is often associated with coronary heart disease, hypertension, kidney disease, and diabetes; it is associated with an annual stroke incidence of 5% [26]. Treatment with beta-blockers, calcium channel blockers, and digoxin as well as anticoagulation is recommended for normalization of the heart rate and for stroke prevention.

Two animal studies, both performed in dogs, have demonstrated that injection of BoNTs into the epicardial fat pad can inhibit the effect of experimental vagal stimulation that could lead to cardiac arrhythmia and atrial fibrillation. Tsuboi et al. [27] have shown that injection of botulinum neurotoxin A into the sinoatrial fat pad prevents reduction of sinus rate caused by vagus nerve stimulation. In another study [28], investigators assessed the short-term effects of botulinum toxin injection into GP of dog's heart and on AF inducibility. Effective refractory period (ERP) and AF inducibility from vagal stimulation were significantly attenuated at 1 week after botulinum toxin injection. This effect dissipated within 2–3 weeks. The above studies illustrate that in canine models, botulinum toxin injection into GP of the heart can temporarily suppress atrial fibrillation.

Recurrence of preexisting atrial fibrillation is a challenge to cardiac surgeons and clinicians after Cardiacbypass graft (CABG) surgery. Pukoshalow et al. [29] investigated the effect of botulinum toxin injections into the GP of human heart in a double blind, placebo-controlled study. Prior to CABG surgery, 60 patients were randomized into toxin and saline groups (30 each). Subjects received injections of either 50 units of incobotulinumtoxinA or saline into each of the four pericardial fat pads (located close to the superior pulmonary vein, (Fig. 1) following thoracotomy. During the first 30 days after surgery, two of 30 patients (7%) in the botulinum toxin group and nine of 30 patients (30%) in the placebo group experienced recurrence of

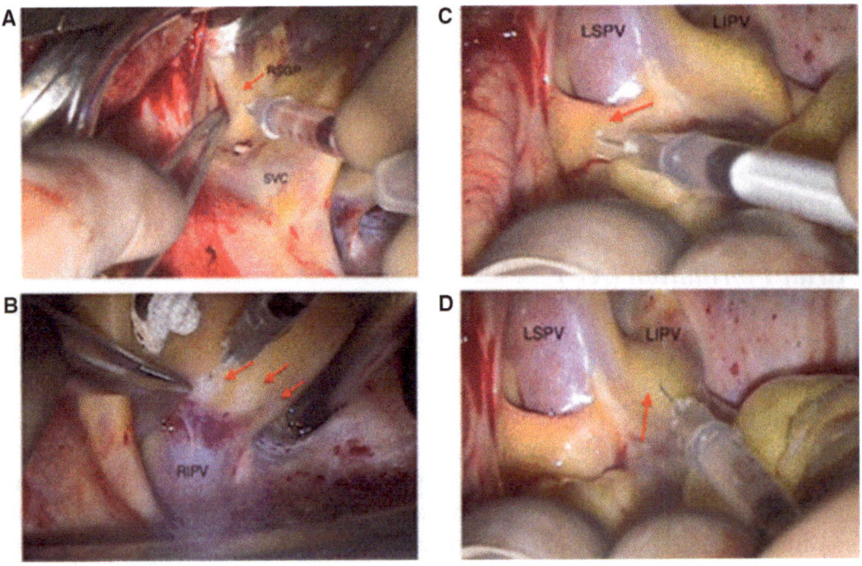

Fig. 1 Site of 4 different epicardial fat pad injections marked with red arrow. LIPV indicates left inferior pulmonary vein; LSPV, left superior pulmonary vein; RIPV, right inferior pulmonary vein; RSGP, right superior ganglionated plexus; RSPV, right superior pulmonary vein; and SVC, superior vena cava. From Pukoshalow et al. Printed with permission from Circulation: Arrhythmia and electorphysiology 2015

atrial fibrillation ($P = 0.024$). After that, up to the 12-month of follow-up, seven of the 30 subjects in the placebo group (27%) and none of the 30 subjects in the botulinum toxin group developed recurrent atrial fibrillation ($P = 0.002$). No patient reported any side effects. The authors concluded that injection of incobotulinumtoxinA into the GP of human heart significantly reduces the incidence of post-CABG atrial fibrillation over 12 months and this treatment is safe with the doses applied in their study (50 units per each of 4 GPs).

Comment

Refractory atrial fibrillation and recurrence of AF after cardiac surgery is an important issue in clinical medicine. Medical and surgical (ablation procedure) approaches are not always successful. Injection of BoNTs into the pericardial GP is a novel approach of potentially significant value, but well-designed clinical trials are needed to prove its efficacy and safety in human subjects.

Autonomic Nervous System: Prevention of Radiation-Induced Damage to the Salivary Gland in Cancer Patients

Radiation to the face and neck often damages the salivary glands and leads to a variety of unpleasant symptoms caused by the salivary glands' dysfunction. Being less protected than the parotid gland, the submandibular gland (SMG) is often more damaged than parotid gland. Submandibular glands provide 60–67% of the unstimulated and 50% of stimulated saliva. There is evidence in animals that injection of BoNTs into the salivary glands prior to irradiation reduces the damage to these glands substantially.

Teymoortash et al. [30] showed that injection of BoNT-A or B into submandibular glands of the rat before irradiation of the gland prevented the marked radiation-induced parenchymal loss and acinar fibrosis compared to the saline-injected rats. The weight of submandibular gland after radiation was also markedly reduced in the saline-injected rats, but not in the BoNT-injected rats ($P = 0.008$).

In another study of irradiated salivary glands, at third day post-irradiation, mice pre-injected with BoNT-A demonstrated 25% reduction in the flow of saliva compared to 50% reduction in the BoNT-untreated mice ($P < .05$). Local neutrophil infiltration, detected by myeloperoxidase staining, was threefold lower for the BoNT-treated mice. At 4 weeks post-irradiation, the saline (control) group showed a 40% reduction in basal SMG weight, compared with a 20% weight reduction in the BoNT group. Histologically, BoNT-pretreated glands showed relative preservation of acinar structures after radiation [31].

In a recent prospective, randomized, placebo-controlled, double-blinded study conducted in human subjects affected by head and neck cancer, investigators assessed safety of BoNT A and B injection into the submandibular gland prior to radiotherapy. Subjects were divided into four groups each consisting of three subjects. The injected doses were 20 units for type A and 750 units for the type B toxin. Injections were safe, but authors found no difference between BoNTs (A or B) and placebo regarding the gland's uptake of technetium pertechnetate or regarding the salivary excretion fraction. The authors concluded that due to the small number of patients, further investigation of various doses and timing of BoNT injection is required for a more precise analysis of toxin's efficacy in humans [32].

Comments

Data in animals indicate that injection of BoNTs into the submandibular gland prior to irradiation of the gland prevents paranchymal damage, gland atrophy, and reduction of salivation. In human, additional studies are needed for assessing the efficacy of BoNTs in this setting.

References

1. Cheng OT, Souzdalnitski D, Vrooman B, Cheng J. Evidence-based knee injections for the management of arthritis. Pain Med. 2012;13:740–53.
2. Mahowald ML, Singh JA, Dykstra D. Long term effects of intra-articular botulinum toxin A for refractory joint pain. Neurotox Res. 2006;9:179–88.
3. Singh JA, Mahowald ML, Noorbaloochi S. Intraarticular botulinum toxin A for refractory painful total knee arthroplasty: a randomized controlled trial. J Rheumatol. 2010;37:2377–86.
4. Singh JA, Mahowald ML, Noorbaloochi S. Intra-articular botulinum toxin A for refractory shoulder pain: a randomized, double-blinded, placebo-controlled trial. Transl Res. 2009;153(5):205–16.
5. Castiglione A, Bagnato S, Boccagni C, Romano MC, Galardi G. Efficacy of intra-articular injection of botulinum toxin type A in refractory hemiplegic shoulder pain. Arch Phys Med Rehabil. 2011;92(7):1034–7.
6. Boon AJ, Smith J, Dahm DL, Sorenson EJ, Larson DR, Fitz-Gibbon PD, Dykstra DD, Singh JA. Efficacy of intra-articular botulinum toxin type A in painful knee osteoarthritis: a pilot study. PMR. 2010;2:268–76.
7. Sun SF, Hsu CW, Lin HS, Chou YJ, Chen JY, Wang JL. Efficacy of intraarticular botulinum toxin A and intraarticular hyaluronate plus rehabilitation exercise in patients with unilateral ankle osteoarthritis: a randomized controlled trial. J Foot Ankle Res. 2014;7(1):9. doi:10.1186/1757-1146-7-9.
8. Wu T, Dong HX, Song Y, Ye Y, Li H. Intra-articular injections of botulinum toxin A for refractory joint pain—a systematic review and meta-analysis. Clin Rehabil. 2017;31:435–43.
9. Kessler RC, Berglund P, Demler O, et al. The epidemiology of major depressive disorder. Results of National Comorbidity Survey Replication (NCS-R). JAMA. 2003;289:3095–105.
10. Finzi E, Wasserman E. Treatment of depression with botulinum toxin A: a case series. Dermatol Surg. 2006;32:645–9.
11. Wollmer MA, de Boer C, Kalak N, Beck J, Götz T, Schmidt T, et al. Facing depression with botulinum toxin: a randomized controlled trial. J Psychiatr Res. 2012;46(5):574–81. doi:10.1016/j.jpsychires.2012.01.027.

12. Hexsel D, Brum C, Siega C, Schilling-Souza J, Dal'Forno T, Heckmann M, Rodrigues TC. Evaluation of self-esteem and depression symptoms in depressed and nondepressed subjects treated with onabotulinumtoxin A for glabellar lines. Dermatol Surg. 2013;39(7):1088–96.
13. Finzi E, Rosenthal NE. Treatment of depression with onabotulinum toxin A: a randomized, double-blind, placebo controlled trial. J Psychiatr Res. 2014;52:1–6.
14. Magid M, Reichenberg JS, Poth PE, Robertson HT, LaViolette AK, Kruger TH, Wollmer MA. Treatment of major depressive disorder using botulinum toxin A: a 24-week randomized, double-blind, placebo-controlled study. J Clin Psychiatry. 2014;75(8):837–44.
15. Finzi E, Rosental NE. Emotional proprioception. Treatment of depression with afferent facial feedback. J Psychiatr Res. 2016;80:93–6.
16. Lee H, Heller AS, van Reekum CM, Nelson B, Davidson RJ. Amygdala-prefrontal coupling underlies individual differences in emotion regulation. NeuroImage. 2012;62(3):1575–81.
17. Hennenlotter A, Dresel C, Castrop F, Ceballos-Baumann AO, Wohlschlager AM, Haslinger B. The link between facial feedback and neural activity within central circuitries of emotion-new insights from botulinum toxin-induced denervation of frown muscles. Cereb Cortex. 2009;19:537–42.
18. Ruhe HG, Booij J, Veltman DJ, Michel MC, Schene AH. Successful pharmacologic treatment of major depressive disorder attenuates amygdala activation to negative facial expressions: a functional magnetic resonance imaging study. J Clin Psychiatry. 2012;73(4):451–9.
19. DeRubeis RJ. Cognitive therapy vs. medications for depression: treatment outcomes and neural mechanisms. Nat Rev Neurosci. 2008;9(10):788–96.
20. Parsaik K, Maskarenhas SS, Hashmi A, Prokop LG, John V, Osusaga O, Singh B. Role of botulinum toxin in depression. J Psychiatr Pract. 2016;22(2):99–110.
21. French J, Gronseth G. Lost in a jungle of evidence: we need a compass. Neurology. 2008;71:1634–8.
22. Gronseth G, French J. Practice parameters of the technology assessments: what they are, what they are not, and why you should care. Neurology. 2008;71:1639–43.
23. Armour JA, Murphy DA, Yuan BX, Macdonald S, Hopkins DA. Gross and microscopic anatomy of the human intrinsic cardiac nervous system. Anat Rec. 1997;247:289–98.
24. Go AS, Hylek EM, Phillips KA, et al. Prevalence of diagnosed atrial fibrillation in adults: national implications for rhythm management and stroke prevention: the AnTicoagulation and Risk Factors in Atrial Fibrillation (ATRIA) study. JAMA. 2001;285(18):2370–5.
25. Pulignano G, Del Sindaco D, Denitza Tinti M, Tolone S, Minardi G, Lax A, Uguccion M. Atrial fibrillation management in older heart failure patients: a complex clinical problem. Heart Int. 2016;11:e41–9.
26. Wolf PA, Abbott RD, Kannel WB. Atrial fibrillation as an independent risk factor for stroke: the Framingham study. Stroke. 1991;22(8):983–8.
27. Tsuboi M, Furukawa Y, Kurogouchi F, et al. Botulinum neurotoxin A blocks cholinergic ganglionic neurotransmission in the dog heart. Jpn J Pharmacol. 2002;89:249–54.
28. Oh S, Choi E, Zhang Y, et al. Botulinum toxin injection in epicardial autonomic ganglia temporarily suppresses. Circ Arrhythm Electrophysiol. 2011;4:560–5.
29. Pokushalov E, Kozlov B, Romanov A, et al. Long-term suppression of atrial fibrillation by botulinum toxin injection into epicardial fat pads in patients undergoing Cardiac surgery-one-year follow-up of a randomized pilot study. Circ Arrhythm Electrophysiol. 2015;8:1334–41.
30. Teymoortash A, Müller F, Juricko J, Bieker M, Mandic R, Librizzi D, Höffken H, Pfestroff A, Werner JA. Botulinum toxin prevents radiotherapy-induced salivary gland damage. Oral Oncol. 2009;45:737–9.
31. Zeidan YH, Xiao N, Cao H, Kong C, Le QT, Sirjani D. Botulinum toxin confers radioprotection in Murine salivary glands. Int J Radiat Oncol Biol Phys. 2016;94:1190–7.
32. Teymoortash A, Pfestroff A, Wittig A, Franke N, Hoch S, Harnisch S, Schade-Brittinger C, Hoeffken H, Engenhart-Cabillic R, Brugger M, Strauch K. Safety and efficacy of botulinum toxin to preserve gland function after radiotherapy in patients with head and neck cancer: a prospective, randomized, placebo-controlled, double-blinded phase I clinical trial. PLoS One. 2016;11(3):e0151316. doi:10.1371/journal.pone.0151316.

Index

B. Jabbari (ed.), *Botulinum Toxin Treatment in Clinical Medicine*,
DOI 10.1007/978-3-319-56038-0

MIX
Papier aus verantwortungsvollen Quellen
Paper from responsible sources
FSC® C105338
www.fsc.org

If you have any concerns about our products,
you can contact us on
ProductSafety@springernature.com

In case Publisher is established outside the EU,
the EU authorized representative is:
Springer Nature Customer Service Center GmbH
Europaplatz 3, 69115 Heidelberg, Germany

Printed by Libri Plureos GmbH
in Hamburg, Germany